Assessment of Neuropsychological Functions in Psychiatric Disorders

ASSESSMENT OF NEUROPSYCHOLOGICAL FUNCTIONS IN PSYCHIATRIC DISORDERS

Edited by
Avraham Calev, D.Phil.

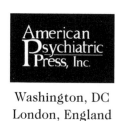

Washington, DC
London, England

Copyright © 1999 American Psychiatric Press, Inc.
ALL RIGHTS RESERVED
Manufactured in the United States of America on acid-free paper
02 01 00 99   4 3 2 1
First Edition

American Psychiatric Press, Inc.
1400 K Street, N.W., Washington, DC   20005
www.appi.org

Library of Congress Cataloging-in-Publication Data
A CIP record is available from the Library of Congress.

British Library Cataloguing in Publication Data
A CIP record is available from the British Library.

To my wife, Gila,
and my children, Hila and Yuval.

Contents

Contributors

BONNIE R. ARONOWITZ, PH.D.
Assistant Professor of Psychology in Psychiatry, Mount Sinai School of Medicine, New York City

SAMITA BANERJEE, B.A.
Teaching Assistant, Department of Psychology, State University of New York at Stony Brook

MARSHA E. BATES, PH.D.
Associate Professor of Research Psychology, Center of Alcohol Studies, Rutgers University, Piscataway, New Jersey

STEFANIE BERNS, PH.D. CANDIDATE
Research Associate, Hillside Hospital; and Doctoral Candidate, City University of New York, New York City

AVRAHAM CALEV, D.PHIL.

Director, Assessment and Counseling Center of Long Island, Smithtown, New York

ANTONIO CONVIT, M.D.

Assistant Professor of Psychiatry, New York University Medical College: N. S. Kline Institute for Psychiatric Research, Orangeburg, New York

KAREN L. DAHLMAN, PH.D.

Assistant Professor, Department of Psychiatry, Mount Sinai School of Medicine, New York City

CONCETTA M. DECARIA, PH.D.

Assistant Professor of Psychology in Psychiatry, Mount Sinai School of Medicine, New York City

SHMUEL FENNIG, M.D.

Director of Outpatient Services, Shalvatah Medical Center, Kfar Sabah, Israel

ELIZABETH A. GAUDINO, PH.D.

Department of Neurology, State University of New York at Stony Brook

AMY GORDON, M.A.

Doctoral Candidate in Clinical Psychology, Drexel University, Philadelphia, Pennsylvania

GREGG E. GORTON, M.D.

Assistant Professor of Psychiatry and Human Behavior, Jefferson Medical College, Philadelphia, Pennsylvania

PHILIP D. HARVEY, PH.D.

Associate Professor of Psychiatry, Mount Sinai School of Medicine, New York City

ERIC HOLLANDER, M.D.

Professor of Psychiatry, Mount Sinai School of Medicine, New York City

JUDITH JAEGER, PH.D., M.P.A.
Associate Professor of Psychiatry, Albert Einstein College of Medicine, Bronx, New York; and Director of Neuropsychological Rehabilitation Research, Hillside Hospital, Glen Oaks, New York

LAUREN B. KRUPP, M.D.
Associate Professor, Department of Neurology, State University of New York at Stony Brook

DONALD W. O'DONNELL, M.P.S.
Neuropsychologist, Pilgrim Psychiatric Center, West Brentwood, New York

DEAN A. POLLINA, PH.D.
Research Associate, Department of Neurology, State University of New York at Stony Brook

THOMAS PRESTON, PH.D.
Research Associate, Department of Neurology, State University of New York at Stony Brook

STEVEN SAMUEL, PH.D.
Clinical Associate Professor of Psychiatry and Human Behavior, Jefferson Medical College, Philadelphia, Pennsylvania

RICHARD SOBEL, M.D.
Clinical Assistant Professor of Psychiatry and Human Behavior, Jefferson Medical College, Philadelphia, Pennsylvania

THOMAS SWIRSKY-SACCHETTI, PH.D.
Clinical Associate Professor of Psychiatry and Human Behavior, Jefferson Medical College, Philadelphia, Pennsylvania

REBECCA TWERSKY-KENGMANA, B.A.
Research Associate and Medical Student, Mount Sinai School of Medicine, New York City

PREFACE

IN RECENT YEARS, neuropsychology has contributed significantly to the understanding of psychiatric disorders. Clinicians and researchers now frequently use neuropsychological evidence in their daily work. This volume encompasses neuropsychological effects of psychiatric disorders. It also provides an overview of clinical assessment of neurocognitive deficits in psychiatric disorders and their attempted treatment, management, and rehabilitation. The book aims to provide clinicians, researchers, and trainees in the fields of psychology and psychiatry with knowledge about neuropsychological functions in psychiatric disorders.

The book is the result of a joint effort of many experts in their fields, each contributing a significant portion of their knowledge of the field. The contributions of Lauren Krupp, M.D., Philip D. Harvey, Ph.D., Antony Bolton, Ph.D., Thomas Preston, Ph.D., Armin Paul Thies, Ph.D., Alan Yasowitz, Ph.D., and Peter Lovell, Ph.D., in the peer review process are acknowledged.

1

CLINICAL NEUROPSYCHOLOGICAL ASSESSMENT OF PSYCHIATRIC DISORDERS

Avraham Calev, D.Phil., Thomas Preston, Ph.D.,
Steven Samuel, Ph.D., and Gregg E. Gorton, Ph.D.

NEUROPSYCHOLOGICAL TOOLS WERE used initially to assess the effects of neurological disease or trauma on cognitive functioning (Heilman and Valenstein 1993; Lezak 1995; Spreen and Strauss 1991). With the advent of brain imaging techniques, neurological dysfunctions were observed in psychiatric illnesses, and neuropsychological evaluation of psychiatric patients became important. In this introductory chapter, we concisely review neuropsychological assessment methods and their application to psychiatric disorders.

◈ PURPOSES OF NEUROPSYCHOLOGICAL ASSESSMENT

Neuropsychological assessment aims to describe different cognitive functions and to understand the biological and functional causes of malfunctions or hyperfunctions to improve management and treatment. To achieve these aims, the following cognitive constructs are assessed.

Global Cognitive Function

Global cognitive function refers to a general level of cognitive ability and is routinely assessed by intelligence tests. This assessment is necessary because the brain is a unitary organ. Different cognitive functions performed by the brain depend on one another and are also affected by overall intelligence. The brain often compensates, to some extent, for damage to a specific function. A global assessment includes only certain central aspects of cognition; nonetheless, it provides a baseline to assess

◆ General deterioration (or dementia) from a premorbid level of functioning
◆ Areas of cognitive deficit or hyperfunction that may be related to brain locations, such as the hemispheres, the different lobes, and other lower brain structures

Executive Function

Executive function consists of the control and organization of behavior by inhibition and planning of responses and results in goal-directed acts. This function has been associated with the prefrontal lobe (including the dorsolateral and orbital cortices). However, findings suggest that other brain parts also may be involved (Lezak 1995). Examples of symptoms related to an executive dysfunction include disinhibition (either hypersexual or hyperaggressive), disorganization, confusion, and perseveration (i.e., repetition of a response beyond a desired point).

Memory Function

Memory function includes the encoding (registration), storage, and retrieval of knowledge.

Long-term memory. Long-term storage has traditionally been associated with the temporal lobes, particularly the hippocampus. Other brain functions, such as executive function, may control memory aspects such as retrieval and thus affect memory. The temporal lobe of the left or dominant hemisphere is associated with verbal memory, and the temporal lobe of the right or nondominant hemisphere is associated with visuospatial memory.

Immediate sensory memory. Immediate sensory (echoic, iconic) memory, lasting for milliseconds, is not well localized and may be associated with the sensory receptive corresponding brain areas.

Short-term memory. Memory that lasts for a few minutes is referred to as short-term memory. For example, during a conversation, a person remembers a question verbatim until he or she answers it. Soon after, the person may forget the details of the question asked. This kind of memory has not been well localized in the brain. Shallice and Warrington (1970) found evidence that a part of the left parietal lobe, at the border of the fissure of Sylvius, is active during this type of verbal memory process.

Working memory. Working memory (Baddeley 1976) uses short-term memory capacity and combines it with long-term and permanent knowledge to perform a task such as writing a composition.

Semantic memory. Semantic memory is a permanent knowledge store including the knowledge of language and grammar rules.

Declarative and nondeclarative memory. All of the above-mentioned memory components are *declarative,* in the sense that a person is aware of them, but *nondeclarative* knowledge also exists. In nondeclarative memory, the person is not aware of, and cannot articulate, his or her knowledge. One such example is *procedural memory,* which includes skills such as bicycle riding or swimming. People perform various movements to achieve these tasks, but the skill requires more than that. People usually cannot describe the knowledge involved in making swimming or bicycle riding balanced and smooth. This knowledge is part of their procedural memory. Another example of nondeclarative memory comes from priming experiments assessing *implicit memory.* An amnesic patient may be unable to remember any list words when tested. When prompted to say any word, however, the patient may unknowingly come up with the correct response. These memory functions are not well localized in the brain.

Language Function

Language function includes the perception of speech and of written language, the production of speech and of written language, and the repetition or articulation of speech, as in vocal reading. Speech perception has been localized at Wernicke's area in the posterior left temporal lobe (planum temporale). The decoding of written language is mediated by the visual (occipital) cortex and the posterior left or dominant parietal lobe. Speech production has been localized at Broca's area in the left frontal lobe. However, motor aspects of speech such as tongue and lip movement are localized at the motor cortex of the frontal lobe. Dysfunctions in this motor area result in slurring of speech, or *dysarthria*. Problems with speech production, speech perception, and language repetition are known as *dysphasia* or *complete aphasia*. Difficulty with or loss of writing ability is called *dysgraphia* or *agraphia*. Exner's area at the foot of the second frontal convolution and the angular gyrus has been implicated in graphic difficulties. *Dyslexia* or *alexia* involves mainly disability in reading skills. *Prosody,* the emotional tone and other emphatic aspects of speech, is attributed to analogous locations of speech in the right or nondominant hemisphere. The varieties and subclassifications of difficulties in speech, writing, and reading are reviewed elsewhere (e.g., Heilman and Valenstein 1993).

Visuospatial and Other Perceptual Functions

Senses have brain interpretation areas. The right or nondominant parietal lobe has been associated with interpretation and representation of visual images. Damage to these areas causes visuoperceptual errors, the most severe form being visuospatial neglect or inattention. In such cases, the patient fails to perceive objects in his or her left visual field. Tactile perceptions, as well as perception of pain and of heat, are localized adjacently at postcentral sulcal parietal areas in both hemispheres, with collateral representation.

Motor, Visuoconstructive, and Praxic Functions

Pure *motor function* is localized at the precentral frontal motor cortex, the motor subcortical regions, and the spinal tract. The cerebellum contributes to smooth movement. Purposeless motor speed, such as tapping speed, has to be supplemented by contributions from visual and executive functions to produce an eye-hand coordinated purposeful act. *Visuomotor speed* thus includes the use of motor function in combination with other functions (at least visuospatial and executive function). *Visuoconstructive ability* includes complex eye-hand coordination to produce either two- or three-dimensional spatial constructs. Skills such as dressing, building with blocks, and cooking are related to *praxic* ability. *Apraxia* or *dyspraxia* means a dysfunction in these skills.

Comment

Despite attempts to localize cognitive functions, they are not well localized, and individuals with atypical brain organization are frequently found. Some neuropsychologists emphasize localization. Others view the brain as one centrally organized organ, putting less emphasis on parts.

◈ METHODS OF NEUROPSYCHOLOGICAL ASSESSMENT

Neuropsychological assessment is usually done by psychologists trained in neuropsychology. Experience in observing and identifying cognitive deficits associated with different brain dysfunctions or injuries helps clinicians make a diagnosis. Observing behaviors and cognitive functions in patients with recent brain injuries, interviewing these patients, and using assessment tools that quantify their difficulties are essential processes in diagnosing neuropsychological deficits. Because deficits become less localized with time, it is important to follow up the emerging neuropsychological picture.

To form a comprehensive neuropsychological picture and to produce a report for other clinicians, several assessment methods must be combined.

In one assessment method, the clinician observes the patient's behaviors and responses in everyday life. Recording unusual or atypical responses associated with certain brain dysfunctions can help to characterize the patient's individualized dysfunction. Observations can also be made during an interview with the patient or during testing.

In a second assessment method, the clinician asks the patient to describe subjectively his or her cognitive failures or difficulties. A survey form can help collect history from the patient and include his or her personal comments. One such form is shown in Table 1–1.

In a third assessment method, collection of information about the history of premorbid and postinjury functioning is done in an interview. Educational, social, occupational, and medical background information is included. Medical information is of special importance. Assessment of vascular problems can help hypothesize what nature of brain dysfunction may be expected. Knowing the patient's medical conditions, such as epilepsy, chronic fatigue syndrome, Alzheimer's disease, or diabetes mellitus, helps the clinician to hypothesize what type of cognitive dysfunction is expected. Structural brain scanning using magnetic resonance imaging (MRI) or computed tomography (CT) is always important. Functional assessment of blood flow and metabolism in the brain includes at least positron-emission tomography (PET) or single photon emission computed tomography (SPECT). These measures evaluate the functioning of deep brain structures. More peripheral cerebral blood flow (CBF) measurements, with or without brain activation (achieved when performing a neuropsychological task during brain scanning), can also be done with resting regional CBF after xenon inhalation. Multichannel electroencephalograms (EEGs) provide mapping of brain function with or without activation of the brain.

Comment

These brain structure and brain function measures have limited use in neuropsychology. They are not sensitive enough and do not detect every instance of damage or dysfunction. If their results are not consistent with neuropsychological test findings suggesting a dysfunction, brain dysfunction still should be suspected. These medical measures should be regarded as aids to understanding causes of neuropsychological malfunctioning. The neuropsychologist's objective is to define patients' cognitive deficits in order to manage and treat them.

In a fourth assessment method, the clinician administers neuropsychological tests. Extensive test batteries, such as the Halstead-Reitan Neuropsychological Test Battery for Children (Reitan and Wolfson 1993) and the Luria-Nebraska Neuropsychological Test Battery for Children (Golden et al. 1985), are available. These comprehensive neuropsycho-

Table 1–1. Initial neuropsychological interview for psychiatric patients

Personal history

Name _____

Address _____

Telephone _____

Sex   M____ F____

Date of birth _____ Age _____

Place of birth _____

Dates of testing _____

Referred by _____Specialty _____

Referral question as stated by referral source _____

_____

Reason for referral as viewed by patient _____

_____

Family physician _____ tel _____

Psychiatrist _____ tel _____

Psychologist_____ tel _____

Neurologist _____ tel _____

Dates of previous psychological/neuropsychological tests _____

_____

Handedness_____

Native language _____

Date of immigration (if any) _____

Marital status_____ Previous marriages _____

Age at first marriage_____ Ages at other marriages _____

Children (ages and names; specify from which marriages)_____

_____

Marital problems/counseling? When? _____

_____

Siblings/their marital status/is the patient a twin? ___

_____

Education _____

High school or other more recent school performance (grades, special classes)_

_____

Number of friends (during high school and now) _____

_____

(continued)

Table 1–1.   Initial neuropsychological interview for psychiatric patients *(continued)*

How often meets with friends _____

How often meets with relatives _____

Occupation _____

Employment history _____

Current employment_____

Source of income_____

Economic status   Very Good/Good/Average/Low/Very Low

Developmental history

In pregnancy: maternal anemia, toxemia, high blood pressure, leg swelling, kidney disease, diabetes, bleeding, heart disease, rubella, thyroid problem, alcohol or drug abuse, Rh, or any other known problem

_____

_____

Length of delivery _____

Type of delivery (cesarean, forceps, vacuum) _____

Induced labor? _____

Special observations in infancy (feeding/activity level)

Developmental milestones:

Age at first step _____

Age at first word_____ Toilet problems? _____

Bed-wetting?_____

Clumsiness? _____

Behavior problems: Excessive shyness/withdrawal _____

Emotional immaturity (impulsiveness, temper tantrums, sleep problems, tics) _

_____

Psychiatric and neurological history

Psychiatric diagnoses/problems (as seen by patient) _____

_____

_____

_____

(continued)

Table 1–1.   Initial neuropsychological interview for psychiatric patients
(continued)

Psychiatric family history (including mainly first-degree blood relatives)

_____

_____

Previous psychotherapy/behavior therapy/counseling_____

_____

_____

Previous psychiatric hospitalizations (date, length, problem at the time) _____

_____

_____

Past alcohol abuse _____

Recent alcohol abuse _____

Past drug abuse (and with which drugs)_____

Present drug abuse (and with which drugs)_____

Previous psychotropic medications/electroconvulsive therapy _____

_____

Present psychotropic medications/electroconvulsive therapy _____

_____

Other past medication use_____

Other current medication use_____

_____

Head injury (details) _____

Loss of consciousness _____

Seizure history _____

Fainting/blackouts _____

Magnetic resonance imaging (MRI)/computed tomography (CT) scan findings _

Positron-emission tomography (PET)/single photon emission computed
tomography (SPECT) findings _____

(continued)

Table 1–1.   Initial neuropsychological interview for psychiatric patients
(continued)

History of diseases that could affect the brain (meningitis, encephalitis, frequent ear infections) _____

History of other serious medical conditions_____

_____

Symptoms

Vision problems/blurred or double vision/spots in vision/seeing things that are not there _____

Hearing problems/ringing in the ears/unusual sounds/hearing things that are not there _____

Change in sense of smell _____

Change in sense of taste_____

Burning skin_____ Tingling skin _____

Difficulty feeling hot and cold_____

Numbness _____

Tremors/shakiness _____

Twitches/spasms _____

Balance problems _____

Dizziness _____

Coordination problems/dropping things _____

Speech problems _____

Reading problems _____

Writing problems_____

Difficulty following a conversation/understanding others _____

Difficulty concentrating (reading a book, watching a movie) _____

Memory problems _____

Periods of confusion/disorientation _____

Difficulty with house chores _____

Getting lost_____

Difficulty remembering time of day _____

Irritability/mood changes_____

(continued)

Table 1–1.   Initial neuropsychological interview for psychiatric patients *(continued)*

Change in ability to get along with close family members _____

Change in social activities _____

Change in work ability _____

Change in frequency of headaches_____

Any pain_____

Change in sex desire _____

Change in weight (time course) _____

Change in appetite (time course) _____

Increased/reduced sleep (time course) _____

Waking at night/early-morning awakening (time course) _____

Sadness/depression (time course)_____

Vomiting/diarrhea/constipation _____

Acute anxieties/panic periods_____

Tenseness _____

Hallucinations _____

Suspiciousness _____

Delusions_____

Feelings of grandeur/special powers _____

Paranoid thoughts_____

logical test batteries have reliability, validity, and subtest comparability problems, however (Lezak 1995). More flexible approaches such as the Boston Process Approach can be used by more experienced clinicians. Most clinical and research neuropsychologists use batteries they build for the purpose of assessing 1) premorbid level of functioning, 2) level of deterioration, and 3) specific areas of either deficit or hyperfunction. Table 1–2 presents a summary of tests commonly used in adults. These tests may constitute such a battery. Because tests that are designed to assess a certain function also assess other functions, they are not "clean"

Table 1–2. Clinically accepted adult neuropsychological tests: cortical locations and functions hypothesized

Test	Frontal Anterior	Frontal Posterior	Temporal	Parietal Anterior	Parietal Posterior	General	R/L	Function
WAIS-III IQ[a] (or WAIS-R)								
Digit Span	X	X		X			L	Repetition
Digit Symbol						X		
Block Design	X	X			X	X	R	Praxis
Object Assembly	X	X			X	X	R	Praxis
WMS-III[b] (or WMS-R)								
Logical Memory			X				L	Memory
Visual Reproduction			X			X	R	Memory
Immediate			X			X		Attention
Delayed			X			X		Memory
CVLT[c]								
Immediate			X				L	Attention
Delayed			X				L	Memory
Benton								
Figures[d]			X		X		R	Memory
Faces[e]			X		X		R	Memory
Rey-Osterrieth[f]								Praxis
Recall[f]			X		X		R	Memory

Test						Laterality	Function
Bender Copying[g]				X		R	Praxis
Recall[g]				X		R	Memory
WCST[h]	X	X			X		Executive
TMT[i] A	X				X		Visual/Motor
B	X				X		Executive
Stroop[j]	X				X		Executive
Category Test[k]	X			X	X	R	Executive
Aphasia Exam[l]	X			X	X	L	Language
Sentence Repetition[m]		X	X			L	Language
Boston Naming[n]		X	X		X	L	Language
COWA[o]	X					L	Language
WRAT-III[p]	X						
Reading	X	X	X		X	L	Language
Reading Comprehension		X	X		X	L	Language
Spelling/Writing	X		X	X		L	Language
Calculation			X			L	Calculation
FTT[q]	X						Motor
SDMT[r]	X		X	X	X		Visual/Motor
Purdue Pegboard[s]	X		X	X	X		Visual/Motor
Cancellation[t]	X	X	X		X		Attention
Two Point Disc[u]	X		X				Tactile
Object Identification[v]	X		X				Tactile

(continued)

Table 1–2. Clinically accepted adult neuropsychological tests: cortical locations and functions hypothesized (*continued*)

Test	Localization								
	Frontal		Temporal	Parietal		General	R/L	Function
	Anterior	Posterior		Anterior	Posterior			
Reitan-Klove Face Hand test[v]				X				Tactile

[a]Wechsler Adult Intelligence Scale—3rd Edition (Wechsler 1997a).
[b]Wechsler Memory Scale—3rd Edition (Wechsler 1997b).
[c]California Verbal Learning Test—Adult Version (Delis et al. 1987).
[d]Benton Visual Retention Test—5th Edition (Sivan 1991).
[e]Benton Facial Retention (Benton et al. 1983b).
[f]Complex Figure Test (e.g., Rey 1941).
[g]Bender Gestalt Test (Koppitz 1975).
[h]Wisconsin Card Sorting Test (Overall and Gorham 1962).
[i]Trail Making Test (Army Individual Test Battery 1944).
[j]Stroop Color and Word Test (Golden 1978).
[k]Halstead-Reitan Battery (Reitan and Wolfson 1993).
[l]Boston Diagnostic Aphasia Examination (Goodglass and Kaplan 1983a).
[m]Multilingual Aphasia Examination (Benton and Hamsher 1989).
[n]Boston Naming Test (Goodglass and Kaplan 1983b).
[o]Controlled Oral Word Association Test (Benton and Hamsher 1989; Semel et al. 1995).
[p]Wide Range Achievement Test—3rd Edition (Jastak and Wilkinson 1993).
[q]Finger Tapping Test (Reitan and Wolfson 1993).
[r]Symbol Digit Modalities Test (Smith 1982).
[s]Purdue Pegboard Test (Gardner and Broman 1985; Tiffin 1968).
[t]Lezak (1995, pp. 388–390 for different variations on test).
[u]Corkin et al. (1970).
[v]Halstead-Reitan Battery (Reitan and Wolfson 1993).

measures. They implicate, by correlational research and clinical observation, certain brain locations as well as other locations with lesser certainty. A test assessing one function (e.g., memory) also assesses another function (e.g., executive function) and global brain functioning. Therefore, the information derived from these measures is not definitive and should be augmented by other cognitive measures, physiological measures, and clinical judgment.

Neuropsychological assessments almost always use commercial products, or so-called off-the-shelf tests, because they are expected to have desirable test characteristics such as standardization on a large, representative sample; validity; and reliability. Clinicians feel more secure when using commercial tests. The best test in this respect is the Wechsler Adult Intelligence Scale—3rd Edition (Wechsler 1997a). It is very well standardized, and subtests comparison is possible (after correcting for reliability). Most other tests do not meet these requirements. For example, widely used tests such as the California Verbal Learning Test (CVLT; Delis et al. 1987) or the Wisconsin Card Sorting Test (WCST; Heaton et al. 1993) have been applied to limited and biased populations with sample sizes not differing from those of small research studies.

Noncommercial tasks developed in research studies, such as those used to assess memory after electroconvulsive therapy (e.g., Calev et al. 1991; Squire 1987) or in schizophrenic patients (Calev 1990), may be as valid as some commercial tests. Furthermore, these noncommercial tasks may have the advantage of assessing cognitive aspects not assessed by commercial tests. Clinicians' judgment is therefore paramount in constructing the test battery. For example, some clinicians would consider it important to use a malingering tool.

After the assessment is completed, a written report for further clinical use is necessary. A comprehensive report includes sections on

◆ Reasons for referral
◆ Background information about the patient's condition, including history, current functioning, and medical findings (including brain imaging and EEG results)
◆ Details of observations that promote the understanding of the disorder or that show the nature of symptomatology
◆ Details of the tests and other tasks administered
◆ Results of the tests and their interpretation
◆ Summary of the impressions based on all information
◆ Recommendations for further assessment, treatment, and rehabilitative management procedures

Interpretation of Test Results

As stated earlier, at least two questions must be answered after test administration. The first question is whether there is a global deterioration in cognitive functioning compared with the premorbid level of functioning. Of the standardized tests that take age and other interfering variables into account, the Wechsler Adult Intelligence Scale (Wechsler 1997a) best answers this question. The Wechsler scales allow comparisons between tests less resistant to cognitive deterioration after trauma or neuropsychiatric illness (such as the Digit Symbol subtest and most other Performance subtests) and more resistant tests (such as the Vocabulary and Information subtests of the Verbal Intelligence section). If the resistant test scores are higher than the less resistant ones, deterioration should be suspected.

Comment 1. This reasoning has serious flaws. For example, if the patient was a truant, nonattentive student in school, his or her "resistant" or "premorbid" scores would be underestimated, because "resistant" scales are affected by education. The clinician thus may observe little or no deterioration even though major deterioration in functioning had occurred. School history is an important variable that should be taken into account in assessing deterioration.

Once deterioration has been established, it does not necessarily mean that it was caused by brain malfunction. Attentional factors (e.g., due to problems such as anxiety) are likely to affect these less resistant tests, thus erroneously suggesting deterioration. The cause of the observed malfunction on the less resistant tests has to be evaluated by assessing both the psychiatric and the neuropsychological status of the patient.

Another question is which specific cognitive functions show a deficit (or possibly a strength) when different functions in the same patient are compared. The clinician can use specific tests to evaluate these deficits (or strengths). Background and medical information collected for the neuropsychological evaluation is also important.

Comment 2. Deficits (or strengths) observed may either be genuine or represent artifacts because of tasks differing in discriminating power. In clinical practice, clinical judgment and experience are needed to avoid mistakes. In research, statistical control (e.g., partialing out, task matching) may be applied instead. Tests differ in their likelihood of detecting a deficit. One standard deviation below the mean or the fourteenth percentile, in one test, usually is not equivalent to one standard deviation below the mean or the fourteenth percentile in another. Moreover, the more items a test has, the greater the deviation from the mean.

For example, on the Controlled Oral Word Association test (a test assessing verbal fluency; Benton and Hamsher 1989), if a patient scores at the fourteenth percentile when using only one stimulus letter, he or she will probably score lower (at about the first percentile) if the test is expanded and made more reliable by allowing use of three stimulus letters. This is because more test items result in better reliability, and better reliability means greater true score variance, which results in better discrimination between impaired and unimpaired patients. In this example, one may not be able to find another test assessing a different function that can be compared with the Controlled Oral Word Association to determine whether the patient's verbal fluency is lower or higher. Very few tests are matched on discriminating power (Chapman and Chapman 1978, 1989). Consequently, clinical judgment is paramount.

This difficulty in interpreting test results is not limited to single cases. Research findings also can be misleading. For example, Calev and Monk (1982) reviewed studies in which no recognition memory deficits were found in schizophrenic patients. When the results of different studies were combined, a deficit in recognition memory *was* found. Thus, nonsignificant results with small samples, if directional and consistent, may mean a small but significant difference.

As mentioned earlier, the best statistically controlled test is the Wechsler Intelligence Scale. Yet, even in this test, reliability differences among subtests make subtest comparisons difficult. The manual now provides guidelines for maximizing comparability. Other neuropsychological tests are far less accurate and usually noncomparable. At present, the comparison of various results and different cognitive functions of one patient is valid only when some of the patient's scores are above the standardized population mean and others are below it. This situation, however, occurs rarely in neuropsychological dysfunctions. Most patients tend to show dysfunctions on most tasks. Future research should aim at constructing more comparable tests.

An additional problem with the assessment of specific deficits or strengths is that many functions are not assessed by neuropsychological tests. Special abilities such as accurate remote calendar calculations, found mainly in autistic individuals with "savant" features, are not well understood in neuropsychological terms. These abilities are not measured by intelligence tests, and most individuals with such extraordinary abilities score in the borderline or mildly retarded range. Similarly, special musical or artistic abilities, although undoubtedly related to brain function, usually are not part of a neuropsychological assessment. The closest that common neuropsychological assessments come in assessing musical talents is the assessment of sound discrimination and sound localization in space. "Utilization behavior," the pathological tendency of an individual to touch objects in sight, is a sign of disinhibition that is not included in most test batteries. Although many functions usually are not evaluated in neuropsychological assessment, optimism is warranted because those functions that are evaluated provide clues for further clinical investigation of nonassessed functions. Despite all the pitfalls, the contemporary use of neuropsychological tests has proved helpful in defining pathologies of many psychiatric and neurological disorders.

◈ NEUROPSYCHOLOGICAL ASSESSMENT IN DIFFERENT POPULATIONS

Assessment of Psychiatric Disorders in Adults

Neuropsychological assessment in psychiatric patients differs from that in other patients, because factors not related to cognition such as psychotic symptoms, level of cooperation, affective state, anxiety, and medications have a substantial effect on the clinical picture. Psychiatric phenomena such as lack of communication, flat affect, and psychotic symptoms, which affect cognitive function, may be a direct result of brain dysfunction. In clinical practice, unlike research (where statistical control of these factors is possible), the clinician must use judgment to evaluate these factors and interpret the results accordingly.

As a general rule, clinicians would like to eliminate irrelevant factors in order to assess patients' status effectively. If a patient is depressed after a stroke, depression can be either a biological result of the stroke or a reactive emotional response to the disabling state. In both cases, controlling the depression is diagnostically necessary to clarify the nature of cognitive deficits caused by the stroke, independent of the depression. After psychotherapy, cognitive therapy, or antidepressant medication treatments, the depression may be alleviated, and the residual deficit caused by the stroke itself may become visible. The cognitive effect of depression can be quantified by deducting cognitive deficits observed without depression from those observed during depression.

In addition to this partialing out method, other methods are used to maximize the effectiveness of neuropsychological evaluation of psychiatric patients. The following guidelines are for the clinician:

♦ Take a comprehensive psychiatric, developmental, and neurological history. Table 1–1 is an instrument that has been designed with this process in mind.

♦ Obtain occupational or school records and a psychological and psychiatric history from the earliest reports possible. Use them to assess the effect of psychiatric history and premorbid cognitive functioning on current functioning.

♦ Administer psychological tests and psychiatric rating scales as part of neuropsychological testing. Personality tests, including an objective test such as the Minnesota Multiphasic Personality Inventory—2 (MMPI-2; Hathaway and McKinley 1989) and a projective test such as the Rorschach (Rorschach 1942), can give a comprehensive view of the patient's psychological profile. Objective tests, however, have at least a 20% risk of error. These instruments are time-consuming, and time is an important factor for clinicians, especially in managed care practices. Alternative brief assessment instruments are available. Although these assessment tools are less sophisticated than longer assessment tools, they provide fairly reliable information. The Hamilton Depression Scale (Hamilton 1960) for inpatients and the Beck Depression Inventory (Beck 1987) for outpatients are valid instruments for assessing depression. If the level of depression is high, more severe cognitive effects may be expected than if the depression is minor (e.g., Calev et al. 1986). The Hamilton Anxiety Scale (Hamilton 1960) can be used to assess anxiety effects on cognitive functioning. The Brief Psychiatric Rating Scale (BPRS; Overall and Gorham 1962) is a useful and quick tool that measures level of psychiatric symptoms. The Global Assessment of Functioning (GAF) scale (American Psychiatric Association 1994) is a useful tool that can compare levels of adaptive daily functioning between recent and prior years. All these measures may have implications for current cognitive functioning.

♦ Follow up and evaluate the patient more than once to assess decline or improvement in cognitive functioning. Global improvement is normally expected after a trauma or an episode of illness. Repeated testing may, however, reveal different effects of time: a decline in a second test may suggest unconscious or conscious malingering (pretending or exaggerating illness), and fluctuations in level of functioning may indicate interference by psychiatric symptoms such as hallucinations or severe depression. If test results vary with BPRS mental health ratings, then the effect of symptoms on cognitive test results will seem certain. Some effects of medications can be assessed by testing the patient with and without medications. However, in most cases, prior research will indicate whether the specific medication the patient is receiving has the potential to cloud test results.

◆ Include, when possible, parallel forms of the same neuropsychological tests, in the same assessment, to evaluate steadiness of response.

◆ Administer more than one test to assess the same function. This method may increase the reliability of results. For example, if the Trail Making Test, Part B (Army Individual Test Battery 1944), performance is high, and the WCST (Heaton et al. 1993) performance is low, then one cannot confirm an executive dysfunction.

◆ Evaluate the possibility that current performance reflects practice effect as a result of prior experience with the same test. This is important if the patient has improved results in the second testing.

◆ Correct for attention and concentration effects. For example, if the patient loses concentration during a memory test in which he or she hears a story and is then asked to recall it, the results may show poor recall or no recall. In this case, memory function is intact, and the results reflect that the patient did not attend to the task. A control assessment of attention and vigilance, as well as the clinician's impressions, is therefore very important to determine the significance of any test results.

◆ Exercise caution in interpreting test results. Clinical neuropsychologists have experience and clinical knowledge that help give meaning to test scores and other information about the patient. Test scores can be misleading. Clinicians often can determine the nature of a specific brain dysfunction from their observations. For example, clinicians expecting behavior and emotional problems may interpret "utilization behavior" as a behavioral malfunction, such as a compulsion. Clinicians considering neurological problems will observe this behavior as response disinhibition, secondary to a prefrontal dysfunction. Clinical observations should outweigh test information. Clinical judgment is thus the most important factor.

Neuropsychological diagnostic ability of clinical psychologists.   Most clinical psychologists do not routinely assess neuropsychological functioning. Yet these clinicians are likely to be the first confronted with patients who have neuropsychiatric difficulties. Because clinical psychologists do administer standard tests and observe patients, their awareness of neuropsychological deficits may be important. Standard psychological tests have neuropsychological significance that can help these clinicians. The Rorschach and the Thematic Apperception Test (TAT) have characteristics that indicate whether brain dysfunction is present. Piotrowski (1937) noted a low level of formed responses, fewer perceived "movement" responses, and fewer commonly seen or "popular" responses in the Rorschach as organic signs. Lezak (1983) suggested that restriction (decrease in number of responses), stimulus-bound responses (responses that stay close to the bare facts), structure-seeking (difficulty in making sense of perceptions), response rigidity (inflexibility in response to changing instructions, stimuli, or test situations), fragmentation (tendency toward concreteness and organizational difficulty), simplification (poorly differentiated whole perceptions), perceptual confusion (logical and spatial confusion), confabulated responses (illogical or inappropriate compounding of discrete perceptions or ideas), and hesitancy and doubt (continuing uncertainty and dissatisfaction about perceptions) all point to possible organic brain dysfunction.

The MMPI and its revised versions, the MMPI-2 and MMPI-A, are commonly used to assess psychological disturbance objectively. Hathaway's early research led him to cluster items into independent groups consisting of 19 *general neurologic,* 11 *cranial nerve,* and 6 *motility and coordination* test items (Colligan et al. 1984). Although further attempts were made to validate organic MMPI scales, they did not hold up to empirical scrutiny.

Therefore, experienced clinicians can use information from standard objective and projective psychological tests to form an impression about organic characteristics of patients, but this diagnosis cannot be definitive. If the clinician forms an impression about an organic dysfunction during personality assessment, he or she should conduct a neuropsychological screening interview (Table 1–1) and a proper neuropsychological evaluation.

Assessment of Psychiatric Disorders in Children

Psychiatric disorders in children are frequently evaluated with neuropsychological testing. Initial forays were marked by attempts to attach an adult "template" to assessment of cognitive function in the developing child. These early efforts tended to ignore the importance of numerous factors differentiating cognitive and emotional development in children from that in adults. We discuss these factors below.

First, children are undergoing constant and dynamic maturational change. Disorders or brain insults that may manifest as loss of function in adult patients may not be immediately apparent in a child who has not yet mastered that particular function. Thus, the cognitive or behavioral consequences of a particular injury may not be apparent in a child until he or she fails to achieve mastery at the appropriate age. Alternatively, a child may not only fail to achieve a developmental milestone but also regress as a result of injury.

Second, cognitive, physical, and behavioral development in children varies significantly. For example, when an average adult is expected to perform within a fairly narrow band on handwriting and drawing tasks, performance outside that band may be considered an indication of injury or disorder. Very young children, however, may show a wide range in terms of the age at which they acquire those skills; moreover, they may advance and regress quite naturally while acquiring them. Thus, poor performance on a graphomotor task in a child does not necessarily indicate a deficit or disorder but may indicate a normal variation in acquisition of skills.

This dynamic and naturally variable development applies to higher-order cognitive functions such as sustained and selective attention, problem-solving, and memory. Children do not clearly establish the capacity to inhibit responses, remain on task, and shift attention flexibly until about age 10 years according to current research (Passler et al. 1985). The capacity to use mnemonic strategies in learning new information also is not established until approximately age 10 or 11 years. Thus, the failure to learn and retrieve information consistently in a young child does not necessarily indicate a disorder (Kail 1984).

Concomitant with the above issues, assertions about the relations between specific brain regions or networks and particular types of cognitive and behavioral manifestations cannot be applied to children simply because they have been supported by research on adults. Because children are evaluated at various points along a dynamic developmental trajectory, it is impossible to localize or lateralize brain dysfunction on the basis of even the most discrete types of cognitive and behavior problems. This point becomes even more apparent when one considers the lack of clear differentiation among neurocognitive functions in children. For example, visuoconstructive skills should not be extracted solely from graphomotor skills. Poor visuoconstructive performance on the Beery Developmental Test of Visual-Motor Integration (VMI; Beery 1989) may be affected by graphic skills rather than more general visuoconstructive skills; performance on tasks that do not involve pencil-paper construction, such as block construction measures, also must be considered.

Third, unlike adults, in children the social environment must be taken into account. Thus, economic factors, family constitution, and emotional stressors in the environment may influence a child's test performance in ways that are unrelated to cognition. A child will likely be less able, for example, to put aside conflict at home and concentrate on a test than will an adult, and the resulting distraction will make interpretation of test results problematic.

Finally, regardless of social context, children vary in terms of behavior to a much greater degree than do adults. A child may be sufficiently intimidated by the testing situation that he or she may perform poorly because of anxiety rather than cognitive deficits. Children are more likely than adults to become fatigued during testing, and the timing of an evaluation during the course of the day may influence results. Children also may be less likely to attach social value to a psychological test and may therefore put less effort into good performance.

All of the above-mentioned factors interact in ways that make careful qualitative and quantitative analysis of children's neuropsychological performance critical for the neuropsychologist. Neuropsychological evaluation in children must identify when a child is most likely to acquire a skill and then consider late acquisition by the child, the family and school context of the child, and personality and behavioral factors that may influence test performance to determine whether neurological impairment is possible. Even with these cautions, the current neuropsychological assessment instruments for children may not completely assess children's strengths and weaknesses (H. G. Taylor and Schatschneider 1992).

However, neuropsychological evaluation in children is useful for a wide array of psychiatric disorders, including disruptive behavior disorders such as attention-deficit/hyperactivity disorder (ADHD) and conduct disorder, specific learning disabilities, tic disorders and Tourette's disorder, anxiety and depressive disorders, and pervasive developmental disorders.

The neuropsychological profile most commonly seen in a particular disorder necessitates the use of tests that are most likely to explain function in that disorder. For example, ADHD often overlaps with disabilities in reading/written language, deficits in motor coordination (graphomotor deficits in particular), difficulty with new learning and short-term retrieval, problems with executive function, and anxiety disorders. A thorough test battery for any child with suspected ADHD would include qualitative and quantitative assessment of function in all of these domains. Alternatively, a child with Asperger's syndrome may have good language skills but specific deficits in visuoperceptive and visuoconstructive performance as well as in his or her capacity to interact warmly and fluently with other people. Careful assessment of these difficulties, with both standardized and nonstandardized instruments, is important. Table 1–3, although not exhaustive, lists the tests that make up a possible pediatric neuropsychological battery.

Although neuropsychological testing per se is useful, a competent clinically oriented neuropsychologist will put significant effort into making recommendations that are relevant and realistic for family, teachers, and helping professionals. The existing tests are not always relevant to the real world in which children live. The neuropsychologist and the medical and educational teams must think together and translate the findings into real-life feasible manipulations and guide parents in a practical way.

◈ RELEVANCE OF NEUROPSYCHOLOGICAL ASSESSMENT TO EVERYDAY LIFE

Neuropsychology has an important research contribution in defining and understanding psychiatric and neurological disorders. However, its ultimate clinical significance pertains to its application. One role of the neuropsychologist is to help in rehabilitation. First, the neuropsychologist may attempt to establish a formal cognitive rehabilitative program (see Jaeger and Berns, Chapter 10, in this volume), targeting areas that need training to allow coping with the demands of everyday life. Such areas include memory, language, attention, and praxis ability. Second, the neuropsychologist may use neuropsychological information when treating a patient with psychotherapy or other behavioral interventions, as shown in the following case example:

> Ms. A, a 24-year-old married woman, had a brain tumor that was successfully removed. After surgery, she experienced perceptual problems and difficulties in focusing her attention. The patient refused a cognitive rehabilitative program, claiming that she was being humiliated when confronted with her cognitive difficulties. Ms. A interpreted her difficulties as "death of her personality" because she felt that she could no longer be a worthy person. She was sad and had poor self-esteem.
>
> Cognitive-behavioral therapy was attempted. In therapy, her residual

Table 1–3.   Pediatric neuropsychological tests

Domain	Tests
General intelligence	Wechsler Preschool and Primary Scale of Intelligence —Revised; Wechsler Intelligence Scale for Children, Third Edition (WISC-III)[1]
	Stanford-Binet Intelligence Scale, 4th Edition[2]
	McCarthy Scales of Children's Abilities[3]
	Kaufman Assessment Battery for Children (K-ABC)[4]
Attention	Digit Span (WISC-III)
	Sentence repetition (Wide Range Assessment of Memory and Learning [WRAML];[5] Stanford-Binet Intelligence Scale, 4th Edition)
	Continuous performance tests[6]
	Go–No-Go paradigm[7]
Language	Peabody Picture Vocabulary Test—Revised[8]
	Receptive One-Word Picture Vocabulary Test[9]
	Expressive One-Word Picture Vocabulary Test—Revised[10]
	Boston Naming Test[11]
	Token Test for Children[12]
	Controlled Oral Word Association Test[13]
	Clinical Evaluation of Language Fundamentals—3rd Edition: Formulated Sentences[14]
	Aphasia screening (Boston Diagnostic Aphasia Examination[15]; Western Aphasia Battery[16])
Achievement	Wide Range Achievement Test, 3rd Edition[17]
	Wechsler Individual Achievement Test[18]
	Peabody Individual Achievement Test—Revised[19]
	Woodcock-Johnson Tests of Achievement—Revised[20]
Sensory/Motor	Sensory testing[21]
	Finger recognition[21]
	Skin writing testing[21]
	Lateral dominance[21]
	Right-left orientation[21]
	Purdue Pegboard Test[22]
	Grooved Pegboard[23]
	Finger Tapping Test[23]
	Grip strength[23]
	Hand movements (K-ABC)[4]

(continued)

Table 1–3.   Pediatric neuropsychological tests *(continued)*

Domain	Tests
Visuoconstructive/ Visual integration	Beery Developmental Test of Visual-Motor Integration[24]/ Bender Visual Motor Gestalt Test[25]
	Rey-Osterrieth Complex Figure or Taylor Figure[26]
	Informal drawings (Draw-A-Person, clock face and bicycle drawing)[27]
	Judgment of Line Orientation Test[28]
	Hooper Visual Organization Test[29]
Learning/Memory	Verbal Selective Reminding Test[30]
	Nonverbal Selective Reminding Test[31]
	California Verbal Learning Test, Children's Version[32]
	WRAML[5]
	Rey/Taylor Recall[26]
	Benton Visual Retention Test, 5th Edition[33]
Executive/Reasoning /Cognitive flexibility/ Working memory	Contingency Naming Test[34]
	Stroop Color and Word Test[35]
	Tower of Hanoi puzzle[36]
	Wisconsin Card Sorting Test[37]
	Category Test[38]
	Raven's Progressive Matrices[39]; Matrix Analogies Test[40]
	Symbol Digit Modalities Test[41]
Adaptive/ Psychosocial/ Behavioral	Vineland Adaptive Behavior Scales[42]
	Child Behavior Checklist and Profile (Parent and Teacher Report Forms)[43]
	Conners' Rating Scales (Parent and Teacher Report Forms)[44]
	Personality Inventory for Children—Revised[45]
	Child Symptom Inventory—4th Edition[46]
	Children's Depression Inventory[47]
	State-Trait Anxiety Inventory for Children[48]
	Revised Children's Manifest Anxiety Scale[49]

[1]Wechsler 1989, 1991.
[2]Thorndike et al. 1986.
[3]McCarthy 1972.
[4]Kaufman and Kaufman 1983.
[5]Adams and Sheslow 1990.
[6]Test of Variables of Attention (Greenberg 1993); Halperin Continuous Performance Test (Halperin et al. 1991).
[7]Trommer et al. 1988, 1991.
[8]Dunn and Dunn 1981.

(continued)

Table 1–3.   Pediatric neuropsychological tests *(continued)*

[9]Gardner 1985.
[10]Gardner 1990.
[11]Goodglass and Kaplan 1983b.
[12]Di Simoni 1978.
[13]Benton and Hamsher 1989; Semel et al. 1995; Spreen and Benton 1977.
[14]Semel et al. 1995.
[15]Goodglass and Kaplan 1983a.
[16]Kertesz 1982.
[17]Wilkinson 1993.
[18]Psychological Corporation 1992.
[19]Markwardt 1989.
[20]Woodcock and Johnson 1989.
[21]Benton et al. 1983a.
[22]Gardner and Broman 1979; Wilson et al. 1982.
[23]Knights and Norwood 1980.
[24]Beery 1989.
[25]Koppitz 1975.
[26]Osterrieth 1944; Rey 1941; L. B. Taylor 1969, 1979.
[27]Lezak 1995.
[28]Benton et al. 1983c.
[29]Hooper 1958; Seidel 1994.
[30]Bushke 1973; Fletcher 1985.
[31]Fletcher 1985.
[32]Delis et al. 1994.
[33]Sivan 1992.
[34]H. G. Taylor and Schatschneider 1992.
[35]Golden 1978.
[36]Borys et al. 1982; Welsh et al. 1991.
[37]Grant and Berg 1993.
[38]Boll 1993.
[39]Raven 1976.
[40]Naglieri 1985.
[41]Smith 1982.
[42]Sparrow et al. 1984.
[43]Achenbach 1991.
[44]Conners 1995.
[45]Wirt et al. 1984.
[46]Gadow 1994.
[47]Kovacs 1992.
[48]Spielberger et al. 1973.
[49]Reynolds and Richmond 1984.

cognitive strengths were reinforced. Some verbal tasks proved her more effective than her husband (who cooperated and attended the session to help his wife). Ms. A's effective care for her newborn baby restored her self-confidence. Further clarifications showed that her self-deprecating attitude following surgery was to be expected from her premorbid personality structure. Ms. A was a perfectionist who strived to meet her mother's expectations of herself.

By redefining her abilities, and using them in family life, she felt in place. Her emotional state gradually improved. Later, she went back to work and produced significant income for her family. Ms. A was, in a sense, lucky because her personality structure and basic aspirations did not change as a result of brain damage. She only needed readaptation to reality. Other patients may not fare that well.

A third way to use neuropsychological information to help patients is through the education of family members, caregivers, and health care professionals. Brainstorming meetings of teams that include professionals and relatives can result in environmental changes that help the patient adapt to his or her disability.

◈ REFERENCES

Achenbach TM: Child Behavior Checklist and Profile (CBCL). Burlington, University of Vermont, 1991

Adams W, Sheslow D: Wide Range Assessment of Memory and Learning (WRAML). Wilmington, DE, Jastak Associates, 1990

American Psychiatric Association: Diagnostic and Statistical Manual of Mental Disorders, 4th Edition. Washington, DC, American Psychiatric Association, 1994

Army Individual Test Battery: Manual of Directions and Scoring. Washington, DC, War Department, Adjutant General's Office, 1944

Baddeley AD: The Psychology of Memory. New York, Basic Books, 1976

Beck AT: Beck Depression Inventory. San Antonio, TX, Psychological Corporation, 1987

Beery K: Beery Developmental Test of Visual-Motor Integration (VMI). Cleveland, OH, Modern Curriculum Press, 1989

Benton AL, Hamsher K deS: Multilingual Aphasia Examination. Iowa City, IA, AJA Associates, 1989

Benton AL, Hamsher K deS, Varney NR, et al: Contributions to Neuropsychological Assessment. New York, Oxford University Press, 1983a

Benton AL, Hamsher K deS, Varney NR, et al: Facial Recognition Test. London, Oxford University Press, 1983b

Benton AL, Hamsher K deS, Varney NR, et al: Judgment of Line Orientation Test. London, Oxford University Press, 1983c

Boll TJ: Children's Category Test. San Antonio, TX, Psychological Corporation, 1993

Borys SV, Spitz HH, Dorans BA: Tower of Hanoi performance of retarded young adults and nonretarded children as a function of solution length and goal state. J Exp Child Psychol 10:611–632, 1982

Bushke H: Selective reminding for analysis of memory and learning. Journal of Verbal Learning and Verbal Behavior 12:543–550, 1973

Calev A: Memory in schizophrenia, in International Perspectives on Schizophrenia. Edited by Weller MPI. London, Libby, 1990, pp 29–41

Calev A, Monk AF: Verbal memory tasks showing no deficit in schizophrenia—fact or artifact? Br J Psychiatry 141:528–530, 1982

Calev A, Korin Y, Shapira B, et al: Verbal and non-verbal recall by euthymic and depressed affective patients. Psychol Med 16:789–794, 1986

Calev A, Nigal D, Shapira B, et al: Early and long term effects of electroconvulsive therapy and depression on memory and other cognitive functions. J Nerv Ment Dis 179:526–533, 1991

Chapman LJ, Chapman JP: The measurement of differential deficit. J Psychiatr Res 14:303–311, 1978

Chapman LJ, Chapman JP: Strategies for resolving the heterogeneity of schizophrenics and their relatives using cognitive measures. J Abnorm Psychol 98: 357–366, 1989

Colligan RC, Osborne D, Swenson WM, et al: The MMPI: development of contemporary norms. J Clin Psychol 40:100–107, 1984

Conners CK: Conners' Parent and Teacher Rating Scales (CPRS/CTRS). North Tonawanda, NY, Multi-Health Systems, 1995

Corkin S, Milner B, Rasmussen T: Somatosensory thresholds. Arch Neurol 23:41–58, 1970

Delis DC, Kramer JH, Kaplan E, et al: California Verbal Learning Test—Adult Version. San Antonio, TX, Psychological Corporation, 1987

Delis DC, Kramer JH, Kaplan E, et al: California Verbal Learning Test—Children's Version (CVLT-C). San Antonio, TX, Psychological Corporation, 1994

Di Simoni F: The Token Test for Children. Allen Park, TX, DLM Teaching Resources, 1978

Dunn LM, Dunn LM: Peabody Picture Vocabulary Test—Revised (PPVT-R). Circle Pines, MN, American Guidance Service, 1981

Fletcher JM: Memory for verbal and nonverbal stimuli in learning disability subgroups: analysis by selective reminding. J Exp Child Psychol 40:244–259, 1985

Gadow KD: Child Symptom Inventory—4th Edition (CSI-4). Stony Brook, NY, Checkmate Plus, 1994

Gardner M: Receptive One-Word Picture Vocabulary Test. Novato, CA, Academic Therapy Publications, 1985

Gardner M: Expressive One-Word Picture Vocabulary Test—Revised. Novato, CA, Academic Therapy Publications, 1990

Gardner RA, Broman M: The Purdue Pegboard: normative data on 1334 school children. Journal of Clinical Child Psychology 8:156–162, 1979

Golden JC: Stroop Color and Word Test. Chicago, IL, Stoelting, 1978

Golden JC, Purisch AD, Hammeke TA: Luria-Nebraska Neuropsychological Battery: Forms I and II. Los Angeles, CA, Western Psychological Services, 1985

Goodglass H, Kaplan E: Boston Diagnostic Aphasia Examination. Boston, MA, Lea & Febiger, 1983a

Goodglass H, Kaplan E: Boston Naming Test, 2nd Edition. Boston, MA, Lea & Febiger, 1983b

Greenberg L: Test of Variables of Attention (TOVA). Los Alamitos, CA, Universal Attention Disorders, 1993

Halperin JM, Sharma V, Greenblatt E, et al: Assessment of the Continuous Performance Test: reliability and validity in a nonreferred sample. Psychological Assessment 3:603–608, 1991

Hamilton M: A rating scale for depression. J Neurol Neurosurg Psychiatry 23:56–62, 1960

Hathaway SR, McKinley JC: Minnesota Multiphasic Personality Inventory—2. Minneapolis, University of Minnesota, 1989

Heaton RK, Chelune CJ, Talley J, et al: Manual for the Wisconsin Card Sorting Test. Odessa, FL, Psychological Assessment Resources, 1993

Heilman KM, Valenstein E: Clinical Neuropsychology, 3rd Edition. New York, Oxford University Press, 1993

Hooper HE: The Hooper Visual Organization Test. Los Angeles, CA, Western Psychological Services, 1958

Kail RV: The Development of Memory in Children, 2nd Edition. San Francisco, CA, WH Freeman, 1984

Kaufman AS, Kaufman NL: Kaufman Assessment Battery for Children (K-ABC). Circle Pines, MN, American Guidance Service, 1983

Kertesz A: Western Aphasia Battery. San Antonio, TX, Psychological Corporation, 1982

Knights RM, Norwood JA: Revised, smoothed normative data on the neuropsychological test battery for children. Mimeograph, Department of Psychology, Carleton University, Ottawa, Ontario, Canada, 1980

Koppitz EM: The Bender Gestalt Test for Young Children: Research and Applications, 1963–1973. New York, Grune & Stratton, 1975

Kovacs M: Children's Depression Inventory (CDI). Tonawanda, NY, Multi-Health Systems, 1992

Lezak MD: Neuropsychological Assessment, 2nd Edition. New York, Oxford University Press, 1983

Lezak MD: Neuropsychological Assessment, 3rd Edition. New York, Oxford University Press, 1995

Markwardt FC: Peabody Individual Achievement Test—Revised (PIAT-R). Circle Pines, MN, American Guidance Service, 1989

McCarthy DA: Manual for the McCarthy Scales of Children's Abilities. San Antonio, TX, Psychological Corporation, 1972

Naglieri JA: Matrix Analogies Test—Expanded and Short Forms. San Antonio, TX, Psychological Corporation, 1985

Osterrieth PA: Le test de copie d'une figure complex: contribution a l'etude de la perception et de la memoire [The complex figure text: contribution to the study of perception and memory]. Arch de Psychologie 30:286–356, 1944

Overall JE, Gorham DR: The Brief Psychiatric Rating Scale. Psychol Rep 10: 798–812, 1962

Passler M, Isaac W, Hynd GW: Neuropsychological development of behavior attributed to frontal lobe functioning in children. Dev Neuropsychol 4:349–370, 1985

Piotrowski Z: The Rorschach inkblot method in organic disturbances of the central nervous system. J Nerv Ment Dis 86:525–537, 1937

Psychological Corporation: Wechsler Individual Achievement Test. San Antonio, TX, Psychological Corporation, 1992

Raven JC: Raven's Progressive Matrices. London, HK Lewis, 1976

Reitan RM, Wolfson D: The Halstead Reitan Neuropsychological Test Battery: Theory and Clinical Interpretation. Tucson, AZ, Neuropsychology Press, 1993

Rey A: L'examen psychologique dans les cas d'encephalopathie tramatique [The psychological exam in the cases of traumatic encephalopathy]. Archives de Psychologie 28:286–340, 1941

Reynolds CR, Richmond BO: Revised Children's Manifest Anxiety Scale (RCMAS). Los Angeles, CA, Western Psychological Services, 1984

Rorschach H: Psychodiagnostics: A Diagnostic Test Based on Perception. Berne, Switzerland, Huber, 1942

Seidel WT: Hooper Visual Organization Test: Preliminary Norms for Children. Los Angeles, CA, Children's Hospital of Los Angeles, unpublished normative data, 1994

Semel EM, Wiig EH, Secord WA: Clinical Evaluation of Language Fundamentals —3rd Edition (CELF-3). San Antonio, TX, Psychological Corporation, 1995

Shallice T, Warrington EK: Independent functioning of verbal memory stores: a neurological study. Q J Exp Psychol 22:261–273, 1970

Sivan A: Benton Visual Retention Test—5th Edition. San Antonio, TX, Psychological Corporation, 1992

Smith A: Symbol Digit Modalities Test: Manual. Los Angeles, CA, Western Psychological Services, 1982

Sparrow SS, Balla DA, Cicchetti DV: Vineland Adaptive Behavior Scales. Circle Pines, MN, American Guidance Service, 1984

Spielberger CD, Edwards CD, Lushene RE, et al: State-Trait Anxiety Inventory for Children (STAIC). Palo Alto, CA, Mind Garden, 1973

Spreen O, Benton AL: Neurosensory Center Comprehensive Examination for Aphasia. Victoria, British Columbia, University of Victoria Neuropsychology Laboratory, 1977

Spreen O, Strauss E: A Compendium of Neuropsychological Tests. New York, Oxford University Press, 1991

Squire LR: Memory and Brain. New York, Oxford University Press, 1987

Taylor HG, Schatschneider C: Child neuropsychological assessment: a test of basic assumptions. Clinical Neuropsychologist 6:259–275, 1992

Taylor LB: Localization of cerebral lesions by psychological testing. Clin Neurosurg 16:269–287, 1969

Taylor LB: Psychological assessment of neurosurgical patients, in Functional Neurosurgery. Edited by Rasmussen T, Marino R. New York, Raven, 1979, pp 165–180

Thorndike RL, Hagen EP, Sattler JM: Guide for Administering and Scoring the Stanford-Binet Intelligence Scale: Fourth Edition. Chicago, IL, Riverside Publishing, 1986

Tiffin J: Purdue Pegboard Examiner's Manual. Rosemont, IL, London House, 1968

Trommer BL, Hoeppner JB, Lorber R, et al: The Go–No-Go paradigm in attention deficit disorder. Ann Neurol 24:610–614, 1988

Trommer BL, Hoeppner JB, Zecker SG: The Go–No-Go Test in attention deficit is sensitive to methylphenidate. J Child Neurol 6:128–129, 1991

Wechsler D: Manual for the Wechsler Preschool and Primary Scale of Intelligence—Revised (WPPSI-R). San Antonio, TX, Psychological Corporation, 1989

Wechsler D: Manual for the Wechsler Intelligence Scale for Children, Third Edition (WISC-III). San Antonio, TX, Psychological Corporation, 1991

Wechsler D: Wechsler Adult Intelligence Scale—3rd Edition (WAIS-III). New York, Psychological Corporation, 1997a

Wechsler D: Wechsler Memory Scale—3rd Edition. San Antonio, TX, Psychological Corporation, 1997b

Welsh MC, Pennington BF, Groisser DB: A normative-developmental study of executive function: a window on prefrontal function in children. Developmental Neuropsychology 5:131–149, 1991

Wilkinson GS: Wide Range Achievement Test—3rd Edition (WRAT-3). Wilmington, DE, Jastak Associates, 1993

Wirt RD, Lachar D, Klinedinst JK, et al: Multidimensional Description of Child Personality: A Manual for the Personality Inventory for Children—Revised (PIC-R). Los Angeles, CA, Western Psychological Services, 1984

Woodcock RW, Johnson MB: Woodcock-Johnson Psycho-Educational Battery—Revised. Allen Park, TX, DLM Teaching Resources, 1989

2

NEUROPSYCHOLOGY OF SCHIZOPHRENIA AND RELATED DISORDERS

Avraham Calev, D.Phil.

SCHIZOPHRENIA IS ONE of the most disabling psychiatric disorders. Epidemiological studies report that the estimated prevalence of schizophrenia is between 0.25% and 1% in the United States and Europe, with minimal cultural variation (Hare 1987; Torrey 1980). Age at onset is in the 20s, although it can vary appreciably. Males may have an earlier age at onset (Stromgren 1987). Low socioeconomic status is related to incidence, possibly because of environmental stress (Dohrenwent and Dohrenwent 1974) or other selective processes. The disease prevents patients from maintaining full employment and requires lifetime care, resulting in an estimated cost of $50 billion a year in the United States alone (Torrey 1988) and accounting for about 25% of all hospital bed occupancy (Davies and Drummond 1990). Mortality rates are high probably because of neglect and difficulty in self-care (Allebeck 1989). In addition to the suffering experienced by individuals with schizophrenia, the disease constitutes a burden on society.

The essential feature of schizophrenia is the presence of positive and negative symptoms for a significant period of time during a 1-month period, with some signs of the disorder persisting for at least 6 months (American Psychiatric Association 1994). Positive symptoms represent a distortion of normal function, and negative symptoms represent a diminution or loss of normal function. Positive symptoms include delusions (erroneous beliefs that usually involve a misinterpretation of perceptions and experiences), hallucinations (false sensory perceptions, in any sensory modality, experienced in a waking state) and disorganized thinking (thought disorder), and grossly disorganized behavior (such as childlike silliness and unpredictable agitation) (American Psychiatric Association 1994). In schizophrenia, auditory hallucinations are the most prominent type. Incoherent speech and loosening of associations are manifestations of disorganized thinking. Negative symptoms include affective flattening (immobile, unresponsive face, with poor eye contact and reduced body language), alogia (brief, laconic, empty replies), and avolition (inability to initiate and persist in goal-directed activities).

Neuropsychological deficits are inherent in the concept of schizophrenia. The modern concept of schizophrenia is attributed to Emil Kraepelin (1919), who first described the disease in 1886. He coined the term *dementia praecox*, implying irreversible and progressive cognitive and behavioral deterioration beginning early in life. Kraepelin described hallucinations, delusions, thought disorder, negativism, avolition, and attention and memory deficits. Emotional incongruity characterized some patients (hebephrenic type), blunted affect characterized some (simple type), and motor disturbance (rigidity or immobility) characterized others (catatonic type). Delusions and persecutory ideas were most prominent in other patients (paranoid type). Implicit in Kraepelin's description was the belief that the disease has an organic pathogenesis.

Eugen Bleuler (1911/1950) later gave the name *schizophrenia* to a disease entity similar to that described by Kraepelin. Unlike Kraepelin's definition, Bleuler's description included nondemented patients and patients whose condition did not necessarily deteriorate early in life. The course of illness could be chronic or characterized by intermittent attacks, "which can stop or retrograde" at any time (Bleuler 1911/1950, p. 8). The illness does not permit "restitutio ad integrum" (i.e., full recovery). The splitting of different psychic functions, such as thinking and feeling, was thought to be the central process of the disease. The term schizophrenia (in Greek) represented this split.

◈ SCHIZOPHRENIC SYMPTOMS

Schizophrenic symptoms, in Bleuler's conceptualization, could be *primary*, resulting directly from the organic disease process, or *secondary*, resulting from adaptation to the disease. Symptoms also could be *fundamental*, present in every case of schizophrenia, or *accessory*, present in some patients only. Only four fundamental symptoms (the four A's) were described:

1. Disturbed *association:* difficulty relating ideas and memories to each other
2. Disturbed *affectivity:* responding with unusual affect (e.g., blunt affect) to emotion-arousing stimuli
3. *Autism:* a predilection toward withdrawal and fantasy
4. *Ambivalence:* the coexistence of opposite impulses, wishes, and ideas

Many accessory symptoms, such as hallucinations, delusions, and catatonia (i.e., decreased motor reactivity culminating in a fixed posture), were described. Of the four fundamental symptoms, only the disturbance of association among ideas or cognition, which results in neuropsychological deficits, was described as primary. Thus, it was the central symptom of the disease.

In this chapter, I review the neuropsychological findings in relation to the etiological hypotheses. Because impaired cognition is a significant sign of schizophrenia, neuropsychological research is of major importance.

◈ EVIDENCE FOR A BIOLOGICAL ETIOLOGY OF SCHIZOPHRENIA

The psychodynamic and psychosocial theories viewed schizophrenia as a social disease, created by circumstances (Laing 1965; Sullivan 1953). However, evidence suggesting genetic transmission emerged at about the same time (Kallman 1946; Rosenthal and Kety 1968). A possible interplay between constitutional predisposition and environmental factors was suggested. The diathesis hypothesis (e.g., Mednick 1970) suggested that only people with a constitutional predisposition will become schizophrenic and that environmental factors, such as stress, are necessary to produce the illness. Later, physical environmental factors, such as toxic processes (e.g., Beaton et al. 1975), vitamin deficiencies (e.g., Hoffer 1971), and viral infections (Hunter et al. 1969), were proposed to cause schizophrenia. The effects of neuroleptic medications on the brain neurotransmitter dopamine led some researchers to suggest that dopamine excess is a causative, or at least a mediating, factor in schizophrenia (Snyder 1976). Other researchers suggested other brain dysfunctions based on neuropsychological deficits in schizophrenia. Attentional deficits suggested abnormal neural arousal mechanisms (e.g., Venables and Wing 1962) and were associated with the amygdala, hippocampus, and reticular formation. R. E. Gur (1978) suggested left-hemispheric dysfunction and overactivation as a possible cause of the behavioral manifestations of the disease.

Newer brain imaging technology indicated stronger evidence for brain abnormality. In some early studies before the mid-twentieth century, researchers observed enlarged brain ventricles with an early, unreliable brain imaging method, namely, pneumoencephalography (e.g., Young and Crampton 1974). However, this evidence was not viewed as credible until Johnstone et al. (1976) first reported enlarged ventricles in a controlled study in England that used modern computed tomography (CT). Later, researchers from the National Institute of Mental Health replicated this finding with CT and more refined magnetic resonance imaging (MRI) techniques (Shelton and Weinberger 1986).

Comment 1: Large Versus Enlarged Ventricles

Note that the size of the brain ventricles, per se, should not be considered the brain dysfunction in schizophrenia. Many schizophrenic patients have smaller ventricles than do nonschizophrenic people, and many healthy people have large ventricles. *Ventricular enlargement* should not be equated with *large ventricle*. Ventricular enlargement is a presumed pathological process of increase in size from a genetically determined premorbid size.

To confirm this hypothesis, Suddath et al. (1990) presented evidence that monozygotic twins with schizophrenia (who are expected to have ventricular size similar to that of their nonschizophrenic twin) had larger ventricles and smaller hippocampi than did their nonaffected twin. Even schizophrenic twins who had average or small ventricle size compared with the general population had larger ventricles than did their healthy siblings. In this study, matched pairs comparisons further showed that the affected twins almost always performed worse than the healthy twins on a neuropsychological test battery (Goldberg et al. 1990b). Cognitive tasks activated cerebral blood flow to a lesser extent in the affected twin's brain (Randolph et al. 1993). These findings suggest a cognitive impairment that may be induced by, or at least concomitant with, a brain structural defect in schizophrenia. The cause of this defect is unknown, but it has been attributed to a toxic or a contagious disease process, and genetic predisposition is assumed to play a role.

Later brain imaging studies suggested that specific sites in the brain of schizophrenic patients may be affected. Brown et al. (1986) and Suddath et al. (1989) found evidence for structural temporal-lobe abnormality—in particular, a larger temporal horn of the left lateral ventricle. These findings have not been satisfactorily replicated, but they are consistent with the hemispheric hypothesis of schizophrenia (R. E. Gur 1978). Findings of structural difference in the corpus callosum may also be associated with the hypothesized hemispheric dysfunction (Casanova et al. 1990; Rossi et al. 1990). Small frontal lobes have been reported in several studies, more recently by Raine et al. (1992). Again, these findings have not been satisfactorily replicated. Localized site damage in the brain of schizophrenic patients is thus not well defined.

Comment 2: Schizophrenia and Influenza

Investigators attempted to define a causative disease process that produced temporal-lobe abnormalities in schizophrenia. The high incidence of schizophrenic babies born during winter (Randolph et al. 1993) suggests an association between schizophrenia and influenza during the second trimester of pregnancy in late fall. The temporal lobe develops during the second trimester. The findings that the temporal brain regions are structurally more severely affected than other brain regions (Brown et al. 1986; Suddath et al. 1989) suggest that a viral infection may cause this brain damage. This finding also explains why schizophrenia usually first manifests in adolescence or early adulthood. At about these ages, the connectivity between affected temporal-lobe structures and the frontal lobe develops (e.g., Elliott and Sahakian 1995), resulting in the first pathological behavioral manifestations of the disease, such as disorganized thinking and behavior, which are frontal in nature.

This evidence for brain abnormality stimulated further behavioral and cognitive studies that investigated neuropsychological functions in schizophrenia.

◈ COGNITIVE AND BRAIN FUNCTIONING IN SCHIZOPHRENIA

Evidence for a Global Cognitive Deficit: Encephalopathy or Dementia?

The term *dementia praecox* stimulated research attempting to show a dementing, or at least encephalopathic, process in schizophrenia. *Encephalopathy* means a static state of poor cognitive ability caused by the disease, whereas *dementia* implies progressive deterioration in cognitive function. Revolutionary evidence came from the same research group (led by Crow) that reported enlarged ventricles. Crow and Mitchell (1975) observed age and time disorientation, suggestive of dementia, in some schizophrenic patients. This tentative finding suggested either static encephalopathy or progressive dementia in schizophrenia.

Evidence for encephalopathy.   Cognitive studies show that healthy subjects outperform schizophrenic patients on almost any cognitive task (Chapman and Chapman 1973). Schizophrenic patients also perform worse than other mentally ill patients, such as those with depression or bipolar affective disorder (e.g., Calev et al. 1995; Goldberg et al. 1993a). These results can be attributed to global cognitive deficit or encephalopathy. However, schizophrenic traits such as lack of motivation, cooperation, concentration, and interest (Chapman and Chapman 1973) also may cause poor cognitive performance, which suggests a functional rather than a neurological cognitive deficit in schizophrenia.

Several studies provide further evidence for a general neurological encephalopathy in schizophrenia. For example, Goldstein (1978) found that schizophrenic patients cannot be reliably discriminated from brain-damaged patients on the basis of neuropsychological test scores. Goldberg et al. (1993b) observed that a group of patients treated with clozapine, whose psychotic and negative symptoms declined over 15 months, showed no improvement in cognitive impairments during treatment. This finding suggests that the cognitive deficits and the behavioral manifestations of the disease are not necessarily dependent and that cognitive deficits are not secondary to negative symptoms. The difficulty in rehabilitating schizophrenic patients may be the result of an irreversible cognitive disability. The positive correlation between ventricular size and degree of generalized cognitive impairment strongly suggests a neurological cause of encephalopathy in schizophrenia (e.g., Lawson et al. 1988).

Roxborough et al. (1993) repeated a previous finding showing an abnormal electroencephalographic (EEG) P300 evoked potential response in schizophrenic patients and in relatives of schizophrenic patients who had neuropsychological deficits. This abnormal response, observed on EEG, suggested that a brain dysfunction results in neuropsychological deficits, even in healthy subjects at greater risk for schizophrenia.

Research evidence indicates that the level of cognitive deficit during schizophrenic illness does not increase over time. This evidence suggests a static encephalopathy rather than progressive dementia. Most cross-sectional studies of schizophrenic patients at two time points or in different age cohorts show no deterioration and suggest a static encephalopathy rather than progressive dementia (e.g., Heaton et al. 1994; Hyde et al. 1994). Older schizophrenic patients are not affected intellectually more than younger patients if normal aging effects are taken into account. Schizophrenic patients show some deterioration after the onset of the disorder (Frith et al. 1991). This deterioration, if real, may be secondary to anxiety about symptoms, the illness itself, and lack of exposure to new learning.

In an epidemiological study (Calev et al. 1995), patients and families reported low intellectual performance during early school years before onset of the illness. The study further showed a statistical correspondence between premorbid elementary school performance (a measure of intelligence) and current intellectual functioning (Calev et al. 1995). Intellectual difficulties thus appear to precede the onset of the disorder, suggesting static encephalopathy rather than progressive dementia.

Evidence for progressive dementia.　　The Kraepelinian concept of schizophrenia suggests that progressive deterioration is involved in schizophrenia. Bilder et al. (1992) and others suggested deterioration mainly on the basis of patients' neuropsychological profile. For example, schizophrenic patients show larger deficits in the Digit Symbol test of the Wechsler Adult Intelligence Scale—3rd Edition (WAIS-III; Wechsler 1997) than in the Vocabulary test. Because Digit Symbol is less resistant to cognitive deterioration and schizophrenic patients show larger deficits on this task, deterioration over time can be inferred. This argument, however, is not very convincing because factors other than a dementing process may cause the observed deficits on these tasks (see Calev et al., Chapter 1, in this volume). These studies thus provide indirect and uncertain evidence for progressive deterioration or dementia. Frith et al. (1991), however, observed deterioration in the first 5 years of illness and a plateau thereafter. This finding requires further replication because it may suggest dementia followed by encephalopathy.

Substantial evidence indicates a generalized cognitive deficit that can represent a biological encephalopathic process, and inconclusive evidence indicates deterioration over time; however, there is room to investigate specific brain functions associated with brain regions implicated in schizophrenia. Executive function has been studied extensively.

Executive or Frontal Function

The behavioral manifestations of schizophrenia are similar to those of prefrontal-lobe disease. Poor planning ability, poor social judgment, flat affect, avolition, anhedonia, a certain degree of perseveration, and a lack of inhibition are all characteristics of schizophrenic patients that can be attributed to a dorsolateral or orbital prefrontal or executive dysfunction. Attentional problems described in schizophrenia (e.g., McGhie 1969; Venables and Wing 1962) also can be attributed to poor frontal or executive function control (Damasio and Anderson 1993; Elliott and Sahakian 1995). Indeed, abundant research confirms such a dysfunction in schizophrenia. Tasks sensitive to executive function, such as the Wisconsin Card Sorting Test (WCST), are poorly performed by schizophrenic patients (e.g., Stuss et al. 1983). Schizophrenic patients tend to perseverate on their responses and not to shift to new solutions when task demands change. They also have large deficits on word and design fluency tasks (e.g., Kolb and Whishaw 1983) and on the "release from proactive inhibition" paradigm, a learning task involving executive control (Randolph et al. 1992).

The finding of abnormal smooth pursuit eye movement (SPEM) in schizophrenia is important, because eye movement is related to central frontal areas more than to the prefrontal cortex. Schizophrenic patients cannot carry out SPEMs, suggesting a qualitative rather than a quantitative difference between schizophrenic patients and healthy control subjects. SPEM is correlated with other neuropsychological measures assessing frontal-lobe function such as verbal fluency (Friedman et al. 1995). Malaspina et al. (1994) reported odor discrimination deficits in 80% of schizophrenic patients, a perceptual orbital dysfunction that was highly correlated with SPEM deficits. These findings, however, have not been replicated satisfactorily.

Comment 1: problems in the neuropsychological findings. The problems with these findings are 1) the possibility of errors when comparing different functions (e.g., Chapman and Chapman 1978), 2) the incomplete specificity of tasks to brain locations, and 3) the general lack of frontal structural impairment in schizophrenic patients.

Although frontal structural impairment usually is not found in schizophrenic patients, measures of brain metabolism provide additional evidence for frontal dysfunction. When tasks that activate the brain are administered with cerebral blood flow measures, schizophrenic patients activate their frontal cortex less than do control subjects (Buchsbaum et al. 1990). Cerebral blood flow and glucose metabolism studies have shown poor activation during administration of the WCST when patients were either medicated or drug free (Berman et al. 1986; Weinberger et al. 1986). In contrast, schizophrenic patients showed normal activation when working on visuospatial perception tasks, such as Raven's Progressive Matrices, involving the right parietal cortex (Berman et al. 1988). However, evidence is contradictory regarding hypofrontal cerebral blood flow and metabolism during rest (R. E. Gur et al. 1995). Therefore, hypofrontality may apply to schizophrenia only during activation.

Comment 2: frontal deficits may relate to brain disease elsewhere. Contradictory results obtained from neuroimaging and activation studies may be caused by the high probability of error in this kind of research. First, interpretation of neuroimaging results involves many steps, each including a chance of error. Second, situational factors such as anxiety level, age, and arousal may affect baseline metabolism. Third, most tasks used for activation purposes lack adequate reliability, construct validity, and matching for difficulty. R. C. Gur et al. (1992), therefore, suggested that future research should follow certain guidelines to ensure that research results are valid.

To resolve the inconsistency in the findings, some investigators have offered theoretical explanations. For example, Elliott and Sahakian (1995) suggested that because there is no similarity between the behavior of schizophrenic patients and patients with frontal-lobe dysfunction who have dorsolateral cortex dysfunction, a modified neurological explanation is needed for schizophrenia. They pointed out that strong corticostriatal connections are found in the brain, particularly with the dorsolateral and orbital prefrontal areas, the striatum innervating the limbic and medial temporal brain regions. These brain connections may act to disrupt frontal-lobe function when other brain regions are in fact dysfunctional. Subcortical and medial temporal defects may thus explain both the excess of subcortically produced dopamine in schizophrenia and a subsequent frontal-lobe dysfunction.

Single photon emission computed tomography (SPECT) provided evidence suggestive of altered D_2 receptor distribution and density within the basal ganglia of schizophrenic patients (Pilowsky et al. 1994). The finding that both left and right hippocampal volumes were related to WCST performance in affected schizophrenic twins, but not in their unaffected twins (Weinberger et al. 1992), indeed suggests that the medial temporal brain pathology, which may directly cause memory impairment, also may affect frontal functions through such brain connections. The expression of the above-mentioned behavioral manifestations and executive dysfunction in adolescence and early adulthood may thus be related to the development of connectivity between prefrontal and limbic-temporal regions, reported to co-occur in adolescence and early adulthood in humans (Breslin and Weinberger 1990).

This theory may be appealing, but little research evidence supports it. Whether executive function is more compromised than other functions such as memory is not clear (Saykin et al. 1991). Other cognitive functions should be examined to explain the neuropsychological dysfunction in schizophrenic patients. Because the temporal lobe has been seriously implicated by neuroimaging studies, memory function may be at least as adversely affected as prefrontal or executive function.

Memory

Clinicians usually do not report memory deficits in their schizophrenic patients. Patients' memory deficits may, however, be too subtle to impress clinicians. For example, some mild memory problems in patients with early Alzheimer's disease do not appear amnesic in a clinical evaluation. Furthermore, many clinicians do not detect memory deficits in amnesic patients after electroconvulsive therapy (ECT). Thus, amnesic phenomena may be overlooked and should therefore be assessed with objective neuropsychological tests.

On a theoretical basis, memory deficits are expected in schizophrenia. The medial temporal lobe—in particular, the hippocampus—frequently has been associated with memory function (Squire 1987); this brain region is also implicated in schizophrenia (Brown et al. 1986; Suddath et al. 1989). Some amnesic patients with temporal-lobe dysfunction are reported to show a tendency for forgetting more quickly than healthy people; this problem is superimposed on their difficulty in learning new information (Squire 1987). These two deficits are described as *anterograde amnesia*. *Retrograde amnesia* refers to forgetting of information learned and retained before a traumatic event, such as illness.

An example of anterograde amnesia is the famous case study of H. M. (e.g., Milner et al. 1968). This patient's temporal lobes were removed because of intractable seizures. Consequently, H. M. had difficulty acquiring new information because of an extremely rapid rate of forgetting. After reading a story, he would be unable to state what had happened in it. Yet, he would want to read it again. H. M. could follow a conversation, and his immediate memory was more or less intact. This could have been because immediate articulatory memory is not located in classical temporal memory regions of the brain but in a parietal site posterior to the sylvian sulcus (Shallice and Warrington 1970). Indeed, most patients with memory problems, such as those with amnesic Korsakoff's syndrome, have intact immediate memory functions. To carry out a conversation, one also must have an intact knowledge base for word and grammar rules, that is, *semantic memory*. This function seemed to be relatively preserved in H. M.'s case.

Schizophrenic patients show some similarity to amnesic patients, such as H. M., in their anterograde memory function. Early studies of memory function in schizophrenia assumed that memory deficits were caused by the symptoms and psychological distress that characterized schizophrenic patients (e.g., Koh 1978). These studies attributed memory deficits to defective encoding processes, secondary to attention difficulties (e.g., see review by Koh 1978), and suggested that schizophrenic patients would have no memory deficits if encoding strategies were compensated for. One method of investigation was the comparison between *recognition* and *recall* memory.

In recognition memory testing, the to-be-remembered material presented at the acquisition stage is presented again at the retrieval stage with other distracting material not presented during acquisition. The patient needs to identify the material that was presented at the acquisition stage. This paradigm contrasts with the recall paradigm in which at retrieval, the patient has to reproduce actively from memory all materials presented, without presentation of the material at retrieval. Some studies showed recall but no recognition memory deficit in schizophrenic patients (Bauman and Murray 1968; Koh et al. 1973). Because recognition requires almost no association in memory compared with recall (Kintsch 1970), investigators concluded that attention difficulties and poor cooperation interfere with the creation of association at encoding, thus disrupting the organization of memory and producing a secondary recall deficit in schizophrenia. The intact recognition memory was attributed to the fact that recognition does not rely on establishing associations in the to-be-remembered material at encoding.

This conclusion, however, was erroneous. First, the finding of no recognition memory deficit was not replicated with severely disturbed patients (Traupmann 1975). Second, Calev and Monk (1982) suggested that the tasks showing no deficit, in fact, did show a recognition memory deficit. When data from different studies were pooled together, recognition memory deficits were apparent. These recognition memory deficits were too small to reach significance in any individual study. Indeed, Calev et al. (1983) found both recall and recognition deficits in long-stay patients with chronic schizophrenia. In another study, Calev (1984a) used recall and recognition tasks matched on their level of difficulty and discriminating power and found both recall and recognition deficits in long-stay patients, with a larger recall deficit. He thus concluded that the schizophrenic associative deficit adds to the nonassociative purer memory deficit. Calev et al. (1983, 1991b) suggested that temporal-lobe dysfunction explains the nonassociative recognition memory deficit in schizophrenia because the recognition memory deficit is little affected by other cognitive functions.

Further evidence suggesting an anterograde memory deficit in schizophrenia, similar to that in amnesic patients with temporal-lobe dysfunction, is rapid forgetting. Calev et al. (1983) attempted to improve the memory deficit in long-stay patients with chronic schizophrenia on the basis of the hypothesis that memory deficits are secondary to symptoms and behavioral manifestations of the disease. To compensate for patients' memory deficits, Calev and colleagues used an orienting task before recall. This task required patients to associate the to-be-remembered words with category labels to organize their memories better at encoding and to compensate for lack of mnemonic organization in order to reach normal levels of recall. After this training, patients' recall performance did improve compared with nonschizophrenic control subjects. This result suggests that once the associative disturbance in schizophrenia is helped at encoding, memory performance will improve. However, the performance of long-stay patients with schizophrenia on the recall task did not reach the recall levels of nonschizophrenic control subjects. This suggested, like the recognition studies, a nonassociative component to the memory deficit of schizophrenic patients that may result from their temporal-lobe dysfunction. Furthermore, recall performance of schizophrenic patients on a retest, 2 days later, showed evidence of rapid forgetting. No floor or ceiling effects were apparent, and immediate and delayed recall were matched on their discriminating power (Chapman and Chapman 1978). These results were replicated with drug-free schizophrenic patients (Calev et al. 1991b).

Another study included schizophrenic, schizophreniform, and schizoaffective patients (Calev, in press). All patient groups that ever had positive symptoms also showed rapid forgetting; those patients who never had positive symptoms did not show rapid forgetting. These findings suggest that the hippocampal temporal-lobe structural abnormality in schizophrenia may cause a mild memory deficit and that florid psychosis may be associated with this memory deficit. Indeed, Nestor et al. (1993) reported a correlation between left temporal-lobe structural abnormality and verbal memory.

Comment: schizophrenia and amnesia. One problem with the findings of rapid forgetting is that they were always observed with the same, or very similar, verbal recall task. Replications with other tasks are important.

Some investigators, impressed by anterograde memory deficits, took this argument further to suggest amnesia in schizophrenia. McKenna et al. (1990) concluded that the severity of memory impairment in schizophrenia suggests amnesia. Saykin et al. (1991) used the residual scores approach (Chapman and Chapman 1989) to control for differences in discriminating power between memory and other cognitive tasks and found that memory tasks were the least well performed by schizophrenic patients of all the tasks. This finding supported the hypothesis that in schizophrenia, memory centers in the brain are affected more than other centers.

A criticism of this study is that scores of various memory tasks were pooled, which indicates little about pure memory function compared with other cognitive functions. Many memory tasks are affected by other functions, such as associative ability, attention, and language. The pooled memory scores are thus diluted and do not assess memory effectively. Although the evidence for a neurological memory dysfunction is strong, the evidence showing that this dysfunction is selectively larger than other neuropsychological dysfunctions in schizophrenia requires further substantiation.

Other Memory Functions

Other memory functions in schizophrenia were also investigated. Schizophrenic patients have a deficit in *working memory* (Goldman-Pakic 1994; Koh 1978), which requires combining immediate memory with basic knowledge (Baddeley 1976). Some investigators suggest that working memory deficits are due to a diminution of overall processing resources (Fleming et al. 1995), as in dementia, whereas other investigators view them as distinct deficits localized at the prefrontal cortex that involve executive function (Park and Holzman 1993). The case for a specific deficit in working memory, however, is weak, because of methodological problems. Strous et al. (1995), for example, studied echoic memory (immediate sensory memory for sound) and found that schizophrenic patients were impaired in their ability to match two tones after an extremely brief delay of 300 msec but were not impaired when there was no delay between tones. This was interpreted as a working memory deficit. Inspection of the data, however, revealed that control subjects showed the same trend as the patients. Lack of immediate and delayed working memory task matching may thus explain the results (Chapman and Chapman 1978). The finding of an echoic memory deficit can, therefore, be attributed to the schizophrenic generalized deficit, or encephalopathy. The differences in discriminating power between the immediate and delayed tasks, which were not matched on their true score variance, shape of distribution, means, and item distributions (Calev and Monk 1982; Chapman and Chapman 1978, 1989), may have erroneously produced the impression of a larger difference between schizophrenic and control subjects at the delayed, more difficult, task.

Schizophrenic patients show *procedural memory* as well as *implicit memory* deficits (Clare et al. 1993; B. L. Schwartz et al. 1992). Semantic memory is also affected, although less than *episodic memory* (memory of information related to a specific duration in time). Because schizophrenic patients have a global deficit or encephalopathy, all aspects of memory may be affected (Elliott and Sahakian 1995). However, memory functions associated with the temporal lobe seem to be more severely affected.

Attention

Attention, unlike executive function and memory, is not well localized in the brain. The large body of attention research in schizophrenia has not contributed substantially to neuropsychological brain localization.

Attention is a broad concept. *Vigilance,* the ability to focus and respond to changes in displayed details as they occur, as assessed by continuous performance or cancellation tasks (see Calev et al., Chapter 1, in this volume), has been operationally defined as attention. The ability to concentrate, listen to questions, and solve arithmetic problems, as in the WAIS-III Arithmetic test, also has been operationally defined as attention. Visuomotor speed, as in the WAIS-III Digit Symbol test, is also taken as an indirect measure of operationally defined attention. Each of these measures focuses on different aspects of attention, and these are poorly intercorrelated. In each study, a different function of attention is assessed.

Despite these problems, clinicians learned a great deal from the study of attention in schizophrenia. McGhie (1969) was one of the first to describe attention problems of nonmedicated patients with acute schizophrenia. Patients reported difficulties absorbing information and felt that too much was happening at the same time for them to absorb. As a result, they tended to become overwhelmed and lose attention. They had difficulty attending to the essential and blocking off unessential stimuli—a dog barking at a distance could be as vivid as the conversation with the therapist. Healthy people can subjectively amplify essential and suppress irrelevant information. This phenomenon is called *filtering.* Schizophrenic patients have difficulty with filtering. After filtering, attentional strategies are applied to categorize the attended information to further processing. This stage of information processing is called *pigeon-holing.* Hemsley and Richardson (1980) showed that schizophrenic patients had a deficit in pigeon-holing. This may be a reason that information is not encoded in a way that enhances memory in schizophrenia.

Different attempts to study and theorize about attention dysfunctions in schizophrenia were made in the 1950s and 1960s (for review, see Nuechterlein 1977). Although attention research helped describe the disease, it did not directly link to the structural abnormalities observed in schizophrenia.

Language

Language function is most characteristic of the human species. Unlike other functions, language involves different brain sites (see Calev et al., Chapter 1, in this volume). Language function is usually located in the left or dominant hemisphere. Broca's area in the frontal lobe controls speech production and the planum temporale, and Wernicke's area in the posterior upper temporal lobe controls speech comprehension. The repetition of language requires activation of a tract connecting these two centers. Exner's area at the foot of the second frontal motor convolution and the angular gyrus in the parietal lobe have been associated with writing. The occipital lobe is responsible for vision, and vision is necessary for reading. The decoding and interpretation of reading materials are associated with the parietal lobe. The temporal lobe may be involved in the interpretation of reading. Analogue areas in the right or nondominant hemisphere are usually associated with prosody (i.e., the affective and other intonations of speech reception and production). The corpus callosum is an important connecting structure between the two hemispheres, necessary for the integration of speech and its emotional or other emphatic content. Damage or dysfunction in various brain areas may thus produce language problems including different forms of aphasia, agraphia, alexia, and speech repetition problems.

Schizophrenic patients show evidence of language problems. Schizophrenic patients speak in a peculiar way. Sometimes they are semi-mute (alogia), which is associated with negative symptoms (Stolar et al. 1994); sometimes they are incoherent, are loose in their associations, and produce new words (neologisms). These phenomena have been attributed to positive symptoms, confusion, and attention problems; however, they may be secondary to brain dysfunction.

Indeed, language functions may appear to be more seriously affected in schizophrenia than other functions. For example, receptive language, associated with the planum temporale, may be more severely affected because of temporal-lobe structural abnormalities in schizophrenia (e.g., Brown et al. 1986). The evidence for left-hemisphere dysfunction caused by its overactivation (e.g., R. E. Gur 1978) also suggests a language dysfunction.

However, the findings to date are that language function, as assessed in neuropsychological studies, is not more severely affected than other functions (Calev et al. 1995; Goldberg et al. 1993a; Hoff et al. 1992). Further research focusing on specific brain locations affecting specific language functions is likely to be revealing.

Motor and Visuomotor Coordination

The consensus is that schizophrenic patients perform most neuropsychological functions poorly. One less disrupted function is pure motor function. This function is often confused with visuomotor function; however, these two functions differ substantially. *Motor function* involves aspects such as motor speed. An example of a motor test is the Finger Tapping Test, which measures motor speed of the right or left index finger. This test involves the motor cortex, the motor tract, and other brain parts related to motion. On this task, schizophrenic patients seem to show only minor deficits (e.g., Calev et al. 1995), compared with other psychotic patients. F. Schwartz et al. (1990) assessed finger tapping speed, along with motor grip strength and finger dexterity, and found that schizophrenic patients performed worse than nonpsychotic subjects but not worse than affective and schizoaffective patients. Gold et al. (1994) found that finger tapping speed of schizophrenic patients was slower than that of temporal-lobe epileptic patients. B. L. Schwartz et al. (1992) found deficits in motor speed as well as in learning procedural motor tasks and suggested a procedural memory deficit in schizophrenia. Yet, in an overview, the motor deficit in schizophrenia seems mild and does not stand out compared with other areas of deficit (Calev et al. 1995; Goldberg et al. 1993c).

Visuomotor function, unlike pure motor function, involves occipital, parietal-spatial, frontal-motor cortex, and other brain areas. It involves coordination of movement using the input from vision. It is considered a sensitive measure of global brain functioning. Examples of such measures are the Symbol Digit Modalities Test (SDMT); the Trail Making Test (TMT), Part A; and the Purdue Pegboard Test. Schizophrenic patients have substantial deficits on these tasks (Bilder et al. 1995; Calev et al. 1995), thus supporting the hypothesized global encephalopathy in schizophrenia.

Visuospatial, Visuoconstructive, and Praxic Functions

Visuospatial functions are usually associated with the right parietal lobe. Visuoconstructive and praxic functions are localized in the posterior frontal lobes and the parietal lobe, which act together. Studies usually show that deficits in all these functions are moderate and do not stand out in schizophrenia (Calev et al. 1995; Goldberg et al. 1993a; Hoff et al. 1992). The findings of normal posterior brain activation during hypofrontality in schizophrenia (Goldberg et al. 1990a) indeed argue for relatively preserved visuospatial and praxic functions. However, results are contradictory. Kolb and Whishaw (1983) reported that constructional and visuospatial functions are more severely affected than other functions in schizophrenia. These results can, however, be criticized because unmatched tasks were used. Studies using unmatched tasks may magnify or reduce deficits disproportionately.

Case for Specific Hemispheric Dysfunction

Following interest in hemispheric differences, R. E. Gur (1978) published the results of her study, which suggested hemispheric aberrations in schizophrenia. She gave schizophrenic subjects tasks requiring simultaneous and successive processing. *Simultaneous processing* is required in tasks performed by the nondominant right hemisphere, such as grasping the shape of a design; *successive processing* is believed to be performed by the dominant left hemisphere and is used in tasks requiring temporal orientation, such as arithmetic or sentence construction. Gur found evidence suggesting a dysfunction producing overactivation of the left hemisphere and argued that this may be caused by right-hemisphere damage that reduces right-hemisphere processing capacity. In line with this evidence, R. E. Gur et al. (1985) reported increased cerebral blood flow in the left hemisphere of schizophrenic patients. R. E. Gur et al. (1987) repeated the finding of high left brain metabolism (consistent with excessive left-hemisphere activation in schizophrenia). They also reported that increased right-hemisphere metabolism and decreased left-hemisphere metabolism (i.e., normalization) were correlated with clinical improvement. The finding of more left-handedness among schizophrenic patients (e.g., R. E. Gur 1977) further supported this finding. Left-handed schizophrenic patients have been found to perform cognitive tasks more poorly than right-handed schizophrenic patients and had larger lateral ventricles (Katsanis and Iacono 1989). Other studies have supported this hypothesis, and hemispheric disparity remains an important research issue in schizophrenia.

Nevertheless, some findings show no major differences in hemispheric function on many tasks (e.g., Calev et al. 1987, 1991a; Gold et al. 1994) and in ratios of left- to right-handedness in schizophrenic patients (Torrey et al. 1993). Some studies found right-hemisphere dysfunction in schizophrenia with standard neuropsychological test batteries specifically designed to assess lateral dysfunction (Oepen et al. 1987). Cutting (1990) reviewed different methods used in detecting hemispheric differences in schizophrenia, including formal cognitive testing, dichotic listening tests, tachistoscopic methods, and tactile perception procedures. He reported that the results are inconclusive and thus disappointing, although this may be partially a result of inefficiency of experimental methods.

Some investigators have suggested that differences in laterality observed in perceptual tasks may be due to differences in allocation of attention (Ragland et al. 1992) and other factors such as effort. Overall, it seems that to date the laterality hypothesis does not have sufficient research support.

Comment. Support for the hemispheric hypothesis in schizophrenia also comes from the finding of abnormal, sometimes reduced, size (Rossi et al. 1990) and, most often, thicker structure of the corpus callosum, which is expected to affect interhemispheric communication (Casanova et al. 1990; Raine et al. 1990). David (1987) found that schizophrenic patients made significantly more errors than depressive and nonschizophrenic control subjects in matching colors across their left and right visual fields. This function may be mediated by the posterior corpus callosum and supports a callosal dysfunction in schizophrenia. Some investigators reported differences in callosal structure between schizophrenic men and women, which suggests a sex and corpus callosum interaction (Raine et al. 1990). However, such findings have not been replicated successfully.

Emotion and cognitive function in schizophrenia. If schizophrenic patients have a lateral or hemispheric brain dysfunction and the reports of normal hemispheric specialization for positive and negative emotion are correct (Heilman et al. 1993), then emotional malfunctioning is to be expected in schizophrenia. The negative symptoms of schizophrenia, such as the flattening of affect, anhedonia, and avolition, do suggest such a component.

Koh et al. (1981) tested the hypothesis that emotion will affect cognition in schizophrenia. They found that adding affective connotation to the to-be-remembered verbal material improved encoding. This suggested that emotional arousal can help schizophrenic patients' cognitive ability. These investigators also found better recall of negative than positive or neutral materials, compared with control subjects. This suggested that negative emotion, possibly mediated by the right hemisphere, interacts with memory performance in schizophrenic patients. In line with this finding, Calev and Edelist (1993) reported that schizophrenic patients forgot positive or neutral information more quickly than negative information, compared with nonschizophrenic control subjects.

David and Cutting (1990) used a chimeric face test with happy and sad faces. The test is known to elicit left-sided perceptual bias in right-handed persons. Schizophrenic patients showed no bias. Depression was associated with reduced bias, and mania was associated with increased bias. The lack of left-sided bias in schizophrenic patients may suggest a hemispheric dysfunction in schizophrenia. However, Kerr and Neale (1993) investigated the ability of schizophrenic patients to perceive facial and vocal emotion in others. Emotional recognition tests were standardized and cross-validated to ensure equivalent discriminating power (Chapman and Chapman 1978). The results suggested that the differences between schizophrenic and nonschizophrenic subjects reflect the schizophrenic patients' generalized cognitive deficit and not a specific deficit in emotion. Although the emotional bias concept in schizophrenia seems appealing, the studies are inconclusive and require additional research.

◆ NEUROPSYCHOLOGY AND SUBTYPES OF SCHIZOPHRENIA

Schizophrenic patients are a diverse group in terms of their symptoms. One reason for this diversity is the past overinclusion of patients in this diagnostic category. A genuine phenomenological heterogeneity also exists in this illness. Some patients are active, but others are withdrawn. Some have florid psychosis, but others show little evidence of hallucinations or delusions. Some patients have average or even higher intelligence, whereas most patients have low-average intelligence. Some can

lead a social life with gainful employment, but others are socially and oc-
cupationally disabled and need permanent hospitalization.

Diagnoses were refined in recent diagnostic systems such as DSM-IV
(American Psychiatric Association 1994) in an attempt to define the disease more accurately. DSM-IV excluded the hebephrenic and simple subtypes and included the "undifferentiated type" (patients who are not
paranoid, disorganized, or catatonic) and the "residual type" (patients
who still have impairments and negative symptoms after recovery from
the prominent symptoms that characterize the acute episode). The diversity in illness manifestations stimulated the division of schizophrenia initially into three, and later into four, subtypes (Kraepelin 1919). Because
these divisions were not satisfactory, other subtyping of schizophrenia
emerged:

1. The most influential division is between *patients with positive and
    negative symptoms suggested as two disease processes* (e.g., Crow
    1980). Positive symptoms include hallucinations, delusions, and
    thought and behavior disorder, and negative symptoms include with-
    drawal, mutism, and poverty of speech. Cognitive impairment, such
    as age and time disorientation, is considered a negative symptom.
    Neuropsychological tests show that negative symptoms are associ-
    ated with greater cognitive impairment (e.g., Stolar et al. 1994), en-
    larged ventricles, and poor premorbid adjustment (e.g., Randolph et
    al. 1993). However, functions may be selectively affected in patients
    with positive symptoms (Calev, in press). It is interesting that posi-
    tive and negative symptoms respond to different kinds of medication.
    Antipsychotic (neuroleptic) medications usually affect positive but
    not negative symptoms. Medications that reduce negative symptoms,
    such as clozapine, do not improve positive symptoms. Both kinds of
    medications have minor cognitive effects (see next section).
2. The distinction between positive and negative symptoms was pre-
    ceded by a distinction between *chronic and acute schizophrenia* and
    *withdrawn (usually chronic) and active (usually acute) schizophre-
    nia* (Venables 1957; Venables and Wing 1962). This theory was sup-
    ported by the observations that acutely ill patients show positive
    symptoms, and chronically ill patients show negative symptoms. The
    neuropsychological findings suggested that acutely ill patients have
    narrow attention and overexclude perceptual details, whereas chron-
    ically ill patients with schizophrenia have broad attention and
    overinclude perceptual details. Note that unlike the distinction be-

tween positive and negative symptoms, the acute-chronic distinction was related to the stage rather than the type of illness. These distinctions, although useful for diagnosis and treatment, do not explain the genesis of schizophrenia and do not seem to define patients in a consistent way.

3. Bilder et al. (1985) and Liddle (1987a, 1987b) attempted to classify schizophrenia as representing *three brain syndromes*. Liddle (1987b) presented evidence from neuropsychological tests that three different brain locations produce three different syndromes: 1) dorsolateral frontal: *psychomotor poverty* consisted of negative symptoms such as flattening of affect, decreased spontaneous movement, and poverty of speech; 2) ventromedial frontal: *disorganization* consisted of formal thought disorder, inappropriate affect, and poverty of speech; and 3) temporal: *reality distortion* consisted of positive symptoms such as delusions and hallucinations. However, replicating these findings was very difficult (Marks and Luchins 1990). Cluster analysis of schizophrenic symptoms identifies more than three subtypes of schizophrenia. Dollfus et al. (1996) observed the above-mentioned three syndromes as subtypes, as well as an additional mixed subtype including both positive and negative symptoms (syndromes 1 and 3 mixed) and a subtype with few symptoms labeled *simple schizophrenia,* which is similar to the residual subtype in DSM-IV.

4. The distinction between *process schizophrenia* and *reactive schizophrenia* is now used rarely. Process schizophrenia represents the Kraepelinian type, characterized by insidious early onset and deteriorating course. Reactive schizophrenia is caused primarily by environmental stress and is reversible. Studies have found differences in neuropsychological functions between these two types (e.g., Randolph et al. 1993); mainly, more severe cognitive deficits are seen in patients with process schizophrenia. Today, the concept of brief reactive psychosis seems to have replaced the concept of reactive schizophrenia.

5. Another distinction is between *paranoid* and *nonparanoid types;* paranoid patients have better cognitive functioning than nonparanoid patients (e.g., Randolph et al. 1993). This distinction also is not very useful in understanding the disease process but has good descriptive value.

6. A recently proposed distinction is between *deficit* and *nondeficit schizophrenia.* Deficit schizophrenia is characterized by greater neu-

rological impairment, negative symptoms that persist beyond episodes, poorer premorbid adjustment, and increased anhedonia
compared with nondeficit schizophrenia. Parietal-lobe function and
deficits in executive function have been associated with the deficit
syndrome. Buchanan et al. (1994) administered an extensive
neuropsychological battery to deficit patients. They performed more
poorly on two executive function tasks: the Stroop Color and Word
Test and the Trail Making Test, Part B. The Mooney Faces Closure
Test, a right parietal measure, was also more severely impaired in
deficit patients compared with nondeficit patients. These findings
are, however, preliminary.

◆ MODIFICATIONS OF COGNITIVE SYMPTOMS IN SCHIZOPHRENIA

Schizophrenic patients are subjected to extensive effects of medication,
hospitalization, and illness symptoms. These factors may contribute to
and modify the neuropsychological profile of schizophrenia. The possible
effects are considered below.

Medications

The evidence seems to converge in showing that neuroleptic medications
do not produce extensive cognitive effects (Cassens et al. 1990; Spohn
and Strauss 1989). However, tardive dyskinesia, characterized by excessive lip, mouth, and other movements that look inappropriate, may
emerge. This disorder is rare in younger adults but has a high incidence
among aged patients. Tardive dystonia is a variant of this disorder, characterized by prolonged or permanent inability to keep muscle tone,
sometimes resulting in severe physical disability. Anticholinergic medications, used to combat parkinsonian symptoms caused by neuroleptics,
seem to have adverse effects on memory (Calev 1984b; Tune et al. 1982).
These effects may be limited, however, to patients who use these drugs
for a short time. Chronically ill patients do not seem to have adverse effects of neuroleptic medication (Nigal et al. 1991). Serotonergic and
other medications affecting negative symptoms, such as clozapine, affect
cognition. Their effects are reported to be mild, however, compared with
the effects of illness (Goldberg and Weinberger 1994; Goldberg et al.
1993b; Lee et al. 1994). These medications seem to result in mild im-

provement on tasks assessing attention, visuomotor speed, and expressive language (such as verbal fluency, considered a negative symptom). However, they seem to have adverse effects on executive function and visual memory (Goldberg and Weinberger 1994). Many schizophrenic patients receive antianxiety and antidepressant medications. (The effects of these medications are reviewed in Calev et al., Chapter 3, in this volume.)

Hospitalization

Institutionalization can be expected to produce cognitive deficits because of the lack of intellectual stimulation. However, studies of hospitalization do not show a significant effect. Harrow et al. (1987), for example, did not observe differences between continuously hospitalized and intermittently hospitalized patients. Johnstone et al. (1981) found no deterioration in Mini-Mental State Exam results as a function of length of hospitalization. Goldstein et al. (1991) analyzed the data of 245 schizophrenic patients to determine the effects of age, education, and length of hospitalization on performance. Hospitalization did not account for a significant proportion of the variance in cognitive test performance.

Illness Symptoms

The effect of illness symptoms on cognition has not been determined definitively by research findings (Gold et al. 1991). Some investigators have suggested that symptoms adversely affect performance. Others suggest that symptoms have no effect because cognitive deficits at the beginning of the illness remain unchanged after years of treatment (Frame and Oltmanns 1982; Gold and Hurt 1990). Moreover, when negative symptoms are reduced with clozapine, cognitive deficits persist (Goldberg et al. 1993b). These findings suggest that schizophrenia causes cognitive deficits and that their modification by illness symptoms is minimal.

Age

Aging is reported to modify cognitive symptoms because of the interaction between schizophrenia and dementia in elderly patients (see Harvey and Dahlman, Chapter 8, in this volume). Additive effects of aging illnesses and schizophrenia thus may be observed in geriatric schizo-phrenic patients.

Cognitive deficits can be modified therapeutically. Reducing use of drugs that cause adverse effects, using drugs that improve cognition, and using cognitive rehabilitative techniques (see Jaeger and Berns, Chapter 10, in this volume) can be combined to improve the cognitive status of patients.

◈ NEUROPSYCHOLOGY OF OTHER PSYCHOTIC DISORDERS

Other psychotic disorders include variants of schizophrenia such as schizoaffective and schizophreniform disorders, brief reactive psychosis, and delusional disorder. The findings of these variants of schizophrenic disorder seem to present a neuropsychological profile similar to that of schizophrenic patients. Calev (in press) found similar memory functioning in schizophrenic, schizoaffective, and schizophreniform patients; patients who were never florid were a far better functioning group. Hoff et al. (1992) reported similar deficits in schizophreniform and schizo-phrenic patients and suggested that chronicity does not affect cognitive performance. Schizophreniform and schizophrenic patients were not distinguished in their frontal and subcortical brain activity assessed with regional cerebral blood flow measures. All patients showed low left frontal activation during WCST administration. Both schizophrenic and schizoaffective patients, but not affective patients, showed memory deficits that were related to poor social skills (Mueser et al. 1991). Some studies, however, found that schizoaffective patients may be somewhat better functioning and have a general cognitive level and insight similar to that of affective patients (e.g., Buhler et al. 1991). These findings suggest no major neuropsychological distinctions among these schizophrenia spectrum disorders.

The research on brief reactive psychosis and delusional disorder is lean compared with schizophrenia spectrum research. Brief reactive psychosis induced by the Gulf War trauma was reported to cause cognitive deficits (Talmon et al. 1992). Lower intelligence was also observed in delusional disorder (Rockwell et al. 1994). Some studies combined different schizophrenia spectrum patients and found deficits similar to those observed in schizophrenia (e.g., Goldberg et al. 1993b). It seems that these disease entities were rarely investigated as distinct entities.

◈ SUMMARY

A structural brain abnormality exists in schizophrenia. It is characterized by at least enlarged ventricles, but medial temporal-lobe dysfunction also may be present, especially in the left side of the brain. Tentative evidence exists for reduced frontal-lobe size and for corpus callosum structural abnormalities.

Ventricular size is correlated with a global cognitive deficit. This deficit is most likely static and has been termed *encephalopathy*. The case for progressive deterioration or dementia is weak. This deficit precludes in most cases normal occupational and marital functioning and defines schizophrenic patients as disabled.

Of the specific localizable brain functions, executive and memory dysfunctions frequently have been implicated as relatively significant. Negative symptoms and lack of life planning are associated with executive dysfunction. Reduced frontal brain metabolism characterizes patients during brain activation. Anterograde memory deficit, including defective encoding into memory and rapid forgetting, is the most specific evidence for a neurologically induced memory dysfunction. Executive dysfunction has been associated with frontal connections to dysfunctional medial temporal and subcortical brain regions. Memory deficit has been directly associated with structural medial temporal-lobe dysfunction. The case for hemispheric dysfunction is equivocal.

Modification of cognitive deficits by antipsychotic and other medications, hospitalization, and illness symptoms is minimal.

Other psychotic nonaffective disorders have not been investigated extensively. At present, schizoaffective and schizophreniform disorders have cognitive similarity to schizophrenia. Delusional disorders and brief reactive psychosis seem to result in milder cognitive deficits.

◈ REFERENCES

Allebeck P: Schizophrenia: a life shortening disease. Schizophr Bull 15:81–89, 1989

American Psychiatric Association: Diagnostic and Statistical Manual of Mental Disorders, 4th Edition. Washington, DC, American Psychiatric Association, 1994

Baddeley AD: The Psychology of Memory. New York, Basic Books, 1976

Bauman E, Murray DJ: Recognition versus recall in schizophrenia. Canadian Journal of Psychology 22:18–25, 1968

Beaton JM, Smithies JR, Bradlet RJ: The behavioral effects of L-methionine and related compounds in rats and men. Biol Psychiatry 10:45–52, 1975

Berman KF, Zec RF, Weinberger DR: Physiological dysfunction in the dorsolateral prefrontal cortex in schizophrenia, II: role of neuroleptic treatment, attention, and mental effort. Arch Gen Psychiatry 43:126–135, 1986

Berman KF, Illowsky BP, Weinberger DR: Physiological dysfunction of dorsolateral prefrontal cortex in schizophrenia, IV: further evidence for regional and behavioral specificity. Arch Gen Psychiatry 45:616–622, 1988

Bilder RM, Mukherjee S, Rieder RO, et al: Symptomatic and neuropsychological components of defect states. Schizophr Bull 11:409–417, 1985

Bilder RM, Lipschuts-Broch L, Reiter G, et al: Intellectual deficits in first-episode schizophrenia: evidence for progressive deterioration. Schizophr Bull 18: 437–448, 1992

Bilder RM, Reiter G, Bates JA, et al: Neuropsychological profiles of first episode schizophrenia (abstract). Schizophr Res 15:111, 1995

Bleuler E: Dementia Praecox and the Group of Schizophrenias (1911). New York, International Universities Press, 1950

Breslin NA, Weinberger DR: Schizophrenia and the normal functional development of the prefrontal cortex. Development in Psychopathology 2:409–424, 1990

Brown R, Colter N, Corsellis JAN, et al: Post mortem evidence of structural brain changes in schizophrenia: differences in brain structure, brain weight temporal horn areas, and parahippocampal gyrus compared with affective disorder. Arch Gen Psychiatry 43:36–42, 1986

Buchanan RW, Strauss ME, Kirkpatrick B, et al: Neuropsychological impairment in deficit vs nondeficit forms of schizophrenia. Arch Gen Psychiatry 51: 804–811, 1994

Buchsbaum MS, Nuechterlein KH, Haier RJ, et al: Glucose metabolic rate in normals and schizophrenics during continuous performance test assessed by positron emission tomography. Br J Psychiatry 156:216–227, 1990

Buhler KF, Gross M, Jurgensen R: Psychometrische Differenzierung schizophrener und schizoaffektiver psychosen. Schweizer Archiv fur Neurologie und Psychiatrie 142:535–552, 1991

Calev A: Recall and recognition in chronic nondemented schizophrenics: use of matched tasks. J Abnorm Psychol 93:172–177, 1984a

Calev A: Recall and recognition in mildly disturbed schizophrenics: use of matched tasks. Psychol Med 14:425–429, 1984b

Calev A: Immediate and delayed recall performance in schizophrenia spectrum patients. Psychopathology (in press)

Calev A, Edelist S: Affect and memory in schizophrenia: negative emotion words are forgotten less rapidly than other words by long-hospitalized schizophrenics. Psychopathology 26:229–236, 1993

Calev A, Monk AF: Verbal memory tasks showing no deficit in schizophrenia—fact or artefact. Br J Psychiatry 141:528–530, 1982

Calev A, Venables PH, Monk AF: Evidence for distinct verbal memory pathologies in severely and mildly disturbed schizophrenics. Schizophr Bull 9:247–264, 1983

Calev A, Korin Y, Kugelmass S, et al: Performance of chronic schizophrenics on matched word and design recall tasks. Biol Psychiatry 22:699–709, 1987

Calev A, Edelist S, Kugelmass S, et al: Performance of long-stay schizophrenics on matched verbal and visuospatial recall tasks. Psychol Med 21:655–660, 1991a

Calev A, Nigal D, Kugelmass S, et al: Performance of long-stay schizophrenics after drug withdrawal on matched immediate and delayed recall tasks. Br J Clin Psychol 30:241–245, 1991b

Calev A, Fennig S, Jandorf L, et al: Factors associated with neuropsychological performance in first-admission psychotic patients (abstract). Schizophr Res 15:111, 1995

Casanova MF, Sanders RD, Goldberg TE, et al: Morphometry of the corpus callosum in monozygotic twins discordant for schizophrenia: a magnetic resonance imaging study. J Neurol Neurosurg Psychiatry 53:416–421, 1990

Cassens G, Inglis AK, Applebaum PS, et al: Neuroleptics: effects on neuropsychological function in chronic schizophrenic patients. Schizophr Bull 16:477–499, 1990

Chapman LJ, Chapman JP: Disordered Thought in Schizophrenia. Englewood Cliffs, NJ, Prentice-Hall, 1973

Chapman LJ, Chapman JP: The measurement of differential deficits. J Psychiatry Res 14:303–311, 1978

Chapman LJ, Chapman JP: Strategies for resolving the heterogeneity of schizophrenics and their relatives using cognitive measures. J Abnorm Psychol 98:357–366, 1989

Clare L, McKenna PJ, Mortimer AM, et al: Memory in schizophrenia: what is impaired and what is preserved? Neuropsychologia 31:1225–1241, 1993

Crow TJ: Molecular pathology of schizophrenia: more than one disease process? BMJ 280:66–68, 1980

Crow TJ, Mitchell WS: Subjective age in chronic schizophrenia: evidence for a subgroup of patients with defective learning capacity? Br J Psychiatry 126:360–363, 1975

Cutting J: Direct examination of hemispheric imbalance in schizophrenia, in Right Cerebral Hemisphere and Psychiatric Disorders. Edited by Cutting J. New York, Oxford University Press, 1990, pp 328–345

Damasio AR, Anderson SW: The frontal lobes, in Clinical Neuropsychology. Edited by Heilman KM, Valenstein E. New York, Oxford University Press, 1993, pp 170–200

David AS: Tachistoscopic tests of colour naming and matching in schizophrenia: evidence for posterior callosum dysfunction? Psychol Med 17:621–630, 1987

David AS, Cutting JC: Affect, affective disorder and schizophrenia: a neuropsychological investigation of right hemisphere function. Br J Psychiatry 156:491–495, 1990

Davies LM, Drummond MF: The economic burden of schizophrenia. Schizophr Bull 14:522–525, 1990

Dohrenwent BP, Dohrenwent BS: Social and cultural influences on psychopathology. Annu Rev Psychol 24:417–452, 1974

Dollfus S, Everitt B, Ribeyre JM, et al: Identifying subtypes of schizophrenia by cluster analysis. Schizophr Bull 22:545–555, 1996

Elliott R, Sahakian BJ: The neuropsychology of schizophrenia: relations with clinical and neurobiological dimensions. Psychol Med 25:581–594, 1995

Fleming K, Goldberg TE, Gold JM, et al: Verbal working memory dysfunction in schizophrenia: use of a Brown-Peterson paradigm. Psychiatry Res 56:155–161, 1995

Frame CL, Oltmanns TF: Serial recall by schizophrenic and affective patients during and after psychotic episodes. J Abnorm Psychol 91:311–318, 1982

Friedman L, Kenny JT, Jesberger JA, et al: Relationship between smooth pursuit eye-tracking and cognitive performance in schizophrenia. Biol Psychiatry 37:265–272, 1995

Frith CD, Leary J, Calhill C, et al: Performance on neuropsychological tests: demographic and clinical correlates of results of these tests. Br J Psychiatry 195 (suppl 13):26–29, 1991

Gold JM, Hurt S: The effects of haloperidol on thought disorder and IQ in schizophrenia. J Pers Assess 54:390–400, 1990

Gold JM, Goldberg TE, Kleinman JE, et al: The impact of symptomatic state and pharmacological treatment on cognitive functioning of patients with schizophrenia and mood disorder, in Handbook of Clinical Trials: The Neurobehavioral Approach. Edited by Mohr E, Brouwers P. Amsterdam, Swets, 1991, pp 185–216

Gold JM, Hermann BP, Randolph C, et al: Schizophrenia and temporal lobe epilepsy: a neuropsychological analysis. Arch Gen Psychiatry 51:265–272, 1994

Goldberg TE, Weinberger DR: The effect of clozapine on neurocognition: an overview. J Clin Psychiatry 55:88–90, 1994

Goldberg TE, Berman KF, Mohr E, et al: Regional cerebral blood flow and cognitive function in Huntington's disease and schizophrenia: a comparison of patients matched for performance on a prefrontal type task. Arch Neurol 47:418–422, 1990a

Goldberg TE, Ragland JD, Torrey EF, et al: Neuropsychological assessment of monozygotic twins discordant for schizophrenia. Arch Gen Psychiatry 47:1066–1072, 1990b

Goldberg TE, Gold JM, Greenberg R, et al: Contrasts between patients with affective disorders and patients with schizophrenia on a neuropsychological test battery. Am J Psychiatry 150:1355–1362, 1993a

Goldberg TE, Greenberg RD, Griffin SJ, et al: The effect of clozapine on cognition and psychiatric symptoms in patients with psychiatric symptoms. Br J Psychiatry 162:43–48, 1993b

Goldberg TE, Torrey EF, Gold JM, et al: Learning and memory in monozygotic twins discordant for schizophrenia. Psychol Med 23:71–85, 1993c

Goldman-Pakic PS: Working memory dysfunction in schizophrenia. J Neuropsychiatry Clin Neurosci 6:348–357, 1994

Goldstein G: Cognitive and perceptual differences between schizophrenics and organics. Schizophr Bull 86:34–60, 1978

Goldstein G, Zubin J, Pogue-Geile MF: Hospitalization and the cognitive deficits of schizophrenia: the influence of age and education. J Nerv Ment Dis 179: 202–205, 1991

Gur RC, Erwin RJ, Gur RE: Neurobehavioral probes for physiologic neuroimaging studies. Am J Psychiatry 49:409–414, 1992

Gur RE: Motoric laterality imbalance in schizophrenia: a possible concomitant of left hemispheric dysfunction. Arch Gen Psychiatry 34:33–37, 1977

Gur RE: Right hemisphere dysfunction and left hemisphere overactivation in schizophrenia. J Abnorm Psychol 87:226–238, 1978

Gur RE, Gur RC, Skolnick BE, et al: Brain function in psychiatric disorders, III: regional cerebral blood flow in unmedicated schizophrenics. Arch Gen Psychiatry 42:329–334, 1985

Gur RE, Resnick SM, Alavi A, et al: Regional brain function in schizophrenia, I: a positron emission tomography study. Arch Gen Psychiatry 44:119–125, 1987

Gur RE, Mozley PD, Resnick SM, et al: Resting cerebral glucose metabolism in first-episode and previously treated patients with schizophrenia relates to clinical features. Arch Gen Psychiatry 52:657–667, 1995

Hare EH: Epidemiology of schizophrenia and affective disorders. Br Med Bull 43:514–530, 1987

Harrow M, Marengo J, Pogue-Geile M, et al: Schizophrenic deficits in intelligence and abstract thinking: influence of aging and long-term institutionalization, in Schizophrenia and Aging. Edited by Miller NE, Cohen GD. New York, Guilford, 1987, pp 133–144

Heaton R, Paulsen JS, McAdams LA, et al: Neuropsychological deficits in schizophrenia: relationship to age, chronicity, and dementia. Arch Gen Psychiatry 51:469–476, 1994

Heilman KM, Bowers D, Valenstein E: Emotional disorders associated with neurological diseases, in Clinical Neuropsychology. Edited by Heilman KM, Valenstein E. New York, Oxford University Press, 1993, pp 461–497

Hemsley DR, Richardson PH: Shadowing by context in schizophrenia. J Nerv Ment Dis 168:141–145, 1980

Hoff AL, Riordan H, O'Donnell DW, et al: Neuropsychological functioning of first-episode schizophreniform patients. Am J Psychiatry 149:898–903, 1992

Hoffer A: Megavitamin B-3 therapy for schizophrenia. Canadian Psychiatric Association Journal 16:499–504, 1971

Hunter R, Jones M, Malleson A: Abnormal CFS total protein and gamma-glubolin levels in 256 patients admitted to a psychiatric unit. J Neurol Sci 9:11–38, 1969

Hyde TM, Nawroz S, Goldberg TE, et al: Is there a cognitive decline in schizophrenia? A cross sectional study. Br J Psychiatry 164:494–500, 1994

Johnstone EC, Crow TJ, Frith CD, et al: Cerebral ventricular size and cognitive impairment in chronic schizophrenia. Lancet 2(7992):924–926, 1976

Johnstone EC, Cunningham Owens DG, Gold A, et al: Institutionalization and the defects of schizophrenia. Br J Psychiatry 139:195–203, 1981

Kallman KJ: The genetic theory of schizophrenia: an analysis of 691 schizophrenic twin index families. Am J Psychiatry 103:309–311, 1946

Katsanis J, Iacono WG: Association of left-handedness with ventricle size and neuropsychological performance in schizophrenia. Am J Psychiatry 146:1056–1058, 1989

Kerr SL, Neale JM: Emotion perception in schizophrenia: specific deficit or further evidence of generalized poor performance? J Abnorm Psychol 102:312–318, 1993

Kintsch W: Models for free recall and recognition, in Models of Human Memory. Edited by Norman DA. New York, Academic Press, 1970, pp 331–373

Koh SD: Remembering of verbal materials by schizophrenic young adults, in Language and Cognition in Schizophrenia. Edited by Schwartz S. Hillsdale, NJ, Lawrence Erlbaum, 1978, pp 55–99

Koh SD, Kayton L, Berry R: Mnemonic organization in young nonpsychotic schizophrenics. J Abnorm Psychol 81:299–310, 1973

Koh SD, Grinker RR, Marusarz TZ, et al: Affective memory and schizophrenic anhedonia. Schizophr Bull 7:292–307, 1981

Kolb B, Whishaw IQ: Performance of schizophrenic patients on tests sensitive to left or right frontal, temporal, or parietal function in neurological patients. J Nerv Ment Dis 171:435–443, 1983

Kraepelin E: Dementia Praecox and Paraphrenia. Translated by Barclay RM. Edinburgh, Scotland, Livingstone, 1919

Laing RD: The Divided Self: An Existential Study of Sanity and Madness. Middlesex, England, Penguin Books, 1965

Lawson WB, Walsman IV, Weinberger DR: Schizophrenic dementia: clinical and computed axial tomography correlates. J Nerv Ment Dis 176:207–212, 1988

Lee MA, Thompson PA, Meltzer HY: Effects of clozapine on cognitive function in schizophrenia. J Clin Psychiatry 55:82–87, 1994

Liddle PF: Schizophrenic syndrome, cognitive performance and neurological dysfunction. Psychol Med 17:49–57, 1987a

Liddle PF: The symptoms of chronic schizophrenia: a reexamination of the positive-negative dichotomy. Br J Psychiatry 151:145–151, 1987b

Malaspina D, Wray AD, Friedman JH, et al: Odor discrimination deficits in schizophrenia: association with eye movement dysfunction. J Neuropsychiatry Clin Neurosci 6:273–278, 1994

Marks RC, Luchins DJ: Relationship between brain imaging findings in schizophrenia and psychopathology: a review of the literature relating to positive and negative symptoms, in Modern Problems of Pharmacopsychiatry: Positive and Negative Symptoms and Syndromes. Edited by Andreasen NC. Basel, Switzerland, Karger, 1990, pp 89–123

McGhie A: Pathology of Attention. Harmonsworth, England, Penguin Books, 1969

McKenna PJ, Tamlyn D, Lund CE, et al: Amnesic syndrome in schizophrenia. Psychol Med 20:967–972, 1990

Mednick SA: Breakdown in individuals at high risk for schizophrenia: possible predispositional perinatal factors. Mental Hygiene 54:50–63, 1970

Milner B, Corkin S, Teuber HL: Further analysis of the hippocampal amnesic syndrome: 14 years follow-up study of H.M. Neuropsychologia 6:215–234, 1968

Mueser KT, Bellack AS, Douglas MS, et al: Prediction of social skill acquisition in schizophrenic and major affective disorder patients from memory and symptomatology. Psychiatry Res 37:281–296, 1991

Nestor PG, Shenton ME, McCarley RW, et al: Neuropsychological correlates of MRI temporal lobe abnormalities in schizophrenia. Am J Psychiatry 150:1849–1855, 1993

Nigal D, Calev A, Kugelmass S, et al: The effect of neuroleptic and anticholinergic drug withdrawal on memory function in chronic long-stay schizophrenics. Ann Clin Psychiatry 3:141–145, 1991

Nuechterlein KH: Reaction time and attention in schizophrenia: a critical evaluation of the data and the theories. Schizophr Bull 3:373–428, 1977

Oepen G, Fungfeld M, Holl T, et al: Schizophrenia—an emotional hypersensitivity of the right cerebral hemisphere. Int J Psychophysiol 5:261–264, 1987

Park S, Holzman PS: Association of working memory deficit and eye tracking dysfunction in schizophrenia. Schizophr Res 11:55–61, 1993

Pilowsky LS, Costa DC, Ell PJ, et al: D2 dopamine receptor binding in the basal ganglia of antipsychotic-free schizophrenic patients. Br J Psychiatry 164:16–26, 1994

Ragland JD, Goldberg TE, Wexler BE, et al: Dichotic listening in monozygotic twins discordant and concordant for schizophrenia. Schizophr Res 7:177–183, 1992

Raine A, Harrison GN, Reynolds GP, et al: Structural and functional characteristics of the corpus callosum in schizophrenics, psychiatric controls, and normal controls: a magnetic resonance imaging and neuropsychological evaluation. Arch Gen Psychiatry 47:1060–1064, 1990

Raine A, Lencz T, Reynolds GP, et al: An evaluation of structural and functional prefrontal deficits in schizophrenia: MRI and neuropsychological measures. Psychiatry Res 54:123–137, 1992

Randolph C, Gold JM, Carpenter CJ, et al: Release from proactive interference: determinants of performance and neuropsychological correlates. J Clin Exp Neuropsychol 14:785–800, 1992

Randolph C, Goldberg TE, Weinberger RW: The neuropsychology of schizophrenia, in Clinical Neuropsychology. Edited by Heilman KM, Valenstein E. New York, Oxford University Press, 1993, pp 499–522

Rockwell E, Krull AJ, Dimsdale J, et al: Late-onset psychosis with somatic delusions. Psychosomatics 35:66–72, 1994

Rosenthal D, Kety SS: The Transmission of Schizophrenia. New York, Pergamon, 1968

Rossi A, Galderisi S, Di Michele V, et al: Dementia in schizophrenia: magnetic resonance and clinical correlates. J Nerv Ment Dis 178:521–524, 1990

Roxborough H, Muir WJ, Blackwood DHR, et al: Neuropsychological and P300 abnormalities in schizophrenics and their relatives. Psychol Med 23:305–314, 1993

Saykin AJ, Gur RC, Gur RE, et al: Neuropsychological impairment in schizophrenia: selective impairment in memory and learning. Arch Gen Psychiatry 48:618–624, 1991

Schwartz BL, Rosse RB, Deutsch SI: Towards a neuropsychology of memory in schizophrenia. Psychopharmacol Bull 28:341–351, 1992

Schwartz F, Carr A, Munich R, et al: Voluntary motor performance in psychotic disorders: a replication study. Psychol Rep 66:1223–1234, 1990

Shallice T, Warrington EK: Independent functioning of verbal memory stores: a neurological study. Q J Exp Psychol 22:261–273, 1970

Shelton RC, Weinberger DR: X-ray computerized tomography studies of schizophrenia: a review and synthesis, in The Neurology of Schizophrenia. Edited by Nasrallah HA, Weinberger DR. Amsterdam, Elsevier, 1986, pp 325–348

Snyder SH: The dopamine hypothesis of schizophrenia. Am J Psychiatry 133:197–202, 1976

Spohn HE, Strauss ME: Relation of neuroleptic and anticholinergic medication to cognitive functions in schizophrenia. J Abnorm Psychol 98:367–380, 1989

Squire LR: Memory and Brain. New York, Oxford University Press, 1987

Stolar N, Berenbaum H, Banich MT, et al: Neuropsychological correlates of affective flattening in schizophrenia. Biol Psychiatry 35:164–172, 1994

Stromgren E: Changes in the incidence of schizophrenia? Br J Psychiatry 150: 1–7, 1987

Strous RD, Cowan N, Ritter W, et al: Auditory sensory ("echoic") memory dysfunction in schizophrenia. Am J Psychiatry 152:1517–1519, 1995

Stuss DT, Benson DF, Kaplan EF, et al: The involvement of the orbito-frontal cerebrum in cognitive tasks. Neuropsychologia 21:235–249, 1983

Suddath RL, Casanova ME, Goldberg TE, et al: Temporal lobe pathology in schizophrenia: a quantitative magnetic resonance imaging study. Am J Psychiatry 43:36–42, 1989

Suddath RL, Christison GW, Torrey EF, et al: Anatomical abnormalities in the brains of monozygotic twins discordant for schizophrenia. N Engl J Med 322: 789–794, 1990

Sullivan HS: The Interpersonal Theory of Schizophrenia. New York, WW Norton, 1953

Talmon Y, Guy N, Naylor K, et al: "Saddam syndrome": acute psychotic reaction during the Gulf-War—renewal of the concept of brief reactive psychosis. Harefuah 123:237–240, 1992

Torrey EF: Civilization and Schizophrenia. New York, Jason Aronson, 1980

Torrey EF: Surviving Schizophrenia. New York, Harper & Row, 1988

Torrey EF, Ragland JD, Gold JM, et al: Handedness in twins with schizophrenia: was Boklage correct? Schizophr Res 9:83–85, 1993

Traupmann KL: Effects of categorization and imagery on recognition and recall by process and reactive schizophrenics. J Abnorm Psychol 84:307–314, 1975

Tune LE, Strauss ME, Lew MF, et al: Serum levels of anticholinergic drugs and impaired recent memory in chronic schizophrenic patients. Am J Psychiatry 139:1460–1462, 1982

Venables PH: A short scale for rating "activity-withdrawal" in schizophrenics. Journal of Mental Science 103:197–199, 1957

Venables PH, Wing JK: Levels of arousal and the subclassifications of schizophrenia. Arch Gen Psychiatry 7:114–119, 1962

Wechsler D: Wechsler Adult Intelligence Scale—3rd Edition (WAIS-III). New York, Psychological Corporation, 1997

Weinberger DR, Berman KF, Zec RF: Physiologic dysfunction of dorsolateral prefrontal cortex in schizophrenia, I: regional cerebral blood flow evidence. Arch Gen Psychiatry 43:114–124, 1986

Weinberger DR, Berman KF, Suddath RL, et al: Evidence for a dysfunction of a prefrontal-limbic network in schizophrenia: an MRI and regional cerebral blood flow study of discordant monozygotic twins. Am J Psychiatry 149: 890–897, 1992

Young IJ, Crampton AR: Cerebrospinal fluid uric acid levels and cerebral atrophy in psychiatric and neurologic patients. Biol Psychiatry 8:281–288, 1974

3

NEUROPSYCHOLOGY OF MOOD DISORDERS

Avraham Calev, D.Phil., Dean A. Pollina, Ph.D.,
Shmuel Fennig, M.D., and Samita Banerjee, B.A.

AFFECTIVE DISORDERS CONSTITUTE a major diagnostic category of mental disorders. Their prevalence is relatively high. Gold et al. (1988) estimated that 13%–20% of the population have depressive symptoms at any given time, and 2%–3% of the population are hospitalized or seriously impaired because of depression. Women are affected at least twice as often as men. The lifetime risk for developing depression is 3%–4% in men and 5%–9% in women. In people older than 65, the diagnosis of depression is more frequent than in younger people, and one in three patients is likely to have depression. Bipolar depression is relatively rare and is estimated to occur in 0.65% of men and 0.88% of women.

Affective disorders have been described throughout history; the modern concepts of these disorders are formulated in DSM-IV (American Psychiatric Association 1994).

◈ DIAGNOSTIC FEATURES

The cognitive symptoms of mood disorders include disturbances of thinking, attention, and reasoning and of psychomotor, executive, and memory functions. Of these disorders, *unipolar depression,* or *major depressive disorder,* is most common. The defining characteristic of the disorder is at least one episode of either depressed mood or loss of interest or pleasure. Significant weight loss or weight gain, insomnia or hypersomnia, psychomotor agitation or retardation, fatigue or loss of energy, feelings of worthlessness or guilt, diminished ability to think or concentrate, and recurrent thoughts of death or suicide are other characteristic features, but all do not occur in every patient.

Bipolar disorder is characterized by at least one manic or mixed episode and depressive episodes. The manic episode is "a distinct period during which there is an abnormally and persistently elevated, expansive, or irritable mood" (American Psychiatric Association 1994, p. 328). The mixed episode meets criteria for both manic and depressive episodes. Inflated self-esteem or grandiosity, decreased need for sleep, greater talkativeness than usual, flight of ideas or a subjective experience that thoughts are racing, distractibility, psychomotor agitation or increased goal-directed activity such as sex or work, and excessive involvement in pleasurable activities with potential future hazards (e.g., buying sprees, sexual indiscretions) are characteristics of a manic episode. Bipolar disorder and major depressive disorder are sometimes accompanied by florid psychotic symptoms such as delusions or hallucinations.

Recent classifications, such in as DSM-IV, also define *dysthymic disorder* and *cyclothymic disorder.* Dysthymic disorder is characterized by a prolonged depressed mood for at least 2 years. The symptoms are of lesser severity than major depressive episode symptoms. Cyclothymic disorder is characterized by at least 2 years with numerous periods of waning and waxing depressive and hypomanic symptoms.

All these disorders result in significant distress or impairment of social, occupational, or other important areas of functioning.

◈ ETIOLOGY

The etiology of these disorders varies. *Organic* or *endogenous* types of affective disorders include stroke or hypothyroidism causing depression; multiple sclerosis causing affective symptoms such as elation or sadness;

and winter depression (seasonal affective disorder) observed in some people in the northern part of the Northern Hemisphere, presumably caused by a lack of light, which affects brain neurotransmitters. Hormonal changes such as occur during menstruation and innate chemical imbalance may also result in endogenous depression. In *reactive* depression, stressful life events, such as losses of loved ones or money, are considered causes. Postpartum depression may have this component but also may have organic (hormonal) causes. The higher frequency of depression reported in older people may have both components, because aging results in both greater organicity and loss of relatives, friends, property, income, physical health, and personal competence.

◆ DIFFERENTIAL DIAGNOSIS

Sometimes depression is mistaken for dementia. Feinberg and Goodman (1984) reported that 5%–15% of initial diagnoses of dementia were later changed to depression. The reverse occurs less frequently. Of patients with an initial diagnosis of major depression, 2.6%–3% are given a diagnosis of dementia later. The term *pseudodementia* refers to severe cognitive impairment resembling dementia in psychiatric disease such as depression (e.g., Wells 1979). Although differentiating dementia from pseudodementia is extremely difficult, pseudodementia quickly reverses with aggressive psychiatric treatments such as electroconvulsive therapy (ECT). However, pure pseudodementia cases are relatively rare, and most researchers and clinicians believe that depression and dementia often coexist (Jones and Reifler 1994). When patients with dementia are depressed, their levels of both activities of daily living (ADL) and cognitive performance decline, suggesting that depression and dementia have additive adverse cognitive effects.

◆ COURSE

The severity of affective disorders varies. Some people have frequent episodes, and others may experience only a single episode. Some patients become so extremely depressed or manic during an episode that they lose control and even show psychotic symptoms. Other patients have milder symptoms.

The purpose of this chapter is to define the cognitive characteristics of mood disorders as well as their modification with changes in mood, severity, and type of illness and treatment. We give special attention to possible etiologies of these disorders.

◈ AFFECTIVE ILLNESS AND THE BRAIN

Structural brain abnormality in affective disorders has not been established definitively, yet abundant evidence shows that brain damage results in depressive or manic symptoms. After stroke, for example, depression (resembling major depressive disorder) occurs in about 40% of patients (Robinson 1997; Starkstein and Robinson 1993). Mania occurs rarely (Robinson 1997). Some investigators believe that the site of the lesion is not very relevant, whereas others indicate specific sites. Gainotti (1972) suggested that right-hemisphere strokes are associated with depression. Conversely, Robinson's research group found that left-hemisphere frontal stroke locations are more likely to result in depression. Their findings indicate that the closer the site of stroke to the left frontal pole, the higher the likelihood of depression. They also reported that the recovery from depression is faster with subcortical than with cortical lesions and that anxious depression is associated more strongly with cortical than with subcortical strokes (Starkstein and Robinson 1993). Depression caused by strokes is similar to other depressive states in its manifestations and is responsive to medications such as serotonergic or tricyclic antidepressants (TCAs) (Lipsey et al. 1986). Most stroke patients recover within a year (Starkstein and Robinson 1993).

Research evidence suggests that other kinds of depression are also associated with brain abnormalities. Depression is more frequently observed in older than in younger patients, which may be interpreted as a result of increasing brain organicity with age. Indeed, structural brain changes have been identified in elderly depressed patients (Coffey et al. 1993; Jacoby and Levy 1980; Zubenko et al. 1990). Coffey et al. (1993) reported that the prevalence of cortical atrophy is about five times greater in patients with depression than in control patients. Reduced frontal-lobe volume and greater frequency of subcortical hyperintensity on magnetic resonance imaging (MRI) were found in patients referred for ECT. Robinson's (1997) findings that left-hemisphere frontal strokes are most likely to result in depression are consistent with the idea of frontal-lobe dysfunction in depression. The changes in neurotransmitter functions, such as of serotonin and noradrenaline, in depressive and bipolar illness thus may be secondary to structural abnormalities.

However, the patients in these studies do not represent depressive patients in general. Stroke patients and patients referred for ECT are usually elderly, very severely disturbed, and resistant to other treatments of depression such as cognitive therapy and antidepressant medications. The findings suggest that an entity of endogenous affective illness is associated with brain lesions or other structural brain changes. These changes, however, do not always correlate with the cognitive disturbances observed in these affective illnesses (Abas et al. 1990; Kellner et al. 1986). Most patients with affective disorders have no structural brain changes, and their disorder may be described as functional.

Comment: Alternative Theories of Brain Dysfunction

Although the above-mentioned evidence suggests that certain intact brain regions, mainly the frontal regions, may protect from depression, an older body of research suggests different brain etiologies of depression. Experimental work with healthy people shows evidence consistent with right-hemispheric specialization for emotional content. For example, unpleasant video material is rated as more unpleasant and produces greater autonomic changes when projected to the visual field controlled by the right rather than the left hemisphere; pleasant material produces converse results (Dimond et al. 1976). Furthermore, electrodermal measures (e.g., Gruzelier 1983) and regional cerebral blood flow measures (Uytdenhoef et al. 1983) taken during depression indicate abnormal lateralization of brain function.

Theoretical formulations based on these findings were attempted. Sackeim et al. (1982) suggested that depression is associated with right-hemisphere silent frontal lesions and euphoria with such lesions in the left frontal regions. The frontal regions were implicated because of their function in expressing feeling. Because this theory is inconsistent with other findings (e.g., poststroke depression; Robinson 1997), some investigators suggested an alternative theory: the right hemisphere processes all kinds of emotional states more than the left hemisphere (e.g., Heilman et al. 1993). The observation that emotions are expressed more intensely on the left side of the face supports this theory (Sackeim et al. 1978).

However, serious failures to replicate hemispheric effects on emotion led to alternative brain dysfunction theories. Heilman et al. (1993) suggested that the basal ganglia and other lower brain structures may be involved in causing depression. Their hypothesis was based on observations of patients with Parkinson's disease (a basal ganglia motor disorder) who have a high incidence of depressive symptoms. However, this hypothesis is even less substantiated than the hemispheric hypothesis. Further, some types of depression may be functional, as a result of transmitter and brain metabolic changes induced by external cognitive and behavioral stimuli, such as loss of a love object, death of a loved one, or inability to pursue life goals.

◈ AFFECTIVE ILLNESS AND COGNITIVE FUNCTIONING

In this section, we describe the specific cognitive dysfunctions observed during depression and mania, in relation to severity, type, and stage of illness and to possible etiological factors. Early studies by pioneers such as Kahn and Pollack, which do not directly contribute to this discussion, are important (e.g., Fink 1979) but are not reviewed here.

One should bear in mind that most studies addressing cognition in these disordered states have serious methodological problems. Clinical issues, such as severity of depression or mania, florid psychosis, medication status, and previous ECT, and other state-dependent variables, may affect findings. Manic and depressive states are associated with variable degrees of patient cooperation at assessment sessions, which is not always controlled. General intelligence is a confounding factor that must be controlled.

Evidence from studies that used measures other than pure cognitive assessment should be treated with caution. Results of neuroimaging studies may be misleading (Brodie 1996; Gur et al. 1992b). First, interpretation of neuroimaging results involves many steps of data processing, increasing the chance of inaccuracy and error. Second, statistical analyses that are applied often disregard important evidence from exceptional images. Third, factors such as situational level of anxiety, gender, age, arousal, and ultradian biorhythms affect baseline and interpretation of results. Fourth, reliability, construct validity, and difficulty of tasks used during neuroimaging for brain activation purposes are not always considered, even though these factors may affect the interpretation of the results. Gur et al. (1992b) suggested that future research should follow certain guidelines to make research results more valid.

Bearing these problems in mind, we focus on neuropsychological functions during depression in the next section.

Cognitive Functions During Depression

Executive/Frontal Functions

Executive/frontal dysfunction has been hypothesized during depression. The existence of structural problems, in frontal more than in other brain areas (e.g., Coffey et al. 1993), suggests such a dysfunction. The findings showing reduction in frontal-lobe metabolism or blood flow (Baxter et al. 1989; Bench et al. 1992; Marinot et al. 1990), although not always consistent (Berman et al. 1993), also support this idea.

Studies that used neuropsychological tasks have addressed the possibility that executive or frontal function is adversely affected in depression. Trichard et al. (1995) reported poor Stroop Test and verbal fluency performance during depression as compared with patients' verbal intelligence. Whereas verbal fluency reversed with the recovery from depression, Stroop Test performance did not totally improve. The authors argued that both left and right frontal-lobe dysfunction characterizes depression and that the right frontal-lobe dysfunction, represented in their study by the Stroop Test, is a persistent marker because it did not totally reverse with the improvement of depression.

Austin et al.'s (1992) finding of impaired memory and impaired Trail Making Test performance also suggested that executive function is impaired in depression. They found that tracking speed and shifting attention on the Trail Making Test were correlated with Hamilton Depression Scale scores, indicating that the severity of depression is directly related to these functions. Note that these investigators divided their patients into endogenous and neurotic (nonendogenous) subtypes and did not observe group effects. This finding suggests that the degree of depression affects cognition more than the type of depression does. In line with this idea, Martin et al. (1991) reported that the Wisconsin Card Sorting Test deficits correlated with symptom severity regardless of whether the diagnosis was dysthymic disorder or major depression.

Dolan et al. (1994) observed a correlation between reduction in frontal cerebral blood flow and both memory and frontal-lobe tasks and hypothesized a medial prefrontal cortex dysfunction in depression.

These studies, however, do not provide sufficiently clear and replicable evidence to suggest that a significant executive or frontal/prefrontal deficit exists in depression.

Memory

A large body of research has focused on memory function in depression. This literature is consistent in showing poor memory during depression in relation to general cognitive functioning (e.g., Bradley et al. 1995; Calev 1996; Calev et al. 1986, 1989a, 1991; Golinkoff and Sweeney 1989; Grossman et al. 1994; Hart et al. 1987; Hertel and Rude 1991; O'Brien et al. 1993; Schmaling et al. 1994; Sweeney et al. 1989; Watts and Sharrock 1987). These deficits are not limited to a few types of depression. Many kinds of depression, including seasonal affective disorder (O'Brien et al. 1993) and chronic fatigue syndrome, result in similar memory deficits (Schmaling et al. 1994).

Some of these deficits are the result of poor encoding caused by poor attention and concentration (e.g., Sweeney et al. 1989). Training patients to focus their attention has resulted in improved memory functioning (Ellis 1991; Hertel and Rude 1991).

Memory deficits also may be caused by a difficulty in organizing the information in a meaningful way so that it can be easily retrieved. If this is the case, patients will not be able to retrieve information easily that is stored in memory, unless organization becomes unnecessary to retrieve it. For example, a recall testing procedure usually does not provide organizational help, but a recognition procedure provides maximal help by presenting the to-be-remembered items (along with other items) at retrieval, making mnemonic organization unnecessary. Depressed patients show better recognition than recall (e.g., Calev and Erwin 1985; Hart et al. 1987; Watts and Sharrock 1987), even when tasks are comparable in their discriminating power (Calev and Erwin 1985). Depressed patients also benefit less at retrieval than control subjects from increased semantic structure in the to-be-remembered material (Watts et al. 1990).

Alternative explanations for depressed patients' retrieval difficulties are also possible. Watts and Sharrock (1987) reported that depressed patients who were given retrieval cues did not improve in free recall. They concluded that retrieval is deficient in depression not because of inability to generate cues but because of other difficulties. The authors attributed the cause to patients' inability to exert effort to use retrieval cues. Note that their findings do not contradict the alternative hypothesis that deficient memory organization results in poor retrieval from memory during depression.

In addition to these memory functions, which have been localized at the medial temporal lobe and the frontal lobes and are implicated in depression, other memory functions that have not been localized to these memory regions in the brain have been studied in depression. One such function is working memory (e.g., Baddeley 1976; see also Calev et al., Chapter 1, in this volume). Channon et al. (1993) studied working memory in depression and concluded that neither the verbal aspect of working memory (articulatory loop) nor the visual-spatial aspect (visual sketch pad) were affected in clinically depressed patients.

However, another memory function unrelated to the classical memory locations in the brain—implicit memory (see Chapter 1)—did show deficits in depression. Bradley et al. (1995) found better priming of words expressing depressive thinking by depressed patients, whether the stimulus primes (first letters of words) were suprathreshold or subthreshold. Their findings suggested that depression is characterized by an implicit memory deficit, as well as by more obvious declarative memory deficits.

Mood and retrieval from memory. Bradley et al.'s (1995) study adds to a large body of research showing that mood affects the content of information retrieved from memory. Healthy subjects retrieve pleasant memories under pleasant circumstances (e.g., Isen et al. 1978; Lloyd and Lishman 1975; Nelson and Craighead 1977), and mood induction techniques can alter the affective content of the information retrieved (e.g., Teasdale and Russell 1983). Depressed patients behave differently. Williams and Scott (1988) observed that depressed subjects' (as defined by testing techniques) responses to negative emotional cues were notably quicker than to positive cues.

Clinically depressed patients seem to behave in a similar way to depressed patients identified by testing techniques. They tend to retrieve unpleasant rather than pleasant memories (Bradley et al. 1995; Lloyd and Lishman 1975). Dunbar and Lishman (1984) presented positive, negative, and neutral word lists to clinically depressed patients and found that although recognition rates were the same for patients and control subjects, depressed patients recognized pleasant material less easily and unpleasant material more easily. Calev (1996) found, contrary to the hypothesis, that severely depressed hospitalized patients recalled positive, negative, and neutral words equivalently, both immediately and after a delay of 48 hours. Calev (1996) speculated that in retrieval during depression, there is a normal recall tendency but that retrieval of past personal information may be colored by emotion. In another study, Danion et al. (1995) did not report a negative emotional bias in both explicit memory (free recall and recognition) tasks and an implicit memory (word stem completion) task. Inconsistent findings reduce the certainty that emotional content affects retrieval of materials from memory during clinical depression.

The emotional bias in the cognition of depressed patients, however, has not been limited to direct memory testing. Inference about memory retrieval bias also comes from other tasks. Gur et al. (1992a) administered facial discrimination tasks to a sample of 14 patients with depression and 14 nondepressed control subjects matched for sex and balanced for age and sociodemographic characteristics. Depressed patients performed more poorly on measures sensitive to happy discrimination and had a higher negative emotional bias. Gur et al. (1992a) suggested that depressed patients are impaired in the ability to recognize facial display of emotions. Conversely, Wexler et al. (1994) found that depressed patients were impaired in recognizing both positive and negative emotional facial displays and were also impaired in hearing both positive and negative words on a dichotic listening task. Wexler et al.'s (1994) findings dispute the idea that depressed patients have selective negative emotional bias and suggest that the bias is against any affective material.

The evidence is not conclusive but suggests that emotional bias affects the retrieval of information during depression. Further research can better clarify the nature of this bias.

Subjective deficits in depression.   Depressed patients report more memory problems than do other patients. Even when depressed patients have no significant memory deficits on cognitive testing (Williams et al. 1987), they still believe their memory function is poor. This may explain the excessive complaints of some depressed patients about long-lasting cognitive effects of ECT on memory (e.g., Calev et al. 1993).

In summary, the memory research in depression defines depression as a state producing encoding difficulties caused by attention difficulties, which can be improved by training strategies. An apparent retrieval deficit produces a disparity between recall and recognition and difficulty in benefiting from organizational structure in the material. Retrieval cues do not always seem to help. Working memory seems intact during depression. Some unconscious biases in memory contents seem to occur.

For example, when priming words by their beginning sounds, patients respond with negative words, suggesting a deficit in implicit memory.

Processing and Attention Allocation Effort

The observation that depressed patients do better on automatic and easy tasks than on more difficult tasks that require effort (Calev et al. 1989b; Hertel and Rude 1991; Roy-Byrne et al. 1986; Tancer et al. 1990; Weingartner et al. 1981) stimulated the hypothesis that depressed patients have limited attentional processing resources and are therefore unable to allocate sufficient resources to tasks that require effort (Kahneman 1973).

A problem in the aforementioned reasoning is that tasks that require effort, such as recalling a long list of shopping items, are by definition more difficult than automatic tasks, such as recalling the alphabet. Because tasks that require effort are more difficult, they are more likely to be reliable and thus show better discrimination between impaired depressed patients and nondepressed control subjects. Therefore, although findings show a larger deficit in tasks that require effort and attention during depression, many findings may not meet methodological standards (e.g., Chapman and Chapman 1978). Some researchers have been aware that their results may be misleading when attributed to effort rather than to discriminating power biases (e.g., Tancer et al. 1990). This criticism does not intend to dispute the observation that depressed patients have serious problems when exerting effort to allocate attention. It intends only to clarify the point that any cognitive difficulties may be more visible when a magnifying glass such as effortful tasks is used.

Right-Hemisphere Functions

The association between depression and nondominant-hemisphere dysfunction has been addressed frequently. Bruder et al. (1981) found increased right ear sensitivity in bipolar patients, as did Yazowitz et al. (1979). Replication efforts, however, have not been consistently successful. Sackeim et al. (1983) supported this argument in their report of left visual field inattention (neglect) for items in cancellation tasks after bilateral ECT, suggesting that successful treatment of depression with ECT reverses a right-hemisphere dysfunction. Electrophysiological studies (e.g., Flor-Henry 1979; Gruzelier and Venables 1974) often have suggested that depression is characterized as a right-hemisphere deficit.

Cornblatt et al. (1989) studied attention in depressed patients and found greater difficulty with spatial than with verbal tasks. Lyness et al. (1994) examined severely depressed patients (score of 17 or higher on the Hamilton Depression Scale) and found that they were impaired on visuomotor coordinated motor speed and visuospatial scanning, suggesting a deficit in right-hemisphere tasks.

Rossi et al. (1990) and Calev et al. (1991) found deficits in Complex Figure Test Copying and Reproduction in severely depressed patients awaiting ECT, which suggests visuospatial difficulties that are related to right-hemisphere function. Deptula et al. (1991) found better verbal than nonverbal recall in depressed patients. They used a post hoc matched tasks check with only 14 control subjects to correct for differences in tasks' discriminating power. Although this is a small sample for such a check, and the check was done after the results were interpreted, this study still raises the possibility of right-hemispheric memory deficits in depression. Similarly, a study of motor performance in women showed that depressed patients had significantly less perseveration with the left hand than did nondepressed subjects (Crew and Harrison 1994). This suggests that the right hemisphere also is functioning better with respect to executive function.

These findings also suggest a lateral dysfunction—visuomotor and visuoconstructive tasks are affected more severely than verbal tasks during depression (e.g., Sackeim et al. 1992). These investigators also observed that during frontal activation (while performing the Wisconsin Card Sorting Test), nondepressed control subjects had increased left parietal blood flow, whereas depressed patients had increased right parietal blood flow. The parietal lobe may be affected because of the perceptual element of these tasks. However, no further evidence supports this specific finding.

Despite the evidence showing that various cognitive functions are better performed by the left than the right hemisphere in depression, this hypothesis has not been proven. First, some studies do not find such hemispheric effects. Calev et al. (1986) used matched tasks methodology and did not find differences in the recall of verbal compared with nonverbal material by depressed patients. Second, studies reporting negative results are less likely to be published, increasing bias. Third, the evidence seems controversial when results are carefully examined. Cutting (1990) reviewed the literature to evaluate the hemispheric hypothesis in depression. He concluded that objective findings of perceptual deficits, attention, memory, movement, speech, thought, and general intelligence do not yield conclusive results. Direct radiological and electrodermal measures yield contradictory results. Robinson's (1997) findings that poststroke depression is associated with left-hemisphere damage question the hypothesis of right-hemisphere dysfunction in depression.

Other Neuropsychological Functions

The global cognitive deficit in depression is likely to present as deficits in almost any cognitive task. Indeed, neuropsychological deficits were observed in depression across many tasks. Comprehensive batteries that are administered during depression tend to show such deficits in visuomotor, visuospatial, executive, memory, attention, motor, tactual perception, and other tasks (e.g., Calev et al. 1995a; Goldberg et al. 1993).

Reversibility and Persistence of
Cognitive Deficits After Depression Abates

Findings suggest reversibility of cognitive deficits in depressive patients. Memory deficits documented in depression disappeared in euthymic mood states (e.g., Calev et al. 1986; Cohen et al. 1982). Moreover, cognitive deficits are directly related to the severity of depression (e.g., Austin et al. 1992; Bornstein et al. 1991; Brown et al. 1994; Sternberg and Jarvik 1976). Calev et al. (1986) found that euthymic bipolar patients visiting a lithium outpatient clinic recalled both verbal and nonverbal materials as well as nonbipolar control subjects, whereas patients in a depressive episode awaiting TCAs or ECT showed marked deficits on both verbal and nonverbal recall. A 23-point intelligence quotient (IQ) difference was found between the two groups, which suggests marked effects of depression on IQ. Calev et al. (1989b) studied oral verbal fluency in response to a letter or a category label. They found that stable bipolar patients performed almost as well as normal control subjects. In patients hospitalized for a manic episode in a testable hypomanic state, depressed patients performed least well. These results suggest that the severity of mood state affects cognition, thus implying reversibility. Studies that report correlations between the severity of depression and specific task performance also suggest reversibility (e.g., Dolan et al. 1994; Martin et al. 1991). The evidence from poststroke depression studies supports the idea that cognitive deficits in depression reverse even if their origin is biological. Left-hemisphere stroke patients with depression show cognitive deficits in language, visuoconstructive skills, and executive function (Bolla-Wilson et al. 1988). However, these deficits improve with the treatment of depression, suggesting that coexisting depression after stroke is associated with increased cognitive deficits (Robinson et al. 1986).

However, findings suggest that irreversible changes in cognitive functioning persist after depression abates. Despite methodological problems such as confounds from the level of education, socioeconomic status, and age, studies have provided valid evidence for persistent deficits. For example, evidence indicates that a substantial minority of depressed patients show irreversible deterioration in occupational, marital, and other daily functions (Tsuang et al. 1979).

Mason (1956) followed up premorbid IQs of veterans, as assessed by their army entrance examination, in patients with schizophrenia and affective illness. Initially, affective patients with both unipolar and bipolar illness had IQs higher than the population norms, and schizophrenic patients had IQs lower than the population norms. At follow-up, depressive patients' IQs were average. This suggested the possibility that the average IQ observed at follow-up was a result of cognitive deterioration. However, no other study repeated this finding.

Sackeim et al. (1992) tested 100 patients in a major depressive episode and 50 nondepressed control subjects, matched on demographic variables and estimates of premorbid IQ, on the Wechsler Adult Intelligence Scale—Revised (WAIS-R; Wechsler 1981). The groups had equivalent Verbal Scale IQ scores, but the depressed patients had significant deficits in Performance Scale IQ. Patients were retested after depression was treated with ECT. IQ improved as depression and the adverse effects of ECT abated, but the disparity between Verbal and Performance Scale IQ did not change. To ensure that this disparity was not caused by psychomotor retardation, which may be an epiphenomenon of depression, patients were reassessed without time constraints on the Performance Scale IQ test. The deficit in Performance Scale IQ score was observed even with this correction. These results suggest that cognitive characteristics in patients with depression are persistent.

Because in a former sample such a discrepancy between Verbal and Performance Scale IQ was also observed in healthy children relatives of bipolar patients, Sackeim et al. (1992) suggested that this Verbal–Performance IQ discrepancy precedes mental illness and marks depressive patients before depression develops. Sackeim et al.'s (1992) results were obtained with severely depressed patients, however, whose initial treatment was unsuccessful and who needed further treatment with ECT.

These patients may have constituted a subgroup of depressed patients with severe chronic illness.

Indeed, a comparison between affective disorder patients admitted to the hospital and schizophrenic patients showed higher IQs in affective disorder patients; IQs in affective disorder patients also did not differ from those in control subjects (Goldberg et al. 1993). In euthymic states, these IQ patterns seem to persist (Calev et al. 1995a). Almost all neuropsychological tests show better performance in affective than in schizophrenic patients (e.g., Calev et al. 1995a; Goldberg et al. 1993), and affective patients' IQs are about normal. These two studies used large test batteries and evaluated executive function, memory, attention, visuomotor and motor speed, visuospatial perception and other sensory functions, and visuoconstructive ability.

Goldberg et al. (1993) also calculated a deterioration index, based on the comparison of reading IQ scores (resistant to cognitive deterioration) with WAIS-R IQ scores (less resistant to cognitive deterioration). They found no deterioration in affective patients, whether bipolar or unipolar. Schizophrenic patients showed deterioration (Goldberg et al. 1993).

McKay et al. (1995) studied psychotic bipolar patients after remission and concluded that most patients had no enduring deficits, but a subgroup of severely ill depressed patients had persistent neuropsychological deficits that did not reverse *ad integrum*. These patients may have been represented extensively in Sackeim and colleagues' (1992) sample. However, Calev et al. (1995a) observed that depressed patients who had been admitted to the hospital with florid psychotic symptoms did not reach normal levels of functioning at a follow-up assessment.

The irreversibility in performance on the Stroop Color and Word Test found by Trichard et al. (1995) in severely disturbed depressive patients also suggests that such patients may have persistent deficits in executive function as well as in Performance Scale IQ and visuoconstructive tasks. The finding of structural brain changes in some depressed patients (e.g., Coffey et al. 1993) suggests that some brain characteristics in affective illness may last beyond the episode of illness or at least that a subgroup of affective patients has organic features and persistent cognitive deficits.

These results are not conclusive. On the one hand, deficits clearly reverse. On the other hand, evidence indicates that deficits persist, especially in severely disturbed samples of patients. There may be two types of depressive patients: 1) those with irreversible features (neuropsychological deficits, MRI abnormalities in frontal brain regions) perhaps caused by organic factors and 2) those without such features, whose cognitive functioning may improve or completely reverse after recovery from depression. Abas et al. (1990) found that 35% of depressed patients continued to show memory impairment after the depressive episode abated. This percentage may, however, be somewhat different in samples other than the one they drew from the Mauldsley and Bethlem Royal Hospital in London. As expected, ventricular-to-brain ratio, a measure of structural brain damage, estimated with computed tomography (CT) scans, correlated with poor performance at high levels of task difficulty.

Cognitive Functions During Mania and Hypomania

Cognitive functioning is more difficult to describe during mania than during depression because manic patients are not cooperative enough to be examined. Perhaps this is the reason that fewer studies use manic patients than depressed patients. Usually hypomanic rather than manic patients are studied.

By definition, mania is characterized by abnormally increased motor behavior with disorganized speech, derailment of thought, elated mood, extreme irritability, thought disorder, and rapid and excessive thought processes. Spontaneous motor activity is clearly increased in mania (e.g., Foster and Kupfer 1975). This clinical picture, however, does not result in hypernormal cognitive functioning. On the contrary, there may be an overall cognitive impairment during mania, despite the fact that overall intellectual functioning is better during mania than during depression. Donnelly et al. (1982) found that a group of bipolar patients had higher IQs when hypomanic than when depressed. Other reports show that IQs of manic patients do not differ from those of euthymic bipolar patients and normal control subjects (e.g., Calev et al. 1989b). IQ during mania thus may be about normal. However, specific neuropsychological impairments may be present during mania. One area that has been studied is attention.

Attention

Although manic patients seem to lack concentration, studies do not tend to find differential deficits in attention. Sax et al. (1995) assessed vigilance with the Continuous Performance Test in patients with pure and mixed mania. Vigilance did not decline in manic patients, unlike the finding in schizophrenic patients, compared with control subjects. Blackburn (1975) reported less distractibility and better ability to retain motor speed in manic patients than in depressed patients. Blackburn found that during remission, manic patients did not differ from depressed patients, suggesting normal functioning during mania.

Some investigators have speculated that manic or hypomanic patients have hypernormal functioning because of good brain activation; however, this is not usually observed. Despite the fast thinking that occurs in mania, patients do not outperform nonmanic persons perhaps because manic patients are more disorganized and unable to maintain attentional sets. Although attention and vigilance deficits during mania appear minimal, some perceptual tasks are not independent of attention and imply hemispheric dysfunction in mania.

Right-Hemispheric Dysfunction

Indications are that in mania, as in depression, the right or nondominant hemisphere shows a dysfunction. Bruder et al. (1994) used dichotic syllable and complex tones to determine that changes in laterality occurred with the remission of the manic state. This result replicated former findings by Bruder's group. The findings suggested that mania is associated with a deficit in right-hemisphere processing of complex tonal information. Increased left-handedness also has been postulated in mania but had not always been observed (e.g., Nasrallah and McCalley-Whitters 1982). Overall, insufficient findings support the hemispheric hypothesis in mania, and further research is needed (Cutting 1990).

Other Neuropsychological Functions

The research on other neuropsychological functions during a manic episode is sparse, and no consistent deficits have been documented in mania and hypomania. This does not mean that no such deficits exist, but it may be difficult to assess cognition in manic states.

Recurrence of Manic Episodes and Cognition

Altshuler (1993) raised the possibility that an ongoing destructive process accompanies the occurrence of each manic episode. A proportion of manic patients with recurring episodes have shown persistent impairment at follow-up (e.g., Dhingra and Rabins 1991; McKay et al. 1995). These findings should be treated as tentative because of the paucity of research evidence. Furthermore, an artifact is possible. Because mania can be induced by organic brain damage, some manic patients and some depressed patients may have persistent cognitive deficits that are not caused by either type of episode.

Cognitive Function Differences Between Bipolar and Unipolar Illness

Studies comparing bipolar and unipolar patients with extensive neuropsychological test batteries do not show consistent cognitive differences in either IQ or other neuropsychological characteristics during depression (e.g., Goldberg et al. 1993) or at follow-up in a euthymic state (e.g., Calev et al. 1995a). Converse findings are the exception. For example, Wolfe et al. (1987) found that during a depressive episode, the bipolar patients in their sample had better verbal fluency and verbal learning than did unipolar patients, and unipolar patients were more careful and generated more correct responses on the verbal fluency tasks than bipolar patients. Bruder et al. (1994) observed that bipolar depressed patients, unlike unipolar patients and nondepressed persons, did not show the normal left visual field advantage for dot enumeration. These findings need replication. Affective disorder patients, therefore, whether bipolar or unipolar, seem to have little or no global cognitive deterioration, with the possible exception of a subgroup of severely depressed treatment-resistant patients who have both organic signs and persistent cognitive deficits.

Cognitive Functioning in Dysthymic and Cyclothymic Disorders

The neuropsychological effects of dysthymia and cyclothymia have not been studied as independent disease processes. Generally, one can expect dysthymia to resemble major depression during the depressive episode (e.g., Martin et al. 1991) and cyclothymia to resemble hypomania. Yet there may be specific markers in these two disease entities that require further research.

Effects of Treatment on
Cognitive Functions in Affective Disorders

As stated above, the effects of manic and depressive states have not always been well controlled in research. Unlike schizophrenia, depression and mania are unlikely to be characterized by long hospitalization; therefore, the medical treatment is the major source of added cognitive effects. During depression, medications affecting brain neurotransmitters, such as noradrenaline and serotonin, are used. ECT and magnetic brain stimulation are also used. In this section, we consider the potential effects of these treatments.

Tricyclic Antidepressants

TCAs, introduced in the 1960s, were frequently used in the 1980s, but their use was reduced with the introduction of serotonergic drugs. TCAs may induce neurocognitive changes in some individuals (Branconnier et al. 1982; Moskowitz and Burns 1986). The few studies that have assessed these effects tend to report cognitive impairments. Memory deficits may be, in some cases, the result of the anticholinergic action of these drugs. One early study investigating the effects of the TCA amitriptyline on memory found that it caused an impairment relative to a placebo group (Lamping et al. 1984). This study is important because depressed subjects who were given amitriptyline had a true reduction in memory rather than a change in response strategy resulting from their depression. This finding was replicated in subsequent studies that used recognition memory for two- and three-syllable words and recall of figures in the Benton Visual Retention Test (Spring et al. 1992). Amitriptyline has also been found to cause deficits on tests of attention and mental speed such as Letter Cancellation and Digit Symbol tasks, suggesting that part of its effect on memory may be the result of a global sedative effect (Curran et al. 1988; McNair et al. 1984).

Other studies that have examined tricyclics for their effects on cognition and memory have had mixed results. For example, imipramine, a tricyclic with anticholinergic properties, was reported to enhance performance on a memory scanning procedure involving sequences of digits (Glass et al. 1981). However, Calev et al. (1989a) found adverse effects of imipramine on learning and retention over a 30-minute period, suggesting that the anticholinergic properties of these drugs are significant. However, some encouraging evidence indicates that stable doses of amitriptyline given to depressed patients do not correlate with measures of verbal memory, digit span, trail making, or verbal fluency (Austin et al. 1992). Some data also suggest that tricyclic medications produce more cognitive impairment in the elderly than in younger subjects (Branconnier et al. 1982).

Monoamine Oxidase Inhibitors

Monoamine oxidase inhibitors (MAOIs) were among the first drugs used to treat depression effectively in humans. Antidepressant action is mainly related to MAO inhibition, which leads to increased bioavailability of norepinephrine and serotonin. At present, MAOI use is limited in the treatment of major depression, in large part because of their adverse medical effects. However, the reversible MAOI moclobemide has shown an antidepressant effectiveness comparable to that of the tricyclic imipramine, with better performance on the Benton Visual Retention Test and Digit Symbol test relative to imipramine (Pancheri et al. 1994). Moclobemide has little or no anticholinergic activity and so does not seem to result in memory impairments stemming from disruption of the cholinergic system (Amado-Boccara et al. 1994; Wesnes et al. 1989).

An important feature of moclobemide is that it does not permanently inhibit the oxidase enzyme (Priest 1990). The development of reversible inhibitors of MAO is important largely because the older "irreversible" MAOIs were associated with more adverse peripheral effects, including hypertensive reactions (Liebowitz et al. 1990; Zimmer 1990). Moclobemide thus seems to have the advantage over antidepressant drugs that result in cognitive impairment or peripheral effects, especially if future research confirms that its antidepressant potency is comparable to that of other commonly used compounds.

Serotonergic Antidepressants

Several new serotonin reuptake blockers are reportedly able to treat depression effectively without substantial effects on cognition (Moskowitz and Burns 1988; Schaffler 1989). Fluoxetine was the first serotonin reuptake inhibitor widely used for the treatment of depression (Raskind 1993). Other selective serotonin reuptake inhibitors (SSRIs) such as sertraline and paroxetine have been introduced recently. Adverse cognitive effects of fluoxetine treatment are rare but have been reported (Hoehn-Saric et al. 1990, 1991; Ramaekers et al. 1995). The mechanisms responsible for these cognitive effects are not known with certainty but resemble those of frontal-lobe dysfunction (Hoehn-Saric et al. 1990). Symptoms include apathy, flat affect, socially inappropriate behavior, and difficulties in planning goal-oriented activities. Decreases in verbal fluency and complex figure reproduction ability, accompanied by a reduction in frontal cerebral blood flow, also have been reported after 4 months of fluoxetine treatment (Hoehn-Saric et al. 1991).

Atypical Antidepressants With Serotonergic and Noradrenergic Effects

Further attempts to augment the mode of action of SSRIs included noradrenaline reuptake inhibiting compounds such as venlafaxine (Ballenger 1996; Moller and Volz 1996). Preliminary findings suggest that electrophysiological markers of human information processing are largely unaffected by venlafaxine (Semlitsch et al. 1993). However, more neuropsychological research is clearly needed before any firm conclusions about the effect of venlafaxine on cognition can be drawn.

Other new antidepressants include mirtazapine, which acts by blocking adrenergic auto- and heteroreceptors, leading to an increase in noradrenaline and serotonin release; and nefazodone, which combines serotonergic reuptake inhibition with the blocking of postsynaptic serotonergic receptors. Nefazodone is pharmacologically different from newer SSRIs. Some evidence suggests that after repeated treatment with nefazodone, dose-related impairment in general cognitive functioning can occur (Van Laar et al. 1995). Specific tests in which nefazodone showed significant impairment included choice response time tasks such as letter matching, memory scanning, and letter-digit differentiation. However, the investigators pointed out that the results are inconclusive, because sensory, motor, and motivational impairments can all affect slowing in response time, and that further research is needed to assess the neuropsychological effects of the newer medications.

Lithium

Lithium is frequently used with both manic and depressed patients. It is also prescribed as maintenance therapy. Findings are inconsistent: some show memory deficits (e.g., Judd et al. 1977), and some dispute these effects (e.g., Smigan and Perris 1983). There are, however, indications that stable bipolar patients do not show significant cognitive deficits after long periods of maintenance therapy with lithium (e.g., Calev et al. 1986).

Benzodiazepines

Although the benzodiazepines have not proven to be effective antidepressants, they have often been combined with tricyclics or MAOIs to produce faster symptomatic relief (Cowley and Dunner 1991). These compounds can impair psychomotor speed and attention, leading to performance deficits across a range of cognitive tasks (Curran et al. 1986). One study reported that diazepam given in combination with amitriptyline resulted in impairments on a paired-associate learning test (Mattila et al. 1989). In contrast, neither diazepam nor amitriptyline given alone resulted in impairments on this test, which suggests an additive effect of these drugs.

Electroconvulsive Therapy

ECT is a very effective treatment of resistant depression, but it affects cognition transiently (e.g., Calev et al. 1993; Squire 1984). In the hours after treatment, patients experience disorientation and soft neurological signs such as headaches, confusion, and psychomotor slowing. These acute effects resolve within hours, and a memory disturbance becomes evident. Patients rapidly forget new information (anterograde amnesia). They also have difficulty remembering events that occurred before treatment (retrograde amnesia). Events that occurred earlier in life are better remembered than events that occurred shortly before treatment. Events that occurred during the treatment course may be lost permanently (Squire 1986; Squire et al. 1981). These effects gradually improve, and at about 6 months after treatment, most researchers agree that memory effects are no longer present. During memory impairment, other cognitive functions are also impaired, although to a lesser extent (Calev et al. 1995b). It is interesting that the cognitive effects of ECT occur at a time when the cognitive effects of depression or mania improve because depression has abated. Thus, usually 6 months after ECT, when the effects of both depression and ECT have resolved, patients function at a better level than before treatment with ECT (Calev et al. 1991).

◈ CONCLUSION

- ◆ Cognitive deficits are associated with affective disorders.
- ◆ Cognitive impairment is more severe during depression than during mania and in both cases is less severe than in schizophrenia.

◆ Cognitive deficits are mood dependent and tend to reverse, for the most part, after the symptoms abate.
◆ Cognitive deficits persist in a subgroup of depressive patients. Deficits have been reported more often in visuospatial and visuoconstructive tasks and in Performance Scale IQ. The severity and frequency of depressive symptoms in these patients are usually high.
◆ The evidence for lateral cognitive effects in both mania and depression, suggesting that affective disorders may be right-hemisphere diseases, is equivocal. The left hemisphere is strongly implicated by recent poststroke research.
◆ The frontal lobes are strongly implicated by brain imaging studies, stroke research, and cognitive task performance of depressed patients.
◆ The theory that depression is specifically characterized by a lack of effortful processing is equivocal. The evidence for a deficit in attention allocation caused by limited effort allocation comes from studies that used tasks that were more demanding and more sensitive to any disruption.
◆ Depressive and manic cognitive symptoms may be affected by medications taken and biological treatments given during depression. Tricyclic and serotonergic medications, lithium, and ECT have been found to affect cognition. Memory and executive function are frequently affected both by these diseases and by medication effects. Future research should control for the effects of medication to better describe the effects of illness itself.

◈ REFERENCES

Abas MA, Sahakian BJ, Levy R: Neuropsychological deficits and CT scan changes in elderly depressives. Psychol Med 20:507–520, 1990

Altshuler LL: Bipolar disorder: are repeated episodes associated with neuroanatomic and cognitive changes? Biol Psychiatry 33:563–565, 1993

Amado-Boccara I, Gougoulis N, Poirier-Littré MF, et al: Effects of antidepressants on cognitive functions: review of the literature. Encephale 20:65–77, 1994

American Psychiatric Association: Diagnostic and Statistical Manual of Mental Disorders, 4th Edition. Washington, DC, American Psychiatric Association, 1994

Austin MP, Ross M, Murray C, et al: Cognitive function in major depression. J Affect Disord 25:21–29, 1992

Baddeley AD: The Psychology of Memory. New York, Basic Books, 1976

Ballenger JC: Clinical evaluation of venlafaxine. J Clin Psychopharmacol 16 (suppl 2):29S–36S, 1996

Baxter LR, Schwartz JM, Phelps ME, et al: Reduction of prefrontal cortex glucose metabolism common to three types of depression. Arch Gen Psychiatry 46: 243–250, 1989

Bench CJ, Friston KJ, Brown RG, et al: The anatomy of melancholia—focal abnormalities of cerebral blood flow in major depression. Psychol Med 22:607–615, 1992

Berman KF, Doran AR, Pickar D, et al: Is the mechanism of prefrontal hypofunction in depression the same as in schizophrenia? Br J Psychiatry 162:183–192, 1993

Blackburn I: Mental and psychomotor speed in depression and mania. Br J Psychiatry 132:329–335, 1975

Bolla-Wilson K, Robinson RG, Starkstein SE, et al: Lateralization of dementia and depression in stroke patients. Am J Psychiatry 146:627–634, 1988

Bornstein RA, Baker GB, Douglass AB: Depression and memory in major depressive disorder. J Neuropsychiatry Clin Neurosci 3:78–80, 1991

Bradley BP, Mogg K, Williams R: Implicit and explicit memory for emotion-congruent information in clinical depression and anxiety. Behav Res Ther 33:755–770, 1995

Branconnier RJ, Cole JO, Ghaxvinan S, et al: Treating the depressed elderly patient: the comparative behavioral pharmacology of mianserin and amitriptyline, in Typical and Atypical Antidepressants: Clinical Practice. Edited by Costa E, Racagni G. New York, Raven, 1982, pp 195–212

Brodie JD: Imaging in clinical psychiatry: facts, fantasies, and other musings. Am J Psychiatry 153:145–149, 1996

Brown RG, Scott LC, Bench CJ, et al: Cognitive function in depression: its relationship to the presence and severity of intellectual decline. Psychol Med 24: 829–847, 1994

Bruder G, Sutton S, Berger-Gross P, et al: Lateralized auditory processing in depression: dichotic click detection. Psychiatry Res 4:253–266, 1981

Bruder GE, Schnur DB, Fereson P, et al: Dichotic listening measures of brain laterality in mania. J Abnorm Psychol 103:758–766, 1994

Calev A: Affect and memory in depression: positive emotion words are remembered better than negative emotion words. Psychopathology 29:71–76, 1996

Calev A, Erwin PG: Recall and recognition in depressives: use of matched tasks. Br J Clin Psychol 24:127–128, 1985

Calev A, Korin Y, Shapira B, et al: Verbal and nonverbal recall by euthymic and depressed affective patients. Psychol Med 16:789–794, 1986

Calev A, Ben-Tzvi E, Shapira B, et al: Distinct memory impairments following electroconvulsive therapy and imipramine. Psychol Med 19:111–119, 1989a

Calev A, Nigal D, Chazan S: Retrieval from semantic memory using meaningful and meaningless constructs by depressed, stable bipolar and manic patients. Br J Clin Psychol 28:67–73, 1989b

Calev A, Nigal D, Shapira B, et al: Early and long term effects of electroconvulsive therapy and depression on memory and other cognitive functions. J Nerv Ment Dis 179:526–533, 1991

Calev A, Pass HL, Shapira B, et al: ECT and memory, in The Clinical Science of Electroconvulsive Therapy. Edited by Coffey CE. Washington, DC, American Psychiatric Press, 1993, pp 125–142

Calev A, Fennig S, Jandorf L, et al: Factors associated with neuropsychological performance in first admission psychotic patients. Paper presented at the International Congress on Schizophrenia Research, Hot Springs, VA, April 1995a

Calev A, Gaudino EA, Zervas IM, et al: ECT and non-memory cognition: a review. Br J Clin Psychol 34:505–515, 1995b

Channon S, Baker JE, Robertson MM: Working memory in clinical depression: an experimental study. Psychol Med 23:87–91, 1993

Chapman LJ, Chapman JP: The measurement of differential deficits. J Psychiatr Res 14:303–311, 1978

Coffey CE, Wilkinson WE, Weiner RD, et al: Quantitative cerebral anatomy in depression: a controlled magnetic resonance study. Arch Gen Psychiatry 50:7–16, 1993

Cohen RM, Weingartner H, Smallberg SA, et al: Effort and cognition in depression. Arch Gen Psychiatry 39:593–597, 1982

Cornblatt BA, Lenzenweger MF, Erlenmeyer-Kimling L: The Continuous Performance Test, Identical Pairs Version, II: contrasting attentional profiles in schizophrenic and depressed patients. Psychiatry Res 29:65–85, 1989

Cowley DS, Dunner DL: Benzodiazepines in anxiety and depression, in Benzodiazepines in Clinical Practice: Risks and Benefits. Edited by Roy-Byrne PP, Cowley DS. Washington, DC, American Psychiatric Press, 1991, pp 35–56

Crew WD, Harrison DW: Functional asymmetry in the motor performance of women: neuropsychological effects of depression. Percept Mot Skills 78:1315–1322, 1994

Curran HV, Shine P, Lader M: Effects of repeated doses of fluvoxamine, mianserin, and placebo on memory and measures of sedation. Psychopharmacology 89:360–363, 1986

Curran HV, Sakulsriprong M, Lader M: Antidepressants and human memory: an investigation of four drugs with different sedative and anticholinergic profiles. Psychopharmacology 95:520–527, 1988

Cutting J: Depressive illness and mania, in The Right Hemisphere in Psychiatric Disorders. Edited by Cutting J. New York, Oxford University Press, 1990, pp 346–376

Danion JM, Kaufmann-Muller F, Grange D, et al: Affective valence of words, explicit and implicit memory in clinical depression. J Affect Disord 34:227–234, 1995

Deptula D, Manevitz A, Yasowitz A: Asymmetry of recall in depression. J Clin Exp Neuropsychol 13:854–870, 1991

Dhingra U, Rabins PV: Mania in the elderly: a 5–7 years follow-up. J Am Geriatr Soc 39:581–583, 1991

Dimond S, Farrington L, Johnson P: Differing emotional response from right and left hemisphere. Nature 261:690–692, 1976

Dolan RJ, Bench CJ, Brown RG, et al: Neuropsychological dysfunction in depression: the relationship to regional cerebral blood flow. Psychol Med 24:849–857, 1994

Donnelly S, Murphee D, Goodwin F, et al: Intellectual function in primary affective disorder. Br J Psychiatry 140:633–636, 1982

Dunbar GC, Lishman WA: Depression, recognition memory and hedonic tone: a signal detection analysis. Br J Psychiatry 144:376–382, 1984

Ellis HC: Focused attention and depressive deficits. J Exp Psychol Gen 120:310–312, 1991

Feinberg T, Goodman B: Affective illness, dementia, and pseudodementia. J Clin Psychiatry 45:99–103, 1984

Fink M: Convulsive Therapy: Theory and Practice. New York, Raven, 1979, pp 107–141

Flor-Henry P: Laterality shifts in cerebral dominance, sinistrality, and psychosis, in Hemispheric Asymmetry of Function in Psychopathology. Edited by Gruzelier J, Flor-Henry P. New York, Elsevier, 1979, pp 3–20

Foster F, Kupfer D: Psychomotor activity as a correlate of depression and sleep in acutely disturbed psychiatric patients. Am J Psychiatry 132:928–931, 1975

Gainotti G: Emotional behavior and hemispheric side of the lesion. Cortex 8:41–55, 1972

Glass RM, Uhlenhuth EH, Hartel FW, et al: Cognitive dysfunction and imipramine in outpatient depressives. Arch Gen Psychiatry 38:1048–1051, 1981

Gold PW, Goodwin FK, Chrousos JP: Clinical and biochemical manifestations of depression. N Engl J Med 319:348–353, 1988

Goldberg TE, Gold JM, Greenberg R, et al: Contrasts between patients with affective disorders and patients with schizophrenia on a neuropsychological test battery. Am J Psychiatry 150:1355–1362, 1993

Golinkoff M, Sweeney JA: Cognitive impairment in depression. J Affect Disord 17:105–112, 1989

Grossman I, Kaufman AS, Mednitsky S, et al: Neurocognitive abilities for a clinically depressed sample versus a matched control group of normal individuals. Psychiatry Res 51:231–244, 1994

Gruzelier J: Disparate syndromes in psychosis delineated by the direction of electrodermal response lateral asymmetry, in Laterality and Psychopathology. Edited by Flor-Henry P, Gruzelier J. New York, Elsevier, 1983, pp 525–538

Gruzelier J, Venables PH: Bimodality and laterality of skin conductance orienting activity in schizophrenics: replication and evidence of lateral asymmetry in patients with depression and disorders of personality. Biol Psychiatry 8: 55–73, 1974

Gur RC, Erwin RJ, Gur RE, et al: Facial emotion discrimination, II: behavioral findings in depression. Psychiatry Res 42:241–251, 1992a

Gur RC, Erwin RJ, Gur RE: Neurobehavioral probes for physiologic neuroimaging studies. Am J Psychiatry 49:409–414, 1992b

Hart RP, Kwentus JA, Taylor JR, et al: Rate of forgetting in dementia and depression. J Consult Clin Psychol 55:101–105, 1987

Heilman KM, Bowers D, Valenstein E: Emotional disorders associated with neurological disease, in Clinical Neuropsychology, 3rd Edition. Edited by Heilman KN, Valenstein E. New York, Oxford University Press, 1993, pp 461–497

Hertel PT, Rude SS: Depressive deficits in memory: focusing attention improves subsequent recall. J Exp Psychol Gen 120:301–309, 1991

Hoehn-Saric R, Lipsey JR, McLeod DR: Apathy and indifference in patients on fluvoxamine and fluoxetine. J Clin Psychopharmacol 10:343–345, 1990

Hoehn-Saric R, Harris GJ, Pearlson GD, et al: A fluoxetine-induced frontal lobe syndrome in an obsessive compulsive patient. J Clin Psychiatry 52:131–133, 1991

Isen AM, Shalker TA, Clark L, et al: Affect, accessibility of material in memory, and behavior: a cognitive loop? J Pers Soc Psychol 36:1–12, 1978

Jacoby RJ, Levy R: Computed tomography in the elderly, 3: affective disorders. Br J Psychiatry 136:270–275, 1980

Jones BN, Reifler BV: Depression coexisting with dementia: evaluation and treatment. Med Clin North Am 78:823–840, 1994

Judd LL, Hubbard B, Janowky DS, et al: The effect of lithium carbonate on the cognitive functions of normal subjects. Arch Gen Psychiatry 34:355–357, 1977

Kahneman D: Attention and Effort. Englewood Cliffs, NJ, Prentice-Hall, 1973

Kellner CH, Rubinow DR, Post RM: Cerebral ventricular size and cognitive impairment in depression. J Affect Disord 10:215–219, 1986

Lamping DL, Spring B, Gelenberg AJ: Effects of two antidepressants on memory performance in depressed outpatients: a double-blind study. Psychopharmacology 84:254–261, 1984

Liebowitz MR, Hollander E, Schneider F, et al: Reversible and irreversible monoamine oxidase inhibitors in other psychiatric disorders. Acta Psychiatr Scand 360 (suppl):29–34, 1990

Lipsey J, Spencer W, Robins P, et al: Phenomenological comparison of post-stroke depression and functional depression. Am J Psychiatry 143:527–529, 1986

Lloyd GG, Lishman WA: Effect of depression on the speed of recall of pleasant and unpleasant experiences. Psychol Med 2:248–273, 1975

Lyness SA, Eaton EM, Schneider LS: Cognitive performance in older and mid-dle-aged depressed outpatients and controls. J Gerontol B Psychol Sci Soc Sci 49:129–136, 1994

Marinot JL, Hardy P, Feline A, et al: Left prefrontal glucose metabolism in the depressed state, a confirmation. Am J Psychiatry 147:1313–1317, 1990

Martin DJ, Oren Z, Boone K: Major depressives' and dysthymics' performance on the Wisconsin Card Sorting Test. J Clin Psychol 47:684–690, 1991

Mason C: Pre-illness intelligence of mental hospital patients. J Consult Clin Psychol 20:297–300, 1956

Mattila M, Mattila MJ, Vrijmoed-de Vries M, et al: Actions and interactions of psychotropic drugs on human performance and mood: single doses of ORG 3770, amitriptyline, and diazepam. Pharmacol Toxicol 65:81–88, 1989

McKay AP, Tarbuck AF, Shapleske J, et al: Neuropsychological functions in manic-depressive psychosis: evidence for persistent deficit in patients with chronic, severe illness. Br J Psychiatry 167:51–57, 1995

McNair DM, Kahn RJ, Frankenthaler LM, et al: Amoxapine and amitriptyline, II: specificity of cognitive effects during brief treatment of depression. Psychopharmacology 83:134–139, 1984

Moller HJ, Volz HP: Drug treatment of depression in the 1990s: an overview of achievements and future possibilities. Drugs 52:625–638, 1996

Moskowitz H, Burns MM: Cognitive performance in geriatric subjects after acute treatment with antidepressants. Neuropsychobiology 15:18–43, 1986

Moskowitz H, Burns MM: The effects on performance of two antidepressants alone and in combination with diazepam. Prog Neuropsychopharmacol Biol Psychiatry 12:783–792, 1988

Nasrallah H, McCalley-Whitters M: Motor lateralization in manic patients. Br J Psychiatry 140:521–522, 1982

Nelson RE, Craighead WE: Selective recall of positive and negative feedback, self-control behaviors and depression. J Abnorm Psychol 86:379–388, 1977

O'Brien JT, Sahakian BJ, Checkley SA: Cognitive impairment in patients with seasonal affective disorder. Br J Psychiatry 163:338–343, 1993

Pancheri P, Delle Chiaie R, Donnini M, et al: Effects of moclobemide on depressive symptoms and cognitive performance in a geriatric population: a controlled comparative study versus imipramine. Clin Neuropharmacol 17: S58–S73, 1994

Priest RG: Moclobemide and the reversible inhibitors of monoamine oxidase antidepressants. Acta Psychiatr Scand 360 (suppl):39–41, 1990

Ramaekers JG, Muntjewerff ND, O'Hanlon JF: A comparative study of acute and subchronic effects of dothiepin, fluoxetine, and placebo on psychomotor and actual driving performance. Br J Clin Pharmacol 39:397–404, 1995

Raskind MA: Geriatric pharmacology: management of late-life depression and the noncognitive behavioral disturbances of Alzheimer's disease. Psychiatr Clin North Am 16:815–827, 1993

Robinson RG: Neuropsychiatric consequences of strokes. Annu Rev Med 48: 217–229, 1997

Robinson RG, Bolla-Wilson K, Kaplan E, et al: Depression influences intellectual impairment in stroke patients. Br J Psychiatry 148:541–547, 1986

Rossi A, Stratta P, Nistico R, et al: Visuospatial impairment in depression: a controlled study. Acta Psychiatr Scand 81:81–101, 1990

Roy-Byrne PP, Weingartner H, Bearer LM, et al: Effortful and automatic cognitive processes in depression. Arch Gen Psychiatry 43:265–267, 1986

Sackeim H, Gur R, Saucy M: Emotions are expressed more intensely on the left side of the face. Science 202:434–436, 1978

Sackeim H, Greenberg M, Weman A, et al: Hemispheric asymmetry in the expression of positive and negative emotions: neurologic evidence. Arch Neurol 39: 210–218, 1982

Sackeim H, Portnoy S, Decina P, et al: Left visual neglect in ECT patients. Biol Psychiatry 19:83–85, 1983

Sackeim H, Freeman J, McElhiney M, et al: Effects of major depression on estimates of intelligence. J Clin Exp Neuropsychol 14:268–288, 1992

Sax KW, Strakowski SM, McElroy SL, et al: Attention and formal thought disorder in mixed and pure mania. Biol Psychiatry 37:420–423, 1995

Schaffler K: Study on performance and alcohol interaction with the antidepressant fluoxetine. Int Clin Psychopharmacol 4 (suppl):15–20, 1989

Schmaling KB, DiClementi JD, Cullum CM, et al: Cognitive functioning in chronic fatigue syndrome and depression: a preliminary comparison. Psychosom Med 56:383–388, 1994

Semlitsch HV, Arderer P, Saletu B, et al: Acute effects of the novel antidepressant venlafaxine on cognitive event-related potentials (P300), eye blink rate and mood in young healthy subjects. Int Clin Psychopharmacol 8:155–166, 1993

Smigan L, Perris C: Memory functions and prophylactic treatment with lithium. Psychol Med 13:529–536, 1983

Spring B, Gelenberg AJ, Garvin R, et al: Amitriptyline, clovoxamine and cognitive function: a placebo-controlled comparison in depressed outpatients. Psychopharmacology 108:327–332, 1992

Squire LR: ECT and memory dysfunction, in ECT: Basic Mechanisms. Edited by Lerer B, Weiner RD, Belmaker RH. Washington, DC, American Psychiatric Press, 1984, pp 156–163

Squire LR: Memory functions as affected by electroconvulsive therapy, in Electroconvulsive Therapy: Clinical and Basic Issues. Edited by Malitz S, Sackeim H. New York, New York Academy of Science, 1986, pp 307–314

Squire LR, Slater PC, Miller PL: Retrograde amnesia and bilateral electroconvulsive therapy: long-term follow-up. Arch Gen Psychiatry 38:89–95, 1981

Starkstein SE, Robinson RG: Depression in cardiovascular disease. Edited by Starkstein SE, Robinson RG. Baltimore, MD, Johns Hopkins University Press, 1993, pp 30–49

Sternberg DE, Jarvik ME: Memory functions in depression. Arch Gen Psychiatry 33:219–224, 1976

Sweeney JA, Wetzler S, Stokes P, et al: Cognitive functioning in depression. J Clin Psychol 45:836–842, 1989

Tancer ME, Brown TM, Evans DL, et al: Impaired effortful cognition in depression. Psychiatry Res 31:161–168, 1990

Teasdale JD, Russell ML: Differential effects of induced mood on the recall of positive, negative and neutral words. Br J Clin Psychol 22:163–171, 1983

Trichard C, Marinot JL, Alagille M, et al: Time course of prefrontal lobe dysfunction in severely depressed in-patients: a longitudinal neuropsychological study. Psychol Med 25:79–85, 1995

Tsuang M, Woolson R, Fleming J: Long-term outcome of major psychoses. Arch Gen Psychiatry 36:1295–1304, 1979

Uytdenhoef P, Portelange P, Jacque J, et al: Regional cerebral blood flow and lateralized hemispheric dysfunction in depression. Br J Psychiatry 143:128–132, 1983

Van Laar MW, Van Willingenburg AP, Volkerz ER: Acute and subacute effects of nefazodone and imipramine on highway driving, cognitive function, and daytime sleepiness in healthy and elderly subjects. J Clin Psychopharmacol 15:30–40, 1995

Watts FN, Sharrock R: Cued recall in depression. Br J Clin Psychol 26:149–150, 1987

Watts FN, Dalgleish T, Bourke P, et al: Memory deficit in clinical depression: processing resources and structure of materials. Psychol Med 20:345–349, 1990

Wechsler D: Wechsler Adult Intelligence Scale—Revised. San Antonio, TX, Psychological Corporation, 1981

Weingartner H, Cohen R, Murphy D, et al: Cognitive processes in depression. Arch Gen Psychiatry 43:265–267, 1981

Wells CE: Pseudodementia. Am J Psychiatry 136:894–896, 1979

Wesnes KA, Simpson PM, Christmas L, et al: The effects of moclobemide on cognition. J Neural Transm 28:91–102, 1989

Wexler BE, Levenson L, Warrenburg S, et al: Decreased perceptual sensitivity to emotion-evoking stimuli in depression. Psychiatry Res 51:127–138, 1994

Williams JMG, Scott J: Autobiographical memory in depression. Psychol Med 18: 689–695, 1988

Williams JM, Little MM, Scates S, et al: Memory complaints and abilities among depressed older adults. J Consult Clin Psychol 55:595–598, 1987

Wolfe J, Granholm E, Butters N, et al: Verbal memory deficits associated with major affective disorders: a comparison of unipolar and bipolar patients. J Affect Disord 13:83–92, 1987

Yazowitz A, Bruder G, Sutton S, et al: Dichotic perception for right hemisphere dysfunction in affective psychosis. Br J Psychiatry 135:224–237, 1979

Zimmer R: Relationship between tyramine potentiation and monoamine oxidase (MAO) inhibition: comparison between moclobemide and MAO inhibitors. Acta Psychiatr Scand 360 (suppl):81–83, 1990

Zubenko GS, Sullivan P, Nelson JP, et al: Brain imaging abnormalities in mental disorders of late life. Arch Neurol 47:1107–1111, 1990

4

NEUROPSYCHOLOGY OF NONPSYCHOTIC, NONAFFECTIVE PSYCHIATRIC DISORDERS

Donald W. O'Donnell, M.P.S., and Avraham Calev, D.Phil.

THE USE OF neuropsychology in schizophrenia and affective disorders has brought increasing insight into these serious and troublesome illnesses (see Calev, Chapter 2, and Calev and colleagues, Chapter 3, in this volume). Neuropsychological research may help investigators better understand and treat other disorders. Keefe (1995) argued that

> When applied properly, a battery of neuropsychological tests yields an understanding of the cognitive and behavioral abilities and weaknesses of an individual or group of individuals. It provides the clinician or investigator with an objective description of what areas of behavior and cognition are likely to be a problem for the psychiatric patient and what areas are not. (p. 7)

Furthermore, identifying differing patterns of neuropsychological deficits within a single diagnostic category might help to differentiate subgroups with possibly differing etiologies but common symptom pictures (Keefe 1995). Such subgroup identification might lead to more focused and better targeted treatments.

In this chapter, we review the literature on neuropsychological studies of DSM-IV (American Psychiatric Association 1994) nonaffective disorders that do not result in psychosis. We used a MEDLINE-assisted literature search to help review the literature on these disorders.

◈ Anxiety Disorders

The neuropsychological literature focused on obsessive-compulsive disorder (OCD) and posttraumatic stress disorder (PTSD).

Obsessive-Compulsive Disorder

OCD is defined in DSM-IV as "recurrent obsessions or compulsions that are severe enough to be time consuming (i.e., they take more than 1 hour a day)" (American Psychiatric Association 1994, p. 417). "*Obsessions* are persistent ideas, thoughts, impulses, or images that are experienced as intrusive and inappropriate and that cause marked anxiety or distress," whereas "*Compulsions* are repetitive behaviors (e.g., hand washing, ordering, checking) or mental acts (e.g., praying, counting, repeating words silently) the goal of which is to prevent or reduce anxiety or distress" (American Psychiatric Association 1994, p. 418). Some degree of insight is evident because at some point in the disorder the person will recognize that the obsessions or compulsions are excessive or unreasonable. OCD is a much more common disorder than previously thought, with an estimated lifetime prevalence of 2.5% (American Psychiatric Association 1994). It is equally common in males and females.

OCD had the greatest body of neuropsychological research literature. This is not surprising given the large amount of evidence suggesting an organic etiology (Lieberman 1984; Turner et al. 1985), including its association with numerous neurological conditions and acquired brain lesions in adulthood (Breiter et al. 1994; George et al. 1989; Laplane et al. 1989; Swedo et al. 1989; Ward 1988; Weilburg et al. 1989). Its successful treatment with medications (Thoren et al. 1980) and brain surgery (Baer et al. 1995; Jenike et al. 1991; Mindus et al. 1994) also supports a possible biological or brain dysfunction in OCD.

In addition, positive magnetic resonance imaging (MRI) and other neuroimaging findings in OCD have been reported (Garber et al. 1989; Scarone et al. 1992). Reports of sleep disturbance (Insel et al. 1982), positive neurological soft signs (Hollander et al. 1990; Stein et al. 1993a), smooth pursuit eye movement dysfunction (Gambini et al. 1992; Sweeney et al. 1992), and electroencephalographic (EEG) findings (Prichep et al. 1993) all point to possible biological factors in OCD. Most studies, reviewed below, implicated the frontal and parietal cortices and the basal ganglia, and the right hemisphere was implicated more often than the left.

These biological findings should be interpreted with caution because they may be either the *cause* or the *product* of the disorder. Despite the strength of the neuropsychological research findings reviewed below, they do not provide a definitive answer as to whether OCD has a biological cause.

Flor-Henry et al. (1979) did an early neuropsychological investigation of OCD with the Halstead-Reitan Neuropsychological Test Battery (Reitan 1979). It suggested a combined frontal, temporal, and parietal dysfunction in most of the 11 obsessive-compulsive patients, compared with 11 nonobsessive control subjects. The results indicated a left-hemisphere dysfunction. The number of subjects was small, and criteria for subject selection were based on pre-DSM-IV (American Psychiatric Association 1987) diagnostic considerations, but this study set the stage for later studies. Insel et al. (1983) attempted to replicate Flor-Henry and colleagues' results with the Halstead-Reitan Battery (HRB) but found only abnormal Tactual Performance Test results in their group of OCD patients, which suggested *right*-parietal-, not left-, hemisphere dysfunction with no evidence of a frontal dysfunction. Insel and colleagues (1983) reported, however, that anxiety and depression were confounding factors.

Malloy (1987) supported the existence of frontal dysfunction by reporting abnormal perseveration scores on the Wisconsin Card Sorting Test (WCST; Heaton 1985). However, Malloy noted that "the group [of OCD patients] that was impaired on the WCST was described as more psychotic, lower functioning, having poorer prognosis, and less intelligent than the unimpaired WCST group" (p. 212). The failure to control for psychosis and intellectual level, both of which can result in poorer WCST scores, is a serious shortcoming of this study. Indeed, a much later study (Abbruzzese et al. 1995) found no difference in WCST performance in 33 OCD patients and 33 non-OCD control subjects carefully matched for age, sex, and educational status (possibly because of elimination of the contributions of intelligence to the WCST performance).

Rosen et al. (1988) and Hollander et al. (1991) evaluated OCD patients with the Benton Visual Retention Test (Benton 1974), Matching Familiar Faces Test (Kagan and Henker 1966), and Stroop Test (Stroop 1935) and found errors in visual memory retention but not in visual recognition or matching. Patients had deficits in shifting between conceptual sets and in inhibiting responses to an irrelevant stimulus dimension. These findings were reported as consistent with a frontal right-hemisphere dysfunction. Diamond et al. (1988) found that OCD patients had abnormal results on the Complex Figure Test, which substantiates the case for a right-hemisphere dysfunction in OCD.

Another study supporting frontal and parietal brain dysfunctions was that of Neziroglu et al. (1988). They reported Tactual Performance Test deficits and poor performance on the Category Test (Reitan 1979) and Finger Oscillation Test (Reitan 1979) in 12 OCD patients, pointing "to a concentration of deficits in the inferior regions of the brain," namely, "the frontal and parietal lobes, and the inferior motor strip between them" (Neziroglu et al. 1988, p. 356). Lateralization findings were not mentioned. This study did not have a comparison control group. The Luria-Nebraska Neuropsychological Battery (LNNB; Golden et al. 1980) (Bellini et al. 1989) did not show significant differences between 10 OCD patients and 10 matched non-OCD control subjects, suggesting no abnormal lateralization in OCD.

Several studies used comprehensive, albeit varying, neuropsychological batteries designed to assess functions such as memory, attention, intelligence, executive skills, and visual-spatial skills. These studies attempted to control more closely for general intellectual functioning and eliminate or control for confounding variables such as coexisting depression and medication status. Head et al. (1989) noted no difference between control subjects and OCD subjects in spatial functioning but did find a deficit in ability to shift cognitive set when using nonverbal materials. Their findings suggested that OCD patients show frontal right-hemisphere deficits. In a study correlating positron-emission tomography (PET) scores with a number of neuropsychological measures, Martinot et al. (1990) found that OCD patients were significantly impaired in measures of memory and attention. PET scores indicated global hypometabolism in OCD subjects; lowered metabolism in the prefrontal lateral cortex corresponded to a greater number of errors on the interference task of the Stroop Test. The authors indicated that "the globality of the hypometabolism suggests a dysfunction of the general activating systems triggering the expression of OCD symptoms" and provide "a further indication of frontal lobe involvement in OCD" (p. 240).

Boone et al. (1991) found no deficits in frontal-lobe functions in a group of OCD patients. However, they noted subtle deficits in visual-spatial abilities and visual memory, suggesting basal ganglia and/or right-hemisphere dysfunction. They also noted greater deficits in these areas in those patients with a family history of OCD. Zielinski et al. (1991) reached a similar conclusion. They found subtle orbital-frontal deficits in their group of OCD subjects suggested by a tendency toward confabulation on the California Verbal Learning Test (CVLT). However, the more glaring deficits were found across several visual-spatial tasks. Moreover, the less amenable to verbal mediation the task was, the more poorly it was performed. These findings suggested a nondominant or subcortical processing deficit, because a high rate of visual-spatial deficits is also found in subcortical disorders such as Tourette's disorder and Parkinson's disease (Chiu et al. 1986).

Aronowitz et al. (1994) used a specifically selected battery of neuropsychological tests and found deficits in visuospatial abilities, shifting, sequencing, and speed of performance, suggesting either a right frontal- and parietal-lobe or a basal ganglia dysfunction, because deficits in shifting, sequencing, and speed could be the result of both frontal-lobe and basal ganglia dysfunction. Aronowitz et al. found that male OCD subjects, relative to non-OCD control males and contrary to the usual noted superiority of males in spatial abilities (Filskov and Castanese 1986), perform more poorly than female OCD subjects on visuospatial and visuoconstructional tasks. Thus, males "comprise a sub-group of OCD patients distinguished by further (right hemisphere) neuropsychological impairment" (Aronowitz et al. 1994, p. 85). However, no other studies have pursued sex differences.

Another finding that supports a basal ganglia dysfunction is that OCD patients also performed more poorly than control subjects on speed tests (Christiansen et al. 1992). That study included 18 nondepressed OCD patients and 18 age-, education-, and gender-matched non-OCD control subjects. Results were equivocal for executive functions and visual-spatial abilities but significant for recent nonverbal memory. A right medial temporal dysfunction was possible. The evidence for executive frontal dysfunction was weak. The authors noted that, as studies have better control for education and intelligence quotient (IQ), the evidence for frontal dysfunction may become less apparent.

On the basis of the evidence for a basal ganglia dysfunction in OCD (Wise and Rapoport 1989), two groups (Hollander et al. 1993; Martin et al. 1993) attempted to contrast the neuropsychological results in patients with OCD and putative basal ganglia disorders, namely, Parkinson's disease and Huntington's disease. Martin et al. (1993) found no significant neuropsychological impairment in their sample of 17 unmedicated OCD patients. However, Martin et al. (1993) acknowledged that some OCD subjects may show significant cognitive disability: "We would suggest that the occasional co-occurrence of OCD and Huntington's disease-like cognitive deficits result from a dysfunction to proximal, but functionally anatomically, and perhaps neurochemically distinct (basal ganglia) systems" (p. 352). Whereas Martin et al. stressed the distinct nature of OCD, Hollander et al. (1993) noted a degree of dysfunction on tasks requiring visuospatial analysis and visual construction in both OCD and Parkinson's disease patients and suggested that both disorders may have common subcortical, frontal-striatal pathways.

Bornstein (1991) noted the genetic relationship and the high incidence of obsessive-compulsive characteristics in Tourette's disorder as well as the higher incidence of tics in OCD patients and assessed 100 patients between ages 6 and 18 years whose symptoms met DSM-III-R (American Psychiatric Association 1987) criteria for Tourette's disorder. Bornstein noted that the higher scores on an OCD rating scale were associated with worse performance on WCST measures; poorer performance was attributable to problems of response maintenance rather than to perseverative tendencies. He suggested indirect influences on frontal function from the basal ganglia and not a frontal-lobe dysfunction per se.

The subjects in Bornstein's (1991) study were children and adolescents, who may not be similar to patients with adult-onset OCD. Indeed, Rapoport's research group (Behar et al. 1984; Cox et al. 1989; Ludlow et al. 1989; Rapoport et al. 1981) found language deficits that "did not resemble any known pattern associated with particular brain pathology" (Ludlow et al. 1989, p. 104) in younger OCD patients and suggested a lack of normal development for laterality. These investigators also reported that on neuropsychological examination, OCD patients show deficits implicating frontal and/or caudate nucleus dysfunction. Higher than expected ventricular enlargement was found in subjects with childhood OCD, and those subjects with ventricular enlargement had more marked central nervous system dysfunction. Longitudinal studies, although costly and difficult to perform, may be more useful in clarifying this developmental issue.

Verbal and language abilities and verbal memory have not been implicated frequently in adult neuropsychological studies of OCD. Martinot et al. (1990) found "global memory impairment," which they attributed to global brain hypometabolism seen in PET scanning and general slowness in information processing. Otto (1992) found that OCD subjects performed significantly below average on verbal memory tasks and suggested that frontally directed aspects of memory might be implicated. The earlier work of Sher et al. (1983, 1984) is cited by Otto, but these were analogue studies that used college students who scored high on the Maudsley Obsessive-Compulsive Inventory and not clinically diagnosed OCD patients. A replication in a clinical sample (Sher et al. 1989) with 13 compulsive "checkers" (people who check frequently) who scored high on the Maudsley Obsessive-Compulsive Inventory—Checking Scale and 12 "noncheckers" from an outpatient clinic showed poorer recall for recently completed actions by the checkers. Checkers tended to have less vivid visual imagery and to use visual imagery to a lesser extent than noncheckers. Checkers also performed significantly worse on the Wechsler Memory Scale (WMS; Wechsler 1945) Visual Reproduction subtest than did noncheckers.

Comment.   Despite the growing number of neuropsychological studies of OCD, the nature of the contributions from brain areas in the right hemisphere, the frontal cortex, and the basal ganglia remains uncertain. The cognitive deficits involving visuospatial processing and attention shifting, sequencing, and speed and the lack of language deficits may suggest a right-hemisphere dysfunction, perhaps affected by subcortical dysfunction. Parietal (perceptual) and frontal (executive) functions may be affected indirectly.

However, this impression is based on studies that have poorly defined and selected subject groups, no comparison groups, inconsistent and often limited neuropsychological batteries, and small sample sizes. Whether patients with psychosis or other neurological conditions were included in the sample is not always clear because exclusion criteria are rarely stated. Early studies usually did not attempt to control for confounding factors such as alcohol abuse, level of depression, use of medications, age at onset of symptoms, and gender.

More recent studies have attempted to address some of these problems, which has allowed for some model building (i.e., to place these results within a framework of already existing theory). Otto (1990, 1992) presented a preliminary cognitive-behavioral model of OCD based on a configuration of neurological and psychological vulnerability.

Systematic and massive data collection is important in defining causes. Wilhelm et al. (1997) used such an approach. They established that the autobiographical memory deficit found in some OCD patients can be attributed to coexistence of depression and not to OCD per se.

Posttraumatic Stress Disorder

PTSD is characterized by having experienced an unusually traumatic event, after which symptoms of increased arousal and avoidance of stimuli associated with the trauma are observed. Depressive and anxiety symptoms occur. PTSD can occur at any age, and lifetime prevalence rates ranging from 1% to 14% have been reported. In studies of high-risk individuals such as veterans, prevalence rates of 3%–58% have been reported (American Psychiatric Association 1994).

PTSD has received less attention in neuropsychological research than OCD has. Some investigators (Archibald and Tuddenham 1965; Burstein 1985) reported a high frequency of complaints of difficulty concentrating in PTSD subjects. Klonoff et al. (1976) investigated two groups of World War II prisoners of war who had been interned in Japan or Europe. They found subjective reports of impaired neuropsychological functioning in 35.5% of the high-stress (interned in Japan) group and 19.0% of the low-stress (interned in Europe) group 30 years later. The high-stress group performed significantly less well than the low-stress group on the HRB Category and Seashore Rhythm Tests and on Trail B of the Trail Making Test (Reitan 1958). These investigators also found significant differences in the Wechsler Adult Intelligence Scale Full-Scale IQ between the high-stress group (mean IQ 111.1) and the low-stress group (mean IQ 118.3). However, with the lack of a control group, the effects of malnutrition and the high incidence of physical disease differing between the internment camps make it difficult to attribute these results to the effects of stress alone.

Gil et al. (1990) first examined cognitive deficits in clinically diagnosed PTSD subjects objectively with a comprehensive neuropsychological battery. The study used PTSD subjects and two control groups: 1) nonpsychotic psychiatric patients and 2) nonpsychiatric control subjects. Results indicated that the two patient groups performed more poorly than the nonpsychiatric control group. Additionally, when a deterioration quotient was computed and when premorbid intellectual functioning was assessed (before army recruitment) and compared with present-day functioning, investigators found that both patient groups functioned alike—both had an appreciable deterioration in overall intellectual functioning. The results of this study are consistent with the view that PTSD patients have a generalized cognitive deficit similar to that of other psychiatric disorders with a comparable level of impairment in everyday life. The results do not support the existence of specific cognitive impairments in PTSD.

In two studies, both with the same samples of Vietnam veterans with combat-related PTSD and non-PTSD control subjects, Bremner et al. (1993, 1995) found that PTSD patients had deficits in short-term memory, consistent with cognitive and neural problems in PTSD. PTSD patients also had smaller right hippocampal volume on MRI. Unlike Gil et al. (1990), Bremner et al. (1993, 1995) did not find a difference in general intellectual functioning between PTSD and control subjects. However, Bremner et al. reported in their second study that reduced right hippocampal volume in PTSD patients (8% smaller) positively correlated with scores on the WMS Logical Memory test. Left hippocampal volume was 3.8% smaller in PTSD subjects than in non-PTSD control subjects, but this difference was not significant. Bremner et al. (1993) drew some parallels between the performance of patients with PTSD and that of patients with temporal-lobe damage. However, these memory deficits may be nonspecific findings in mentally ill patients in general. The high rate of comorbidity for alcohol abuse in PTSD subjects, unlike that in the Gil et al. study, may have confounded the findings of smaller hippocampal volume and short-term memory deficit in PTSD patients.

Another study that supports a neurological or neuropsychological dysfunction in PTSD is that of Gurvits et al. (1993). They found a significant number of neurological soft signs in a group of 27 Vietnam veterans whose condition met the criteria for PTSD compared with a group of 15 male Vietnam veterans without PTSD.

However, not all studies support a cognitive and neurological dysfunction in PTSD. Yehuda et al. (1995) compared scores of 20 male combat veterans with PTSD with those of 12 non-PTSD subjects on the Wechsler Adult Intelligence Scale—Revised (WAIS-R; Wechsler 1981) and the CVLT and found that PTSD patients had normal abilities in attention, immediate memory, cumulative learning, and proactive interference from previous learning. No significant difference on measures of global intellectual functioning was found between the two groups. However, evidence of a cognitive deficit remained. The PTSD group showed substantial retroactive interference on the CVLT, resulting in a significant decline in retention following exposure to an intervening word list.

Comment. Although some studies suggest general cognitive and neurological impairment in PTSD, this evidence should be regarded as inconclusive until more studies are completed. The number of studies is small, the number of subjects in each study is small, and alcohol abuse and other disorders often co-occur. In addition, most subjects are male.

Like OCD, PTSD is considered a biological disorder by some investigators (B. A. van der Kolk, R. E. Fisler: "The Biological Basis of Post-Traumatic Stress," unpublished manuscript, 1993); therefore, further neuropsychological investigations must be conducted. Wolfe and Charney (1991) noted that neuropsychological evaluation in PTSD can help 1) assess complaints of cognitive dysfunction in this disorder, 2) identify possible PTSD co-occurring brain damage, 3) discriminate PTSD from related syndromes, and 4) provide a most valuable guide in planning treatment for patients with this disorder. Assuming that it is possible that early childhood trauma predisposes individuals to mental disorders or directly results in adult disorders, such studies may be important in understanding psychopathology in general and psychopathology of childhood in particular.

Unlike OCD, PTSD is defined by environmental stress as the primary cause. PTSD "can develop in individuals without any predisposing conditions, particularly if the stressor is . . . extreme" (American Psychiatric Association 1994, p. 427). Biological findings such as small hippocampi (Bremner et al. 1993, 1995) thus are difficult to interpret. They may be predisposing factors or a result of the biological development of PTSD. To control for possible errors, PTSD research should include 1) control for identified independent variables affecting research results, 2) differentiation between state and trait factors affecting neuropsychological condition, 3) consideration of the family history of subjects studied, 4) determination of clinical significance of brain atrophy identified, and 5) attention to secular trends such as birth or cohort effects.

◈ SOMATOFORM DISORDERS

Somatoform disorders have in common "the presence of physical symptoms that suggest a general medical condition and are not fully explained by a general medical condition, by the direct effects of a substance, or by another mental disorder" (American Psychiatric Association 1994, p. 445). The few published neuropsychological studies of somatoform disorders did not use DSM-III-R or DSM-IV criteria, and only studies of "hysteria" (corresponding to the DSM-IV diagnosis of somatoform disorder) and conversion disorder are available. "Conversion disorder involves unexplained symptoms or deficits affecting voluntary motor or sensory function that suggest a neurological or other general medical condition," whereas hysteria (somatization disorder) "is a polysymptomatic disorder that begins before age 30 years, extends over a period of years, and is characterized by a combination of pain, gastrointestinal, sexual, and pseudoneurological symptoms" (American Psychiatric Association 1994, p. 445). Both disorders are more common in women than in men.

Bendefeldt et al. (1976) evaluated attention and memory functions in 17 psychiatric patients (7 men and 10 women) who had a primary diagnosis of hysterical conversion reaction. A control group of 8 men and 9 women was selected from nonpsychotic, nonalcoholic, and nonorganic psychiatric patients residing on the same wards from which the conversion patients were chosen. Bendefeldt et al. found that "in comparison to controls, hysteria patients display heightened suggestibility, increased field dependency, impairment in recent memory and diminished vigilance or attention" (p. 1254). Although no specific brain region was suggested, the authors believed that these results were consistent with some brain dysfunction.

Flor-Henry et al. (1981) used an extensive battery of psychological measures in 10 patients with the "stable syndrome of hysteria" and 10 nonpsychiatric control subjects and reported that 90% of the hysteria patients had abnormal neuropsychological scores, whereas all control subjects were in the normal range. The hysteria group had essentially bilateral, right equal to left, anterior cerebral dysfunction and greater nondominant than dominant hemispheric posterior cerebral dysfunction. Flor-Henry et al. argued that both hysteria in the female and psychopathy in the male are the result of dominant frontal-temporal dysfunction; these two syndromes are equivalent, "the gender determining the manifestation" (p. 615).

Few investigators attempted to be more specific in localizing brain dysfunction. Lawrence and Morton (1980) found a connection between hysteria and increased field dependence (i.e., the degree to which an individual's interpretation of events occurring within a perceptual field is governed by the surrounding frame of reference) in a group of 17 female psychiatric patients who scored high on the Minnesota Multiphasic Personality Inventory (MMPI; Hathaway and McKinley 1951) Hysteria scale. (Field dependence is typically measured by having the subject attempt to adjust a luminous rod to a vertical position when surrounded by a slightly tilted luminous square viewed in a darkened room.) The hysterical subjects took significantly longer to complete the Embedded Figures Test, a measure of field dependence, than did a comparison group of 17 female psychiatric patients who scored high on the MMPI Psychasthenia scale. Note that this perception task may be associated with right-hemisphere function.

Indeed, in a 1984 theoretical article, Miller noted an association between conversion disorders and the right hemisphere. She suggested that the right hemisphere, the brain stem reticular formation, and the second somatosensory area might all contribute to somatoform disorders. Because studies also report conversion symptoms and psychogenic pain more frequently on the left side of the body (Galin et al. 1977; Mersky and Watson 1979; Stern 1977), the association with right-hemisphere function is intriguing, especially so because the right hemisphere is often cited to be "verbally inarticulate," to be responsible for affective information processing, and to mediate unconscious processes independently of the left hemisphere, allowing for unconscious, nonverbal conflicts to be expressed via somatic disturbance (Galin 1974). Unfortunately, no data support these speculations.

Comment. Although a general cognitive impairment may be found in somatoform disorders, the research is meager and inconclusive as to more specific effects.

◈ DISSOCIATIVE DISORDERS

According to DSM-IV, "the essential feature of the Dissociative Disorders is a disruption in the usually integrated functions of consciousness, memory, identity, or perception of the environment" (American Psychiatric Association 1994, p. 477). Most of the neuropsychological research on these disorders has focused on multiple personality disorder (MPD).

Multiple Personality Disorder

MPD (or dissociative identity disorder) is "characterized by the presence of two or more distinct identities or personality states that recurrently take control of the individual's behavior accompanied by an inability to recall personal information that is too extensive to be explained by ordinary forgetfulness" (American Psychiatric Association 1994, p. 477). A recent sharp rise in reported cases of MPD in the United States may be because mental health professionals are more aware of the disorder or because the syndrome has become more common. The disorder is diagnosed three to nine times more frequently in females than in males.

Several studies have established a connection between seizure disorders, especially temporal-lobe seizures, and MPD (Ahern et al. 1993; Benson et al. 1986; Mesulam 1981; Rosenstein 1994; Schenk and Bear 1981). Mathew et al. (1985) found increased right temporal cerebral blood flow, suggesting functional overactivity in one of the personalities in an MPD subject they studied. Saxe et al. (1992) found increased perfusion of the left temporal lobe in another patient with MPD. In support of a temporal-lobe dysfunction in MPD, Teicher et al. (1993) and Yutaka et al. (1993) reported that childhood physical and sexual abuse was associated with increased scores on a limbic dysfunction checklist and also resulted in increased EEG abnormalities most often localized to fronto-temporal areas.

Despite the increased interest in MPD and the above-noted studies strongly implicating temporal-lobe involvement in at least some cases of MPD, very few neuropsychological investigations have been published. Rosenstein (1994) reported neuropsychological data on two subjects with MPD; he found above-average intelligence with significant WAIS-R Verbal and Performance Scale IQ discrepancies and impairment in free recall. Rosenstein noted that both subjects had a 24-point or greater difference between WAIS-R Verbal and Performance Scale IQs, although in opposite directions. He noted that in each subject, one hemisphere was markedly dominant over the other. This finding supports the theory of Ahern et al. (1993) that in MPD "dominance of one hemisphere over the other is associated with pre and post-ictal temporolimbic activity" (Rosenstein 1994, p. 225). In line with motivational forgetting or repression, Rosenstein argued that the impaired recall of information found in his two subjects "reflected problems in the retrieval of learned information as opposed to a deficit in encoding or retention" (p. 224).

Two studies of memory across different personalities in the same person with MPD found greater transfer of information of nonemotional than emotional stimuli across personalities (Ludwig et al. 1972) and reported that information acquired by one personality can facilitate the performance of another on tests that do not require explicit recollection of a prior learning episode (Nissen et al. 1988). A third study (Schacter et al. 1989) assessed within-personality memory function and found a profound deficit in autobiographical memory for information acquired before age 10 years in a 24-year-old woman with MPD, unlike the findings in organic amnesia. These observations suggest motivated repression of memories. At times, one personality represses the other.

Depersonalization

Depersonalization "is characterized by a persistent or recurrent feeling of being detached from one's mental processes or body" (American Psychiatric Association 1994, p. 477).

A literature search found only a single case study of depersonalization involving neuropsychological evaluation. Hollander et al. (1992) reported a case of a 22-year-old man with depersonalization disorder who was evaluated with a brief neuropsychological battery and also underwent EEG and neuroimaging. The patient had a mild visual memory deficit based on four errors on the Benton Visual Retention Test. EEG indicated left temporal and frontal overactivation. Neuroimaging showed impaired perfusion in the left caudate nucleus and increased heterogeneous activity in the posterior frontal areas. The left hemisphere thus may be overactivated in depersonalization disorders, resulting in higher verbal than visual ability. Further experimental research is obviously needed.

Dissociative Amnesia and Fugue States

Dissociative (or psychogenic) amnesia is "characterized by an inability to recall important personal information, usually of a traumatic or stressful nature, that is too extensive to be explained by ordinary forgetfulness" (American Psychiatric Association 1994, p. 477). Fugue involves sudden, unexplained travel away from home accompanied by amnesia, confusion, or the assumption of a new identity.

Neuropsychological investigations of psychogenic amnesias and fugues are limited to a few case studies. The relative rarity and often sudden and unexpected appearances of such patients, along with the need to carefully rule out deliberate feigning of amnesia, make prospective studies of large samples difficult and probably impossible.

Schacter et al. (1982) reported a 21-year-old man who could not remember any identifying information about himself. This patient's amnesia cleared the next day when a funeral scene on television reminded him of his grandfather's recent death. Neuropsychological examination during and after his amnestic period found intact visual scanning, visual constructional ability, and manual dexterity, as well as normal performance on tasks requiring attention and abstract reasoning. WAIS Full-Scale IQ was 102 during amnesia and 108 after it. The WMS Memory Quotient was 82 during amnesia and 100 afterward. A computed tomography (CT) scan revealed evidence of previous right-temporal-lobe damage.

Schacter used experimental measures of memory and found that this patient's access to semantic (public) information was not impaired during the amnestic period. The patient's ability to retrieve episodic (personal) memories improved substantially after rather than during amnesia. Schacter concluded that functional retrograde amnesia involves a differential impairment of semantic and episodic memory and that retrograde amnesia may be organized primarily along affective rather than temporal dimensions. This is unlike organic amnestic disorders, in which retrieval of recent memories is more impaired than retrieval of older memories; in functional, dissociative amnesias, memories may be more easily accessed depending on how emotionally pleasant they are.

Kapur (1991) reported a case of transient 5-day psychogenic amnesia with essentially normal postamnesia neuropsychological findings, including normal performance on verbal and nonverbal recall and recognition tasks and remote memory. This patient, however, had a tendency for poorer verbal memory than nonverbal memory. On a recognition memory test designed to test memory for public events occurring over the prior 6 months, including the 5-day period of amnesia, the patient performed perfectly, showing a distinction between personal and public memory. Kapur suggested that such a distinction may be useful in differentiating cases of organic from dissociative amnesia.

Domb and Beaman (1991) reported a case of psychogenic amnesia in a 58-year-old man.

> Mr. A was tested during a period of total amnesia and loss of personal identity. His WAIS Full-Scale IQ was 87 (low-average intelligence), with Performance Scale IQ (95) higher than Verbal IQ (82). His WMS Memory Quotient was only 66 because he scored poorly on subtests of personal and current information and of orientation. His memory for passages was also very deficient, but memory for visual designs, ability to repeat strings of digits, and ability to learn word-pair associations were intact. However, on this last task, Mr. A could not learn any of the difficult, nonassociated word pairs such as dark-crush.

Through a process of taking Mr. A to important places in his life, he did recover his identity and remembered that his wife had died recently and that he had been depressed and contemplating suicide before losing his memory. Repeated testing with the WMS after recovery of his memory resulted in an improvement of 10 points, but the same inability to learn hard word-pair associations remained.

Saling (1991) noted in a letter to the editor that this inability to learn difficult word-pair associations in Domb and Beaman's Mr. A "is frequently seen in patients with organic amnesias of bilateral hippocampal origin" and suggested that "some cases of functional retrograde amnesia represent massive psychological elaboration around a kernel of organic involvement" (p. 585). Note that the case cited by Schacter et al. had right temporal damage on a CT scan. O'Donnell and Calev (1993) also reported a head injury in a young male who developed psychogenic retrograde amnesia after successful rehabilitation and recovery of memory.

Comment.   Because the dissociative disorders share a disruption in consciousness and memory, the frequent neuropsychological reports of temporal-lobe/hippocampal involvement are consistent with a temporal-lobe/limbic dysfunction (Barr et al. 1990; Milner 1968). Yet it is clear that additional psychogenic factors are essential.

◈ IMPULSE-CONTROL DISORDERS

"The essential feature of Impulse-Control Disorders is the failure to resist an impulse, drive, or temptation to perform an act that is harmful to the person or to others" (American Psychiatric Association 1994, p. 609). The individual may feel an increasing sense of tension or arousal before committing the act, and following the act he or she may or may not have feelings of regret, self-reproach, or guilt.

With the exception of Rugle's (1990) and Rugle and Melamed's (1993) studies (described below), all reports of neuropsychological investigations of the impulse-control disorders have involved case studies.

Pathological Gambling

Pathological gambling is "persistent and recurrent maladaptive gambling behavior that disrupts personal, family, or vocational pursuits" (American Psychiatric Association 1994, p. 615). It may affect as many as

1%–3% of the adult population. Approximately two-thirds of pathological gamblers are males.

Rugle and Melamed (1993) compared 33 white male non-substance-abusing pathological gamblers with 33 white male nonaddicted control subjects on a childhood behavior checklist and on nine measures of attention (such as Symbol Digit Modalities Test; Smith 1973), learning, and memory (across both visual and auditory modalities), as well as on tests of executive function (such as the WCST). Their findings indicated that gamblers had significantly higher ratings on both self-report and collateral report childhood questionnaire measures of attention-deficit/hyperactivity disorder (ADHD)–like behaviors. Gamblers also had lower scores than control subjects on all measures of attention, including all measures of frontally mediated attention processes. This study supports the hypothesis that attention deficit may be a risk factor for the development of impulse-control disorders.

Pyromania

Pyromania is an apparently rare disorder "characterized by a pattern of fire setting for pleasure, gratification, or relief of tension" (American Psychiatric Association 1994, p. 609). Incidents of fire setting "are episodic and may wax and wane in frequency" (American Psychiatric Association 1994, p. 614).

Calev (1995) presented a case study of a 70-year-old man who set fires and underwent neuropsychological testing with repeated neuropsychological evaluation 4 years later. Testing was consistent with left frontal dysfunction and showed evidence of deterioration in frontal functioning between the first and the second evaluation, suggestive of frontal-lobe dysfunction in pyromania.

Kleptomania

"Kleptomania is characterized by the recurrent failure to resist impulses to steal objects not needed for personal use or monetary value" (American Psychiatric Association 1994, p. 609). "Kleptomania is a rare condition that appears to occur in fewer than 5% of identified shoplifters. It appears to be much more common is females" (American Psychiatric Association 1994, p. 613).

Chiswick (1976) published a case study of a 66-year-old woman convicted for shoplifting who had depression and blackouts. Skull X ray identified a right parietal calcified mass. No neuropsychological evaluation was done, and the author concluded that the shoplifting was related to her depression. The author commented on the "remote possibility" that the episode of shoplifting might have occurred during a psychomotor seizure.

A second case of shoplifting associated with a neurological condition was reported by Mendez (1988). A 66-year-old man with multiinfarct dementia had CT and MRI scans that showed damage in the left frontal and left parietotemporal areas and other areas with loss of volume that suggested earlier strokes. This man scored in the mildly demented range on the Mini-Mental State Exam, WCST, the Porteus Maze Test (Porteus 1959), and a frontal-lobe test of verbal fluency. Mendez stated that both neuropsychological investigation and neuroimaging provided evidence of frontal disturbance and that this patient's shoplifting was suggestive of behavior seen in some frontally impaired individuals who feel compelled to pick up an object when they see it, a phenomenon labeled *utilization behavior* (Lhermitte 1983).

McIntyre and Emsley (1990) reported a 52-year-old woman who was arrested for shoplifting. She was later found to have normal-pressure hydrocephalus caused by aqueduct stenosis. She showed poor judgment and other features of dementia. No neuropsychological results were reported. Her treatment by ventriculoperitoneal shunt resulted in resolution of dementia, and no further episodes of stealing occurred.

Trichotillomania

Trichotillomania is the "recurrent pulling out of one's hair for pleasure, gratification, or relief of tension that results in noticeable hair loss" (American Psychiatric Association 1994, p. 609).

In a study cited earlier in this chapter, Martin et al. (1993) used an additional control group of 11 trichotillomania patients, along with a nonpsychiatric control group, when investigating neuropsychological functioning in OCD. Trichotillomania patients did as well as nonpsychiatric control subjects on all neuropsychological measures and, in fact, showed significantly greater learning than both the nonpsychiatric control and the OCD groups.

Comment. Because of the paucity of studies and almost total lack of controlled studies, definitive statements regarding neuropsychological functioning in the impulse-control disorders are not possible. However, Rugle and Melamed's (1993) controlled study and several case studies have suggested a frontal dysfunction as a contributory factor in impulse-control disorders. In this context, it is worth noting that a study (Stein et al. 1993b) found increased soft signs associated with impaired WCST performance, suggestive of frontal-lobe executive dysfunction, in a group of 28 patients with either borderline personality disorder or antisocial personality disorder (disorders sometimes viewed as showing poor control) compared with a group of healthy control subjects (see DeCaria et al., Chapter 5, in this volume). Reports of diminished serotonergic functioning in the frontal lobes of persons who commit suicide also point to a major role of frontal dysfunction in impulse dyscontrol. However, it is not clear why frontal dysfunction sometimes does not result in impulse dyscontrol and why it occurs in one disorder rather than another.

◈ SEXUAL AND GENDER IDENTITY DISORDERS

In the sexual and gender identity disorders literature, only pedophilia has been investigated in neuropsychological studies.

Pedophilia

Pedophilia is the desire to have sexual contact with children. Disordered brain functioning has been associated with such dysfunctional sexual behaviors. An extreme example is Klüver-Bucy syndrome, which follows bilateral ablation of the anterior temporal lobes. Lishman (1968) reported 8 cases of head injury (in a larger sample of 144 head-injured patients showing psychiatric disability) that resulted in disordered sexual behavior, typically involving increased sexual activity without regard for sexual partner. Those lesions most often involved the orbital cortex of the frontal lobes. The role of such lesions in pedophilia must be determined.

Regestein and Reich (1978) reported four cases of pedophilic behavior following illnesses that resulted in cognitive impairment. These four married men were, before their illness, reported to be sexually normal without pedophilic behavior. In one patient, psychological testing was consistent with a right-frontal-lobe deficit (the patient had undergone a right frontal craniotomy for a meningioma). Two additional patients developed pedophilic behaviors after undergoing multiple cardiac resuscitation and presumed episodes of cerebral hypoxia. The fourth subject, who had cognitive dysfunction presumed related to vestibular neuronitis, developed such behavior after consuming alcohol and/or central nervous system depressants. All shared "an incapacitating lack of initiative plus a loss of control over emotional responses" (Regestein and Reich 1978, p. 797).

Graber et al. (1982) examined six mentally disordered sex offenders, three rapists and three pedophilic patients, with regional cerebral blood flow and the LNNB. All three pedophilic patients (in contrast to one of the rapists) had abnormal test results suggesting brain dysfunction. Two of the three pedophilic patients had LNNB results that indicated a dysfunction in the frontal and temporal areas, resulting in disinhibitory syndrome.

Scott et al. (1984) compared a group of 22 forcible sexual assaulters (essentially rapists) with a group of 14 pedophiles and a control group of 31 subjects without sexual criminal history by administering the LNNB. Scott et al. (1984, p. 1118) found "that in the pedophile group 39% met criteria for diagnosing brain dysfunction, 29% performed in the borderline range and 36% were neuropsychologically normal." The percentage of control subjects with two or more scales above their critical value (i.e., brain dysfunction) was not reported, and no attempt was made to relate results to brain areas. Scott et al. suggested that in some pedophilic patients, cerebral dysfunction may be a contributing factor. The behavior in some pedophilic patients may be caused by a combination of poor judgment and poor impulse control, possibly "a consequence of deficits in the cortical structures of the limbic system" (Scott et al. 1984, p. 1118).

Comment. In summary, neuropsychological studies of pedophilia are extremely limited, but the results suggest that a brain dysfunction in frontal, temporal, and limbic areas may play a part in its genesis.

◈ EATING DISORDERS

"The Eating Disorders are characterized by severe disturbances in eating behavior" and include two specific diagnoses: anorexia nervosa and bulimia nervosa (American Psychiatric Association 1994, p. 539). Anorexia nervosa is characterized by a refusal to eat and thus to maintain a minimally normal body weight. Bulimia nervosa is characterized by repeated episodes of binge eating followed by inappropriate compensatory behaviors such as self-induced vomiting, misuse of laxatives or diuretics, use of stimulants as appetite suppressants, fasting, or excessive exercise.

Bulimic patients maintain a more or less normal weight, whereas anorexic patients are typically morbidly underweight. Common to both disorders is a distorted body image with undue emphasis on the significance of shape and weight in self-evaluation.

The prevalence of anorexia nervosa among females in late adolescence and early adulthood is 0.5%–1.0% and of bulimia nervosa is 1%–3%. Both disorders are much more frequent in females.

The few neuropsychological studies on eating disorders suggest a right-hemisphere dysfunction in bulimic and anorexic patients, but this finding is by no means conclusive. Moreover, the literature is hindered by small sample sizes and limited neuropsychological batteries. Findings are also confounded by frequent comorbidity with other psychiatric disorders and by the nutritional status of subjects.

Anorexia Nervosa

Fox (1981) tested 15 subjects with anorexia (14 female, 1 male) with a neuropsychological screening battery. These patients had lowered attention and concentration abilities compared with a control group without anorexia but not when compared with a group of mixed psychiatric control subjects. Eleven of the 15 patients with anorexia were administered the Wide Range Achievement Test (WRAT) Arithmetic subtest; these WRAT Arithmetic performances were one standard deviation below the mean. Citing additional evidence of impaired ability to copy complex geometric designs, the author raised the possibility of constructional dyspraxia and underlying visual-spatial dysfunction, suggestive of compromised right-hemisphere functioning. Fox speculated that the distorted awareness of one's body in anorexia nervosa may be related to a right-hemisphere syndrome.

Hamsher et al. (1981) found impaired neuropsychological functioning in 9 of 20 patients with anorexia prior to treatment. The tasks most often impaired were those involving short-term visual memory and reaction time. The authors believed that the deficits found were not related to a specific localized brain dysfunction but were the result of a generalized attentional problem. In this regard, Small et al. (1983) found that in a group of successfully treated patients with anorexia, weight gain was correlated with scores on the WAIS Arithmetic and Digit Span tests, which suggests that improved clinical status in patients with anorexia is related to improved attentional abilities.

Maxwell et al. (1984) used a more comprehensive battery, including the Halstead-Reitan Neuropsychological Test Battery, WAIS-R, and WMS, to evaluate three women ages 19, 30, and 69. The investigators found a cognitive pattern suggesting increased reliance on left-hemisphere processing because all three subjects showed above-average verbal and academic skills but impaired spatial skills. This finding suggested a spatial reasoning right-hemisphere deficit and increased reliance on left-hemisphere cognition. The authors also noted that the increased incidence of anosognosia (the inability to recognize illness) in right-hemisphere lesions may explain why patients with anorexia refuse to see themselves as ill. Maxwell et al. favor, however, an explanation of hemispheric imbalance in function rather than a right-hemisphere lesion as the underlying deficit in patients with anorexia, because no reports of anorexia nervosa following right-hemisphere lesions are known. In addition, they noted that the 90% incidence of female patients with anorexia and the greater verbal than spatial skills that females show developmentally may be contributing factors to increased reliance on left-hemisphere cognition.

Maxwell et al. (1984) pointed out, however, that all three of their subjects were depressed at the time of testing and that visual-spatial processing impairment has been associated with both clinical and normal depressive states. They also noted, when discussing motor strength tests, that "the two older anorexics were weak relative to controls, probably due to their emaciated state" (p. 39). Clearly, the possible confounding of nutritional status with neuropsychological test performance was not controlled and could account for the results.

Jones et al. (1991) compared 30 underweight patients with anorexia with 20 long-term weight-restored patients with anorexia, 38 normal-weight patients with bulimia, and 39 control subjects with no eating disorders. They found that the underweight patients with anorexia performed more poorly on tasks of executive function, verbal abilities, memory, and visuospatial abilities, suggesting generally poor attentional abilities. However, the absolute differences in scores between the three eating disorder groups and the control group were small, suggesting "subtle rather than frank cognitive difficulties" (p. 711).

Bulimia Nervosa

McKay et al. (1986) administered the LNNB to 30 bulimic patients and 30 matched control subjects. The investigators found that the bulimic patients performed more poorly on the Motor and Pathognomonic clinical scales and on the Right Frontal Localization scale than did the control subjects. The common element in these results seemed to be a significantly poorer performance on the drawing speed factor. Although these results are consistent with those of the Fox and Maxwell et al. anorexia studies, it may be inappropriate to focus on "right frontal dysfunction" in bulimic patients without a large body of supportive research, because findings such as slow drawing speed may also be affected by motivational, nutritional, and medication factors. Also, most of the subjects in the McKay et al. study had symptoms that met criteria for at least one other DSM-III (American Psychiatric Association 1980) disorder.

The authors did attempt to control for coexisting affective disorder and nutritional status by comparing 16 of the bulimic patients with affective disorder with 14 without affective disorder and by comparing 11 of the bulimic subjects who were 12 pounds or more under ideal body weight with 13 subjects at or above ideal body weight. No significant differences were found for the two body weight subgroups, but the affective disorder subgroup tended to perform more poorly than the nonaffective subgroup on the Rhythm and Memory scales, suggesting that affective disorder in bulimia produced greater attention deficit.

Horne et al. (1991) addressed the issue of disturbed body image in eating disorders by administering the Wechsler Intelligence Scales for Children—Revised (WISC-R) or WAIS-R with a short battery of neuropsychological instruments to a large group of patients admitted to an inpatient eating disorder program. Of interest is that in patients who had a distorted body image, a significant discrepancy was found between Verbal and Performance Scale IQ; the Performance Scale IQ was less than the Verbal Scale IQ. These results suggest that a subgroup of patients with eating disorders has a diminution in right-hemisphere functioning and that these patients are most likely to experience distorted body awareness. Results of the other neuropsychological measures were reported to be negative, equivocal, or explainable by diminished energy level and depression. However, the Tactual Performance Test also supported the suggestion of right-hemisphere dysfunction in patients with eating disorders who had a distorted body image.

Comment. Despite evidence for right-hemisphere and posterior dysfunction, studies consistently find that the neuropsychological deficits in patients with eating disorders are not dramatic. Confounding factors limit understanding of the possible deficits in the eating disorders. Variables such as comorbid disorders, depression, and nutritional status are often present.

◙ SLEEP DISORDERS

Of the sleep disorders, breathing-related sleep disorder has been fairly extensively studied with neuropsychological tools. Other disorders seem not to have raised a significant research interest.

Breathing-Related Sleep Disorder

Breathing-related sleep disorder is defined as "sleep disruption, leading to excessive sleepiness or insomnia, that is judged to be due to abnormalities of ventilation during sleep" (American Psychiatric Association 1994, p. 567). Neuropsychological studies have focused on sleep apnea (the cessation of breathing), which often lasts 10–30 seconds, can occur frequently during the night, and characterizes this disorder. Sleep apnea can result in hundreds of arousals lasting 1–3 seconds. The next day the patient does not remember waking up so many times (Flemons and Tsai 1997). This disorder can occur at any age, but prevalence increases with age. Adult prevalence has been estimated at 1%–10% (American Psychiatric Association 1994), increasing to about 30% after age 65 (Shepard 1988).

Patients with sleep apnea complain of problems such as poor concentration and memory (Bonnet 1993; Jennum et al. 1993). Studies completed during the 1980s (Findly et al. 1986; Fix et al. 1982; Greenberg et al. 1987; Yesavage et al. 1985) reported cognitive deficits associated with sleep apnea, most often manifested in poor attention, poor memory, and visual constructive difficulties. Other studies (Hayward et al. 1992; Stone et al. 1994) have found no cognitive dysfunction in sleep apnea patients. Telakivi et al. (1993) found no correlation between cognitive testing and either daytime sleepiness or oxygen blood levels in a group of 31 "highly trained professionals" who were referred for suspected or diagnosed sleep apnea. They explained this negative finding by referring to an "ill suited neuropsychological test battery" for detecting deficits in sustained concentration and attention typical of this type of sleep apnea.

Some studies have attempted more ambitious methodologies. Bedard et al. (1991) compared 10 patients with moderate apnea, 10 patients with severe apnea, and 10 control subjects without apnea to try to differentiate the separate contributions of increased daytime sleepiness (caused by frequent nighttime arousal) and hypoxemia (i.e., lowered blood oxygen saturation caused by cessation of breathing) to cognitive dysfunction. They found deficits in general intelligence (on the WAIS-R), in psychomotor speed (on the Purdue Pegboard Test; Purdue Research Foundation 1948), and in executive function (assessed with the Trail Making Test, the maze test of the WISC-R, and planning in copying the Rey-Osterrieth design; Osterrieth 1944). Severity of hypoxemia was related to severity of deficits. Impairments in measures of vigilance (assessed with the Digit Symbol subtest of the WAIS-R) and memory (assessed with the Logical Memory subtest of the WMS) were related to increased daytime sleepiness. The authors concluded that "dampening of general intellectual performances, as well as . . . specific deficits in executive function" (p. 960) may be attributed to the severity of respiratory impairment, whereas attentional deficits and deficits in memory function may be related primarily to decreased daytime vigilance. Bedard et al. (1991, 1993) further suggested that this neuropsychological pattern is consistent with either a "frontal lobe insufficiency" (Bedard 1991, p. 960) caused by hypoxemia or a subcortical dysfunction caused by brain stem anoxia. The anoxia may result in either actual subcortical damage or a neurotransmitter dysfunction.

Additional support for the hypothesis of executive frontal dysfunction in patients with sleep apnea is provided by the work of Naegele et al. (1995). They administered "frontal lobe related tests" to a group of 17 patients with sleep apnea and a group of 17 control subjects without sleep apnea matched for age, verbal IQ, and educational level. Patients with apnea performed more poorly on tests of short-term and working memory, in both the verbal and the visual domains. Long-term memory results were also significantly lower in patients, but no evidence for rapid forgetting emerged. The lack of rapid forgetting suggests an executive frontal dysfunction rather than an amnesic/temporal-lobe problem. Performance of sleep apnea patients on executive function tests such as the WCST, Tower of Toronto test, and verbal fluency tests again suggested frontal dysfunction. Naegele et al. (1995) concluded that patients with sleep apnea "do have deficits in their executive function . . . " (p. 49) but to a lesser degree than patients with cortically damaged frontal lobes.

An important question is whether the cognitive changes caused by sleep apnea are a permanent disability or temporary and reversible symptoms. Some degree of improvement in cognitive functions, such as concentration and verbal and spatial memory (Borak et al. 1996; Valencia-Flores et al. 1996), has been observed after sleep apnea was treated with continuous positive airway pressure (CPAP). Other studies report that deficits seem to persist after this treatment (Bedard et al. 1993; Montplaisir et al. 1992). Further study is needed to determine definitively whether the deficits are reversible.

Comment. Although these findings are intriguing, controlled studies are needed to confirm results and substantiate any theoretical formulations made thus far. Flemons and Tsai (1997) pointed out that "by and large, investigators have used different methodologies, different control populations, and probably different recruitment strategies to obtain their study populations" (p. S752). Failure to account for variables such as coexisting depression and the inclusion of subjects with dementia in the study of elderly patients make interpretation of reported cognitive deficits problematic. The findings that sleep apnea results in cognitive deficits and that daytime sleepiness results in different cognitive deficits than does hypoxemia need further substantiation, and the suggestion that these deficits are reversed with treatment of sleep apnea needs further investigation.

◈ CONCLUSION

Table 4–1 shows the locus of suggested brain dysfunction of the reviewed disorder. The brain areas most often implicated in the neuropsychological literature of the nonpsychotic, nonaffective disorders are the temporal and frontal lobes. Lesions to these two areas have been noted to cause "prominent alterations in personality" (Blumer and Benson 1975). Moreover, because of extensive connections with the rest of the brain and because it is the most recently developed phylogenetically, the prefrontal cortex is the brain area most vulnerable to disruption, even by nonfocal pathology (Goldberg and Bilder 1987). This table must be considered tentative because each disorder is represented by limited neuropsychological data. Some DSM-IV disorders are represented by case studies only, and some are not represented by any neuropsychological studies. We hope this chapter will provide the impetus for more systematic neuropsychological study of these serious disorders. With further study, the neuropsychological findings in these disorders can be used to improve management, treatment, and rehabilitation in patients, as in other disorders (see Jaeger and Berns, Chapter 10, in this volume). Future

Table 4–1. Brain areas implicated by neuropsychological studies of disorders

Disorder	Brain areas
Anxiety disorders	
OCD	Frontal
	Basal ganglia
	Right hemisphere
PTSD	Temporal/limbic area
	Global
Dissociative disorders	
MPD	Temporal lobe
	Overdominance of one hemisphere over another (L > R or R > L)
Depersonalization	Left temporal/frontal
Dissociative amnesia/fugue	Temporal lobe
Somatoform disorders	
Conversion	Frontal/temporal
	Right hemisphere
Hysteria	Frontal/temporal
	Right hemisphere
Impulse-control disorders	
Pathological gambling	Frontal
Pyromania	Frontal
Kleptomania	Frontal
	Global
Trichotillomania	None
Sexual disorder	
Pedophilia	Frontal
	Frontal/temporal
Sleep disorders	
Breathing-related sleep disorder	Frontal/general

Note. OCD = obsessive-compulsive disorder; PTSD = posttraumatic stress disorder; MPD = multiple personality disorder; L = left; R = right.

research may provide guidelines for specific management techniques for each disorder as neuropsychological knowledge accumulates.

◈ REFERENCES

Abbruzzese M, Ferri S, Scarane S: Wisconsin Card Sort Test performance in obsessive-compulsive disorder: no evidence for involvement of dorsolateral prefrontal cortex. Psychiatry Res 58:37–43, 1995

Ahern G, Herring A, Tackenberg J, et al: The association of multiple personality and temporo-limbic epilepsy. Arch Neurol 50:1020–1025, 1993

American Psychiatric Association: Diagnostic and Statistical Manual of Mental Disorders, 3rd Edition. Washington, DC, American Psychiatric Association, 1980

American Psychiatric Association: Diagnostic and Statistical Manual of Mental Disorders, 3rd Edition, Revised. Washington, DC, American Psychiatric Association, 1987

American Psychiatric Association: Diagnostic and Statistical Manual of Mental Disorders, 4th Edition. Washington, DC, American Psychiatric Association, 1994

Archibald HC, Tuddenham RD: Persistent stress reaction after combat: a 20 year follow-up. Arch Gen Psychiatry 12:475–481, 1965

Aronowitz BR, Hollander E, DeCaria C, et al: Neuropsychology of obsessive-compulsive disorder: preliminary findings. Neuropsychiatry Neuropsychol Behav Neurol 7(2):81–86, 1994

Baer L, Rauch SL, Ballantine T, et al: Cingolotomy for intractable obsessive-compulsive disorder. Arch Gen Psychiatry 52:384–392, 1995

Barr WB, Goldberg E, Wasserstein J, et al: Retrograde amnesia following unilateral temporal lobectomy. Neuropsychologia 28:243–255, 1990

Bedard MA, Montplaisir J, Richer F, et al: Obstructive sleep apnea syndrome: pathogenesis of neuropsychological deficits. J Clin Exp Neuropsychol 13: 950–964, 1991

Bedard MA, Montplaisir J, Richer F, et al: Persistent neuropsychological deficits and vigilance impairment in sleep apnea syndrome after treatment with continuous positive airway pressure (CPAP). J Clin Exp Neuropsychol 15:330–341, 1993

Behar D, Rapoport J, Berg CJ, et al: Computerized tomography and neuropsychological test measures in adolescents with obsessive-compulsive disorder. Am J Psychiatry 141:363–369, 1984

Bellini L, Massioni R, Palladino F, et al: Neurofunctional assessment of obsessive-compulsive disorder (OCD): a neuropsychological study. Research Communications in Psychology, Psychiatry and Behavior 14:73–83, 1989

Bendefeldt F, Miller LL, Ludwig AM: Cognitive performance in conversion hysteria. Arch Gen Psychiatry 33:1250–1254, 1976

Benson DF, Miller BL, Signer SF: Dual personality associated with epilepsy. Arch Neurol 43:471–474, 1986

Benton AL: The Revised Visual Retention Test, 4th Edition. New York, Psychological Corporation, 1974

Blumer D, Benson DF: Personality changes with frontal and temporal lobe lesions, in Psychiatric Aspects of Neurologic Disease. Edited by Benson DF, Blumer D. New York, Grune & Stratton, 1975, pp 151–170

Bonnet MH: Cognitive effects of sleep and sleep fragmentation. Sleep 16 (8 suppl):S65–S67, 1993

Boone KB, Anarth J, Philpott L, et al: Neuropsychological characteristics of non-depressed adults with obsessive-compulsive disorder. Neuropsychiatry Neuropsychol Behav Neurol 4(2):96–109, 1991

Borak J, Cieslicki JK, Kojiej M, et al: Effect of CPAP treatment on psychological status in patients with severe obstructive sleep apnea. J Sleep Res 5:123–127, 1996

Bornstein RA: Neuropsychological correlates of obsessive characteristics in Tourette syndrome. J Neuropsychiatry Clin Neurosci 3:157–162, 1991

Breiter HC, Filpek PA, Kennedy DN, et al: Retrocallosal white matter abnormalities in patients with obsessive-compulsive disorder. Arch Gen Psychiatry 51:663–664, 1994

Bremner JD, Scott TM, Delaney RC, et al: Deficits in short-term memory in post-traumatic stress disorder. Am J Psychiatry 150:1015–1019, 1993

Bremner JD, Randall P, Scott TM, et al: MRI-based measurement of hippocampal volume in patients with combat-related post-traumatic stress disorder. Am J Psychiatry 152:973–981, 1995

Burstein A: Post-traumatic flashbacks, dream disturbance, and mental imagery. J Clin Psychiatry 46:374–378, 1985

Calev A: Pyromania and executive/frontal dysfunction. Behavioral Neurology 8:163–169, 1995

Chiswick D: Shoplifting, depression and an unusual lesion (a case report). Med Sci Law 16(4):266–268, 1976

Chiu HC, Mortimer JA, Slager U, et al: Pathologic correlates of dementia in Parkinson's disease. Arch Neurol 43:991–995, 1986

Christiansen KJ, Kim SW, Dysken MW, et al: Neuropsychological performance in obsessive-compulsive disorder. Biol Psychiatry 31:4–18, 1992

Cox CS, Fedio P, Rapaport JL: Neuropsychological testing of obsessive-compulsive adolescents, in Obsessive-Compulsive Disorders in Children and Adolescents. Edited by Rapoport JL. Washington, DC, American Psychiatric Press, 1989, pp 73–86

Diamond BM, Albrecht W, Borison RL: Neuropsychology of obsessive-compulsive disorders (abstract 215). Society of Biological Psychiatry Scientific Program, Montreal, Canada, 1988

Domb Y, Beaman K: Mr. X—a case of amnesia. Br J Psychiatry 158:423–425, 1991

Filskov SB, Castanese RA: Effects of sex and handedness on neuropsychological testing, in Handbook of Neuropsychology, Vol 2. Edited by Filskov SB, Boll TJ. New York, Wiley, 1986, pp 198–212

Findly L, Barth TT, Powers DC, et al: Cognitive impairments in patients with obstructive sleep apnea and associated hypoxemia. Chest 90:686–690, 1986

Fix AT, Golden CJ, Daughton D, et al: Neuropsychological deficits among patients with chronic obstructive pulmonary disease. Int J Neurosci 16:99–105, 1982

Flemons WW, Tsai W: Quality of life consequences of sleep disordered breathing. J Allergy Clin Immunol 99:S750–S756, 1997

Flor-Henry P, Yeudall LT, Koles ZJ, et al: Neuropsychological and power spectral EEG investigations of obsessive-compulsive syndrome. Biol Psychiatry 14:119–130, 1979

Flor-Henry P, Fromm-Auch D, Tapper M, et al: A neuropsychological study of the stable syndrome of hysteria. Biol Psychiatry 16:601–626, 1981

Fox CF: Neuropsychological correlates of anorexia nervosa. Int J Psychiatry Med 11:285–290, 1981

Galin D: Implications for psychology of left and right cerebral specialization. Arch Gen Psychiatry 31:572–583, 1974

Galin D, Diamond R, Braff D: Lateralization of conversion symptoms: more frequent of the left. Am J Psychiatry 134:578–580, 1977

Gambini O, Abbruzzese M, Scarone S: Smooth pursuit and saccadic eye movements and Wisconsin Card Sort Test performance in obsessive-compulsive disorder. Psychiatry Res 48:191–200, 1992

Garber JH, Ananth JV, Chiu LC, et al: Nuclear magnetic resonance study of obsessive-compulsive disorder. Am J Psychiatry 146:1001–1005, 1989

George MS, Kellner CH, Fossey MD: Obsessive-compulsive symptoms in a patient with multiple sclerosis. J Nerv Ment Dis 177:304–305, 1989

Gil T, Calev A, Greenberg D, et al: Cognitive functioning in post-traumatic stress disorder. J Trauma Stress 3:29–45, 1990

Goldberg E, Bilder RM Jr: The frontal lobes and hierarchical organization of cognitive control, in The Frontal Lobes Revisited. Edited by Perecman E. New York, IRBN Press, 1987, pp 159–187

Golden CJ, Hammeke TA, Purisch AD: Manual for the Luria-Nebraska Neuropsychological Battery. Los Angeles, CA, Western Psychological Services, 1980

Graber B, Hartmann K, Coffman JA, et al: Brain damage among mentally disordered sex offenders. J Forensic Sci 27:125–134, 1982

Greenberg GD, Watson RK, Deptula D: Neuropsychological dysfunction in sleep apnea. Sleep 10:254–262, 1987

Gurvits TV, Lasko NB, Schachter SC, et al: Neurological status of Vietnam veterans with chronic post-traumatic stress disorder. Neuropsychiatry Neuropsychol Behav Neurol 5:183–188, 1993

Hamsher K des, Halmi KA, Benton AL: Prediction of outcome on anorexia nervosa from neuropsychological status. Psychiatry Res 4:79–88, 1981

Hathaway SR, McKinley JC: The Minnesota Multiphasic Personality Inventory Manual, Revised. New York, Psychological Corporation, 1951

Hayward L, Mant A, Eyland A, et al: Sleep disordered breathing and cognitive function in a retirement village population. Age Ageing 21:121–128, 1992

Head D, Bolton D, Hymas N: Deficits in cognitive shifting ability in patients with obsessive-compulsive disorder. Biol Psychiatry 25:929–937, 1989

Heaton R: Wisconsin Card Sorting Test. Odessa, TX, Psychological Assessment Resources, 1985

Hollander E, Schiffman E, Cohen B, et al: Signs of central nervous system dysfunction in obsessive-compulsive disorder. Arch Gen Psychiatry 47:27–32, 1990

Hollander E, Liebowitz MR, Rosen WG: Neuropsychiatric and neuropsychological studies in obsessive-compulsive disorder, in The Psychobiology of Obsessive-Compulsive Disorder. Edited by Zohar J, Insel T, Rasmussen S. New York, Springer, 1991, pp 126–145

Hollander E, Carrasco JL, Mullen LS, et al: Left hemisphere activation in depersonalization disorder: a case report. Biol Psychiatry 31:1157–1162, 1992

Hollander E, Cohen L, Marcus R, et al: A pilot study of the neuropsychology of obsessive compulsive disorder and Parkinson's disease: basal ganglia disorder. J Neuropsychiatry Clin Neurosci 5:104–107, 1993

Horne RL, Van Vactor JC, Emerson S: Disturbed body image in patients with eating disorders. Am J Psychiatry 148:211–215, 1991

Insel TR, Gillin JC, Moore A, et al: The sleep of patients with obsessive-compulsive disorder. Arch Gen Psychiatry 39:1372–1377, 1982

Insel TR, Donnelly EE, Lalakea ML, et al: Neurological and neuropsychological studies of patients with obsessive-compulsive disorder. Biol Psychiatry 18:741–751, 1983

Jenike MA, Baer L, Ballantine T, et al: Cingulotomy for refractory obsessive-compulsive disorder. Arch Gen Psychiatry 48:548–555, 1991

Jennum P, Hein HO, Suadicani P, et al: Cognitive function and snoring. Sleep 16: S62–S64, 1993

Jones BP, Duncan CC, Brouwers P, et al: Cognition in eating disorders. J Clin Exp Neuropsychol 13:711–728, 1991

Kagan J, Henker BA: Developmental psychology. Annu Rev Psychol 17:1–50, 1966

Kapur N: Amnesia in relation to figure-states—distinguishing a neurological from a psychological basis. Br J Psychiatry 159:872–877, 1991

Keefe RSE: The contribution of neuropsychology to psychiatry. Am J Psychiatry 152:6–15, 1995

Klonoff H, McDougall G, Clark C, et al: The neuropsychological, psychiatric and physical effects of prolonged and severe stress: 30 years later. J Nerv Ment Dis 163:246–252, 1976

Laplane D, Lavasseur M, Pillon B, et al: Obsessive-compulsive and other behavioral changes with bilateral basal ganglia lesion. Brain 112:699–725, 1989

Lawrence DM, Morton V: Associating embedded figures test performance with extreme hysteria and psychasthenia MMPI scores in a psychiatric population. Percept Mot Skills 50:432–434, 1980

Lhermitte F: Utilization behaviour and its relation to lesions of the frontal lobe. Brain 106:237–255, 1983

Lieberman J: Evidence for a biological hypothesis of obsessive-compulsive disorder. Neuropsychologia 11:14–21, 1984

Lishman WA: Brain damage in relation to psychiatric disability after head injury. Br J Psychiatry 114:373–410, 1968

Ludlow CL, Bassaich CJ, Connor NP, et al: Psycholinguistic testing in obsessive-compulsive adolescents, in Obsessive-Compulsive Disorder in Children and Adolescents. Edited by Rapoport JL. Washington, DC, American Psychiatric Press, 1989, pp 87–106

Ludwig AM, Brandsma JM, Wilber CB, et al: The objective study of a multiple personality. Arch Gen Psychiatry 26:298–310, 1972

Malloy P: Frontal lobe dysfunction in obsessive-compulsive disorder, in The Frontal Lobes Revisited. Edited by Berecman E. New York, IRBN Press, 1987, pp 207–223

Martin A, Pigott TA, Lalonde F, et al: Lack of evidence for Huntington's disease-like cognitive dysfunction in obsessive-compulsive disorder. Biol Psychiatry 33:345–353, 1993

Martinot JL, Allilaire JF, Mazoyer BM, et al: Obsessive-compulsive disorder: a clinical, neuropsychological and positron emission tomography study. Acta Psychiatr Scand 82:233–242, 1990

Mathew RJ, Jack RA, West WS: Regional cerebral blood flow in a patient with multiple personality. Am J Psychiatry 142:504–505, 1985

Maxwell JK, Tucker DM, Townes BD: Asymmetric cognitive functioning in anorexia nervosa. Int J Neurosci 24:37–44, 1984

McIntyre AW, Emsley RA: Shoplifting associated with normal-pressure hydrocephalus: a report of a case. J Geriatr Psychiatry Neurol 3:229–230, 1990

McKay SE, Humphries LL, Allen ME, et al: Neuropsychological test performance of bulimic patients. Int J Neurosci 30:73–80, 1986

Mendez MF: Pathological stealing in dementia. J Am Geriatr Soc 36:825–826, 1988

Mersky H, Watson GD: The localization of pain. Pain 7:271–280, 1979

Mesulam M: Dissociative states with abnormal temporal lobe EEG. Arch Neurol 38:176–181, 1981

Miller L: Neuropsychological concepts of somatoform disorders. Int J Psychiatry Med 14:31–63, 1984

Milner B: Disorders of memory after brain lesions in man: material-specific and generalized memory loss. Neuropsychologia 6:175–179, 1968

Mindus P, Rasmussen SA, Linquist C: Neurosurgical treatment for refractory obsessive-compulsive disorder: implications for understanding frontal lobe function. Neuropsychiatry Neuropsychol Behav Neurol 6:467–477, 1994

Montplaisir J, Bedard MA, Richer F, et al: Neurobehavioral manifestations of obstructive sleep apnea syndrome before and after treatment with continuous positive airway pressure. Sleep 15:S17–S19, 1992

Naegele B, Thouvard V, Pepin JL, et al: Deficits of cognitive executive functions in patients with sleep apnea syndrome. Sleep 18(11):43–52, 1995

Neziroglu FN, Penzel FI, Vasquez J, et al: Neuropsychological studies in obsessive-compulsive disorder (abstract). Psychopharmacology 96 (suppl):356, 1988

Nissen MJ, Ross TL, Willingham DB, et al: Memory and awareness in a patient with multiple personality disorder. Brain Cogn 8:21–38, 1988

O'Donnell DW, Calev A: A case of "double amnesia"? Sixth Annual New York State OMH Research Conference, Albany, NY, December 1993

Osterrieth PA: Le test de copie d'une figure complex [The complex figure text]. Archives de Psychologie 30:206–256, 1944

Otto M: Neuropsychological approaches to obsessive-compulsive disorder, in Obsessive-Compulsive Disorders: Theory and Management, 2nd Edition. Edited by Jenike MA, Bear L, Minichiello WE. Chicago, IL, Year Book Medical, 1990, pp 132–148

Otto M: Normal and abnormal information processing: a neuropsychological perspective on obsessive-compulsive disorder. Psychiatr Clin North Am 15:825–848, 1992

Porteus SD: The Maze Test and Clinical Psychology. Palo Alto, CA, Pacific Books, 1959

Prichep LS, Mas F, Hollander E, et al: Quantitative electroencephalographic subtyping of obsessive-compulsive disorder. Psychiatry Res 50:25–32, 1993

Purdue Research Foundation: Examiner's Manual for the Purdue Pegboard. Chicago, IL, Science Research Associates, 1948

Rapoport J, Elkins R, Langer D, et al: Childhood obsessive-compulsive disorder. Am J Psychiatry 138:1545–1553, 1981

Regestein QR, Reich P: Pedophilia occurring after onset of cognitive impairment. J Nerv Ment Dis 166:794–798, 1978

Reitan RM: Validity of the Trail Making Test as an indication of organic brain damage. Percept Mot Skills 8:271–276, 1958

Reitan RM: Halstead-Reitan Neuropsychological Test Battery. Tucson, AZ, Neuropsychology Laboratory, University of Arizona, 1979

Rosen WG, Hollander E, Stannick V, et al: Task performance variables in obsessive-compulsive disorder (abstract). J Clin Exp Neuropsychol 10:73, 1988

Rosenstein LD: Potential neuropsychologic and neurophysiologic correlates of multiple personality disorder. Neuropsychiatry Neuropsychol Behav Neurol 7:215–229, 1994

Rugle L: Neuropsychological Assessment of Attention Deficit Disorder in Pathological Gamblers. Dissertation, Kent, OH, Kent State University, 1990

Rugle L, Melamed L: Neuropsychological assessment of attention problems in pathological gamblers. J Nerv Ment Dis 181:107–112, 1993

Saling M: Psychogenic amnesia (letter). Br J Psychiatry 159:585, 1991

Saxe GN, Vasile RG, Hill TC, et al: SPECT imaging and multiple personality disorder. J Nerv Ment Dis 180:662–663, 1992

Scarone S, Colombo C, Livian S, et al: Increased right caudate nucleus size in obsessive-compulsive disorder: detection with magnetic resonance imaging. Psychiatry Res 45:115–121, 1992

Schacter DL, Wang PL, Tulving E, et al: Functional retrograde amnesia: a quantitative case study. Neuropsychologia 20:523–532, 1982

Schacter DL, Kihlstrom JF, Kihlstrom LC: Autobiographical memory in a case of multiple personality disorder. J Abnorm Psychol 98:508–514, 1989

Schenk L, Bear D: Multiple personality and related dissociative phenomena in patients with temporal lobe epilepsy. Am J Psychiatry 138:1311–1316, 1981

Scott ML, Cole JK, McKay SE, et al: Neuropsychological performances of sexual assaulters and pedophiles. J Forensic Sci 29:1114–1118, 1984

Shepard JW: Aging and sleep apnea, in Central Nervous System Disorders of Aging: Clinical Interventions and Research. Edited by Strong R, Gibsinwood W, Burke WG. New York, Raven, 1988, pp 127–148

Sher KJ, Frost RO, Otto R: Cognitive deficits in compulsive checkers: an exploration study. Behav Res Ther 21:357–363, 1983

Sher KJ, Mann B, Frost RO: Cognitive dysfunction in compulsive checkers: further explorations. Behav Res Ther 22:493–502, 1984

Sher KJ, Frost RO, Kushner M, et al: Memory deficits in compulsive checkers: replication and extension in a clinical sample. Behav Res Ther 27:65–69, 1989

Small A, Madero J, Teagno L, et al: Intellect, perceptual characteristics and weight gain in anorexia nervosa. J Clin Psychol 39:3780–3782, 1983

Smith A: Symbol Digits Modality Test Manual. Los Angeles, CA, Western Psychological Services, 1973

Stein DJ, Hollander E, Chan S, et al: Computed tomography and neurological soft signs in obsessive-compulsive disorder. Psychiatry Res 50:143–150, 1993a

Stein DJ, Hollander E, Cohen L, et al: Neuropsychiatric impairment in impulsive personality disorder. Psychiatry Res 48:257–266, 1993b

Stern DB: Handedness and the lateral distribution of conversion reactions. J Nerv Ment Dis 164:122–128, 1977

Stone J, Morin CM, Hart RP, et al: Neuropsychological functioning in older insomniacs with or without obstructive sleep apnea. Psychol Aging 9:231–236, 1994

Stroop JR: Studies of interference in serial verbal reactions. J Exp Psychol 18:643–662, 1935

Swedo SD, Rapoport JL, Cheslow DL, et al: High prevalence of obsessive-compulsive symptoms in patients with Sydenham's chorea. Am J Psychiatry 146:246–249, 1989

Sweeney JA, Palumbo DR, Halper JP, et al: Pursuit eye movement dysfunction in obsessive-compulsive disorder. Psychiatry Res 42:1–11, 1992

Teicher MH, Glod CA, Surrey J, et al: Early childhood abuse and limbic system ratings in adult psychiatric outpatients. J Neuropsychiatry Clin Neurosci 5:301–306, 1993

Telakivi T, Kajaste S, Partinen M, et al: Cognitive function in obstructive sleep apnea. Sleep 10:674–675, 1993

Thoren PA, Asberg M, Berilson L, et al: Clomipramine treatment of obsessive-compulsive disorder, II: biochemical agents. Arch Gen Psychiatry 37:1289–1295, 1980

Turner SM, Beidel DC, Nathan RS: Biological factors in obsessive-compulsive disorders. Psychol Bull 97:430–450, 1985

Valencia-Flores M, Bliwise DL, Guilleminault C, et al: Cognitive function in patients with sleep apnea after acute nocturnal nasal continuous positive airway pressure (CPAP) treatment: sleepiness and hypoxemia effects. J Clin Exp Neuropsychol 18:197–210, 1996

Ward CD: Transient feelings of compulsion caused by hemispheric lesions: three cases. J Neurol Neurosurg Psychiatry 51:266–268, 1988

Wechsler D: A standardized memory scale for clinical use. J Psychol 19:87–95, 1945

Wechsler D: WAIS-R Manual. New York, Psychological Corporation, 1981

Weilburg JB, Mesulum M-M, Weintraub S, et al: Focal striatal abnormalities in a patient with obsessive-compulsive disorder. Arch Neurol 46:233–235, 1989

Wilhelm S, McNally RJ, Baer L, et al: Autobiographic memory in obsessive-compulsive disorder. Br J Clin Psychol 36:21–31, 1997

Wise SP, Rapoport JL: Obsessive-compulsive disorder: is it basal ganglia dysfunction?, in Obsessive-Compulsive Disorder in Children and Adolescents. Edited by Rapoport JL. Washington, DC, American Psychiatric Press, 1989, pp 327–346

Wolfe J, Charney DS: Use of neuropsychological assessment in post-traumatic stress disorder. Psychological Assessment 3:473–480, 1991

Yehuda R, Keefe SE, Harvey PD, et al: Learning and memory in combat veterans with post-traumatic stress disorder. Am J Psychiatry 152:137–139, 1995

Yesavage J, Bliwise D, Guileminault C, et al: Preliminary communication: intellectual deficit and sleep related respiratory disturbance in the elderly. Sleep 8:30–33, 1985

Yutaka I, Teichner MH, Glod CA, et al: Increased prevalence of electrophysiological abnormalities in children with psychological, physical and sexual abuse. J Neuropsychiatry Clin Neurosci 5:401–408, 1993

Zielinski CM, Taylor MA, Juzwin KR: Neuropsychological deficits in obsessive-compulsive disorder. Neuropsychiatry Neuropsychol Behav Neurol 4:110–126, 1991

5

NEUROPSYCHOLOGY OF CHILDHOOD MENTAL DISORDERS: INTEGRATION OF PHENOMENOLOGICAL, NEUROBIOLOGICAL, AND NEUROPSYCHOLOGICAL FINDINGS

Concetta M. DeCaria, Ph.D., Bonnie R. Aronowitz, Ph.D., Rebecca Twersky-Kengmana, B.A., and Eric Hollander, M.D.

IN THIS CHAPTER, we provide an overview of prominent childhood mental disorders described within a neuropsychological framework. This perspective suggests that development is linked to genetic and environmental factors that may interfere with normal brain development. Childhood mental disorders provide a unique contribution to this book because many of them have neurodevelopmental bases relative to adult psychiatric disorders.

Neuropsychological function and child development may be viewed within the context of cognitive functions and associated neural representations. Vulnerability of a particular cognitive or functional system depends on brain location as well as the phylogenic and ontogenic development of that particular area. Five cognitive systems that jointly reflect overall functioning include phonological processing, executive function, long-term memory, social cognition, and spatial reasoning (Pennington 1991a). Phonological processing is associated with the posterior and premotor portion of the left temporal lobe (perisylvian fissure). Executive function is linked to left and right prefrontal lobes. Long-term memory is subserved by the medial temporal lobe (hippocampus, amygdala). Social cognition is associated with the cingulate gyrus, the orbital frontal area, and the posterior right hemisphere. Spatial reasoning is also subserved by the posterior right hemisphere. Each function has a unique developmental profile that begins in infancy and progresses through adolescence or later. Disturbances in the normal development of these brain areas may contribute to compromised cognitive function manifest in the childhood mental disorders discussed in this chapter. These disorders are described in the context of a neuropsychological framework and include 1) learning disorders (reading, mathematics, and writing disorders), 2) pervasive developmental disorders (autism and Asperger's disorder), and 3) attention-deficit/hyperactivity disorder (ADHD). Obsessive-compulsive disorder (OCD) is also included in this chapter, although it is not primarily a childhood mental disorder, because recent findings suggest that neuropsychiatric, neuropsychological, and neuroanatomical abnormalities are found in children and adolescents. We thus discuss OCD as a prototype of other childhood neuropsychiatric disorders, such as Tourette's disorder, as a childhood mental disorder. Diagnostic, phenomenological, neurobiological, and neuropsychological characteristics of each of these disorders are highlighted. Assessment and treatment issues are summarized.

◈ LEARNING DISORDERS

Learning disorders are characterized by a substantial decrease in academic functioning, relative to one's chronological age, education, and level of assessed intelligence, that significantly interferes with academic achievement or daily living activities associated with those specific skills (American Psychiatric Association 1994). Learning disorders must be differentiated from changes in academic achievement that occur as a result of 1) normal variation, 2) inadequate teaching and opportunity for learning, 3) cultural factors, 4) visual or auditory impairment, 5) neuropsychiatric disorders (e.g., mental retardation, pervasive developmental disorders), and/or 6) neurological or medical conditions.

The intelligence quotient (IQ)–academic achievement discrepancy in a learning disorder is quantified by a difference of at least 2 standard deviations (SD) between IQ and academic achievement test scores. Although this approach is frequently used to classify learning disorders, it may inflate the prevalence of learning disorders, particularly in reference to a child with a very high IQ whose academic achievement level is average. Another method to identify learning disorders is use of a cutoff score of 1.5 SD (seventh percentile) below the mean on an academic achievement test. Whereas this approach eliminates an inappropriate learning disorder classification of a very bright child who performs in the average range academically, it may classify a borderline mildly retarded child as having a learning disorder because academic achievement test scores are likely to fall below the seventh percentile cutoff point. A third approach combines the first two methods described, thereby requiring both a significant IQ-achievement discrepancy and an academic achievement test score below the seventh percentile (Barkley 1990).

Specific learning disorders include reading disorder, mathematics disorder, and disorder of written expression (American Psychiatric Association 1994). They frequently co-occur with attention-deficit, disruptive behavior, and depressive disorders (10%–25%) (American Psychiatric Association 1994). In the United States, approximately 5% of public school students have a learning disorder, which frequently persists into adulthood (American Psychiatric Association 1994). Often, adults present with more subtle, masked deficits than do children. As underlying neurobiological bases are becoming more apparent, it is easier to understand why these disorders do not always resolve during childhood. For example, evidence indicates neuroanatomical and physiological abnormalities in dyslexic patients (Duffy and McAnulty 1990; Galaburda et al. 1985, 1994). Neurobiological findings in children with learning disorders and residual effects into adulthood are detailed in this chapter. We review neuropsychological profiles and assessment tools used to identify specific learning disorders. We discuss specific treatment approaches for each of these disorders and, when available, highlight intervention strategies that differ for children and adults. For example, repetitive and multimodal treatment approaches often used with children may not remediate adult learning disabilities.

Academic achievement heavily depends on the integrity of language development and communication skills. As such, learning disorders and communication disorders overlap. Each learning disorder is linked to one or more language functions, including expressive language, receptive language, and phonology (development of speech sounds). Certain cognitive functions that underlie language development and communication similarly underlie the acquisition of reading, writing, and mathematics skills. A general discussion regarding the relationships between learning disorders and communication disorders is beyond the scope of this chapter. However, the role of language function in each learning disorder is described.

Psychiatric problems may develop as a consequence of learning disorders. These disorders may be accompanied by low self-esteem, depression, withdrawal, and increased levels of anxiety (Eliason and Richman 1988; McConaughy and Ritter 1986; Rosenthal 1973). Children with learning disorders are likely to be rejected by their peers (Gresham and Reschly 1986; Stone and La Greca 1990). As these children grow into adulthood, problems related to self-perception and social acceptance frequently manifest (Johnson and Blalock 1987). In one study, the psychological profiles of adults with learning disorders attending either a rehabilitation program or a university were assessed by the Minnesota Multiphasic Personality Inventory—2 (MMPI-2). Significant factors included social isolation, poor self-concept, self-doubt, extreme restlessness, fear, obsessive thoughts, and extreme self-criticism (Gregg et al. 1992). Suicidality among adults with learning disabilities has also been described (Bigler 1989). Acute and chronic stress and anxiety often manifest, and effective coping mechanisms are often unavailable. Comprehensive treatment planning for social-related issues of adults with learning disorders should include an assessment of intellectual ability, academic functioning, learning style, emotional stability, and vocational abilities and interests (Gregg and Hoy 1990). Clinicians may need to teach strategies for managing overall anxiety before vocational planning is begun (Gregg et al. 1992).

Reading Disorder

Diagnostic Criteria and Definition

Reading disorder, also known as *dyslexia,* is characterized by substantially delayed achievement in reading relative to one's age, education, and assessed level of intelligence (American Psychiatric Association 1994).

Primary symptoms include problems in reading and spelling, with difficulty in phonological coding of written language. These difficulties have been associated with impairment in language processes including articulation, naming, verbal short-term memory, and long-term memory (Pennington 1991b). Distortions, substitutions, or omissions may occur when reading orally, whereas slowness and comprehension errors occur in both oral and silent reading (American Psychiatric Association 1994). Reading problems also may involve word discrimination and word sequencing difficulty (Arnold 1990). Further, deficits in mathematics, attention, and visuospatial abilities have been associated with reading disorder. Finally, emotional symptoms, such as anxiety, depression, and reluctance or refusal to attend school, as well as somatic complaints, such as headaches and stomachaches, may accompany the cognitive deficits. These behavioral markers may be early warning signs of problems rooted in academic achievement (Pennington 1991b).

Prevalence

In the United States, the overall prevalence estimate of reading disorders in school-age children is 4% (American Psychiatric Association 1994), with estimates as high as 30% for children in urban areas (Eisenberg 1978). The male-to-female ratio based on clinical samples is approximately 4:1 (DeFries 1989). However, family samples and an epidemiological sample reflect little gender difference, with male-to-female ratios of 1.5:1.8 (DeFries 1989) and 1:1 (Shaywitz et al. 1990), respectively.

Etiology

Reading disorders have been associated with both environmental and genetic factors. A relationship between pre- or perinatal adverse events and the development of reading disorders has been hypothesized (Galaburda 1993). In addition, an association between large family size and low socioeconomic status (SES) and reading difficulties has been implicated (Badian 1984). One predictor of reading skill development is level of phoneme awareness (i.e., aural perception of letters). Early phoneme awareness was significantly related to later reading skills, independent of age, IQ, and maternal education (Maclean et al. 1987). The link between phoneme awareness and SES may be related to decreased preschool exposure to language-related activities (Wallach et al. 1977).

Investigations of genetic factors associated with reading disorders include measures of 1) familiality (i.e., increased rates of a characteristic or disorder found in first-degree relatives of those affected), 2) heritability (primarily assessed by twin studies), 3) modes of genetic transmission, and 4) gene locations. Familial risk ranges from 35% to 40% (Finucci et al. 1976; Naidoo 1972; Volger et al. 1985), compared with a 5%–7% risk for children without an affected parent. Further, evidence indicates a decreased risk for daughters compared with sons of affected parents (Volger et al. 1985). These findings underscore the importance of examining family history as a first-pass method of identifying children at high risk for reading disorder. Heritability of reading disorders has been estimated to be as high as 50% (DeFries et al. 1987), independent of heritability of IQ. More specifically, heritability of phonological coding strongly influenced heritability of a reading disorder (93%) (Olson et al. 1989). Genetic heterogeneity has been suggested in the transmission of reading disorders (Finucci et al. 1976; Lewitter et al. 1980). Gene location studies suggest genetic heterogeneity (S. D. Smith et al. 1990), with evidence for linkage between reading disorder and chromosome 15 markers in a small percentage of families (S. D. Smith et al. 1983).

Pathology and Neuropsychological Function

Reading disorder has been associated primarily with abnormalities of left-hemisphere development. Postmortem studies of the brains of eight dyslexic persons showed symmetry of the planum temporale, the superior posterior surface of the temporal lobes (Galaburda and Kemper 1979; Galaburda et al. 1985), relative to asymmetry (left > right) more frequently found in the posterior left hemisphere of nondyslexic control subjects. This part of the left hemisphere incorporates Wernicke's area, which is associated with phonological processing (i.e., letter-sound correspondence). Because reading disorder has been most consistently linked to deficits in phonological processing, it may be associated with abnormalities in left-hemispheric planum temporale. Postmortem studies by this group revealed abnormalities of neuronal arrangement, most frequently found in the left perisylvian areas but not consistently across all cases.

Magnetic resonance imaging (MRI) studies have also shown planum temporale abnormalities in planum asymmetry in dyslexic patients compared with nondyslexic control subjects (Larsen et al. 1990; C. M. Leonard et al. 1993) and in planum asymmetry/length in dyslexic patients compared with control subjects without dyslexia and those with ADHD (Hynd et al. 1990). Moreover, significant relationships were found between phonological processing and planum symmetry in the dyslexic group (Larsen et al. 1990). The incidence of bilateral cerebral anomalies was higher in dyslexic patients than in nondyslexic control subjects (C. M. Leonard et al. 1993). Thus, the most consistent neuropathological findings associated with reading disorder are left-hemisphere, temporal-lobe abnormalities, focusing on patterns of planum temporale asymmetry that have been linked to deficits in phonological coding processes in dyslexic patients. However, factors such as age, sex, and overall brain size may greatly contribute to group differences or the lack thereof. For example, Schultz et al. (1994) reported that in contrast to their initial findings of smaller left-hemispheric structures in dyslexic patients relative to control subjects, when subsequent analyses controlled for these factors, no significant differences were found in surface area and planum temporale symmetry. The most robust finding reflected sex differences, such that every morphometric measure was larger for boys than for girls. These authors suggested that differences in subject characteristics as well as procedural differences in MRI studies contribute to discrepant findings of analyses of morphological brain measures in children.

Studies have used positron-emission tomography (PET) and cerebral blood flow measures to assess brain activation during reading and language tasks. The rate of regional cerebral metabolic activity in frontal and occipital areas (Gross-Glenn et al. 1991) and in the medial temporal lobe differed between dyslexic patients and nonimpaired control subjects (Hagman et al. 1992). Cerebral blood flow studies have reported differences in left superotemporal activation (Flowers et al. 1991) and posterior portions of the planum (Rumsey et al. 1992), further suggesting different physiological activation patterns in the brains of dyslexic patients relative to nondyslexic individuals.

Developmental Course

Early warning signs of what may later develop into dyslexia may be observed during preschool years. These problems may include delayed onset of speech acquisition, articulation, naming (e.g., colors, letters), word finding, letter transposition, and verbal sequencing (Pennington 1991a). Phonological processing skills (phoneme discrimination, sequencing) appear to be highly correlated with later-developed reading skills (Wagner and Torgesen 1987). Table 5–1 lists the developmental course, problems, and assessments of cognitive function associated with later-developing reading disorders in preschool children (Goldman 1988). If normal language production and comprehension are not acquired by age 2½ years, then a language evaluation should be recommended.

Dyslexia is commonly diagnosed during first or second grade when formal reading instruction occurs. In children with reading disorders who have high IQs, the disorder may not be readily apparent until fourth or fifth grade when language-related demands increase (American Psychiatric Association 1994). As a result of difficulty understanding others and/or expressing oneself verbally, behavior problems (e.g., acting out, social withdrawal) may manifest. During adolescence, reading difficulties may affect performance on timed tests as well as the completion of homework assignments (Pennington 1991a). However, the course of the disorder into adolescence and adulthood varies, ranging from increased deficits in some dyslexic patients to compensated deficits in others. Most individuals with reading disorders fall into the mid-range, with a course of a continuous lag. Nevertheless, having a reading disorder does not preclude the development of a fulfilling and successful life. Early identification and intervention may further enhance one's developmental course. IQ was a good predictor of recovery potential in dyslexic patients whose developmental reading disorders were treated and diagnosed early (Kurzweil 1992). For dyslexic patients with low IQs, concurrent cognitive and reading therapy maximized remedial efforts.

Neuropsychological Patterns and Assessments

Deficits in phonological processing skills have been most consistently and empirically targeted as the primary dysfunction associated with reading disorder (Vellutino 1979) compared with visual-perceptual processing skills, which also have been associated with this disorder (Mattis et al. 1975; Petraukas and Rourke 1979). More specifically, primary deficits include difficulty with word recognition related to impairment in the use of phonological codes. As a result, reading becomes a slow, mechanical process, affecting reading comprehension skills and spelling accuracy and fluency. An interaction between phonemic awareness and verbal short-term memory/name recall has been found to be related to reading skill development and deficits (Pennington et al. 1990, 1991).

Table 5–1. Developmental course, problems, and assessments of cognitive function associated with later-developing reading disorders in preschool children

Development	Problems	Assessments
Auditory attention 5–6 Weeks: actively scans in response to stimuli; sustains attention to human voice	Phonemic discrimination Morphological endings Semantics Discrimination of intonation changes Low frustration tolerance Distractibility Impulsivity Social immaturity	Observe differences in response to structured standardized tests (e.g., Goldman-Fristoe-Woodcock Auditory Skills Test Battery subtest) Auditory selective attention Unstructured play sessions
Auditory perception 2 Months: discriminates voice of mother from stranger 3–7 Months: differentially responds to specific words/contexts of familiar person; prepares for speech sound discrimination	Language Discrimination Rate Sequencing	Goldman-Fristoe-Woodcock Test of Auditory Discrimination Goldman-Fristoe-Woodcock Auditory Skills Test Battery
Auditory memory Infants: have recognition memory, not recall 2 Years: acquires mental representation and recall	Word retrieval Following directions Retelling stories	Age 3 years and older: Binet Sentence Memory Detroit Test of Learning Aptitude • Auditory Attention Span for Unrelated Words • Oral Directions

(continued)

Table 5–1. Developmental course, problems, and assessments of cognitive function associated with later-developing reading disorders in preschool children (*continued*)

Development	Problems	Assessments
3–5 Years: uses semantic categories (e.g., animals, clothes) to organize recall 6–7 Years: labels/rehearses information asked to recall	Word-finding difficulties (predictive of decoding problems) Memory function interrelated with attention, motivation, and anxiety	Kaufman Assessment Battery for Children • Auditory Memory Slingerland Pre-reading Screening Test (Kindergarten) Jansky Predictive Reading Index • Naming (Kindergarten) Clinical Evaluation of Language Functions (CELF) • Word Confrontation
Symbolic representation 18–24 Months: is able to symbolize	Expressive language Receptive language	Present child with more/less symbolic toys Observe level of symbolic play Significant discrepancy between level of symbolic play and verbal symbolic representation (word meanings) suggests possible language delay

Conceptualization
Develops concepts of object, self, body, space, time, attributes, and relationships
Pragmatic aspects of language
Cause-and-effect relationships with integration of these concepts

All aspects of language development

Rule out general intellectual retardation
Look for specific areas of strengths and weaknesses
Infancy
  Bayley Scales of Infant Development
  Cattel Infant Intelligence Scale
  Denver Developmental Screening Test
Preschool
  Goodenough Draw-a-Person Test
  Illinois Tests of Psycho-Linguistic Abilities (ITPA)
  • Visual Reception, Visual Association, and Manual Expression
  Leiter International Performance Scale
  Wechsler Preschool and Primary Scale of Intelligence—Revised (WPPSI-R)
  McCarthy Scales of Children's Abilities
  Boehm Test of Basic Concepts
  Piagetian Tasks for the Preoperational Stage

(continued)

Table 5–1. Developmental course, problems, and assessments of cognitive function associated with later-developing reading disorders in preschool children (*continued*)

Development	Problems	Assessments
Word meanings	Delayed or deviant language development: child may lose presymbolic words and does not develop higher-level words at 18–24 months	WPPSI-R
10–15 Months: words are presymbolic (10–15 words)		Token Test
18–24 Months: words become social symbols		Peabody Picture Vocabulary Test—Revised
2 Years: uses 200–400 words	Semantic disorders (receptive language): difficulty with links between words/ grammatical structures and meanings, independent of conceptual problems	ITPA
3 Years: uses 900–1,000 words		• Auditory Reception, Auditory Association, Verbal Expression
4 Years: uses 1,500 words		CELF
6 Years: uses 2,500 words	Difficulty comprehending/ using concepts regarding logical relationships (e.g., "if-then"; "all-some")	• Word Classes, Linguistic Relationships, Relationships and Ambiguities
	Difficulty with relationship regarding logical operations (i.e., comparative, familial, spatial, temporal sequencing)	Boston Naming Test
		Expressive One-Word Picture Vocabulary Test
	Verbal analogies	Jansky Predictive Index
	Word-finding	• Naming

| **Syntax and morphology**
$1\frac{1}{2}$ to 4 or 5 Years: uses well-developed grammatical/phonological rules | Phonologic syntactic syndrome:
Difficulty mastering rules of phonology and grammar
Substitutions/inversions in speech articulation
Very limited use of functional words/very simple syntactic construction
Often accompanied by dysarthria/dyspraxia
Syntactic-pragmatic syndrome (less common)
Deficits in syntactic/pragmatic use of language
Variable phonology/prosody; responds to simple commands, not "why" questions
Syntactic deficits linked to attention and memory deficits | Assess spontaneous language in natural setting, particularly ages 2–4 years
CELF
• Grammatical Understanding
ITPA
• Grammatical Closure
Token Test
Test of Language Development
• Grammatical Understanding
Binet Sentence Repetition
Detroit Tests of Learning Aptitude
• Auditory Attention Span for Unrelated Syllables |

(continued)

Table 5–1. Developmental course, problems, and assessments of cognitive function associated with later-developing reading disorders in preschool children (*continued*)

Development	Problems	Assessments
Pragmatics Communicative function of language First appears when baby cries as regulatory function 2–3 Months: has mutual/ alternating gaze and vocalization with parent 9–12 Months: purposefully uses eye contact, gesture, and vocalizations 12–18 Months: points to indicate needs (correlated with extent of child's early vocabulary)	Syntactic-pragmatic Semantic pragmatic	No structured, standardized assessment exists Use thorough history and observation of child in different settings (home, school) with different people (parents, siblings, peers)

Assessments necessary to confirm the diagnosis of dyslexia include tests of intelligence, academic achievement, language, and other cognitive functions to identify the loci of the reading disorder. Suggested tests are listed in Table 5–2 to aid in identification and discrimination of underlying deficits associated with dyslexia in school-age children, adolescents, and adults.

In adults with subtle dyslexic difficulties, confrontational naming, sentence repetition, word fluency (phonologically based), and phonologically oriented memorization task deficits are common (Denckla 1993). Felton et al. (1990) found that performance on rapid naming, phonological awareness, and nonword reading tasks was significantly impaired in a well-characterized group of 115 adult dyslexic patients relative to healthy control subjects when age and socioeconomic status were controlled for in statistical analyses. Capacity for finger localization (Badian et al. 1990) and diminished memory performance (DeRenzi and Lucchelli 1990) also have been identified as predictors for the persistence of reading disorder into adulthood.

Treatment

Nonpharmacological treatment.   Phonological and visual-perceptual deficits have been associated with dyslexia. Remedial efforts have been directed toward retraining cognitive functions associated with the presumed nature of the underlying problem and/or "teaching to strengths" as a compensatory mechanism.

Because phonological coding is believed to be a primary process in the development of reading skills (M. J. Adams 1990; Clark 1988), phonics-based remedial efforts are critical. Moreover, prerequisite phoneme awareness training is essential, especially with younger children who have reading disorders. Although many dyslexic patients have deficits in phonological coding, some may still be able to learn these skills, albeit more slowly, via sustained and systematic instruction. A variety of effective standardized instructional methods address specific components or an integration of associated deficits related to phonological coding problems (see Pennington 1991a, p. 75). However, the effectiveness of remediating cognitive deficits is controversial because underlying genetic and neurological factors may be associated with reading disorder in many dyslexic patients. Thus, it may be difficult to train or remediate cognitive functions associated with impaired or dysfunctional cortical areas (Hynd and Cohen 1983).

Table 5–2.   Neuropsychological assessments for validation and discrimination of reading disorder in children, adolescents, and adults

Test	Normed for ages	Functions assessed
Wechsler Intelligence Scale for Children, Third Edition (WISC-III; Wechsler 1991)	6-0—16-11	Verbal and nonverbal intelligence
Wechsler Adult Intelligence Scale— Revised (WAIS-R; Wechsler 1981)	16–74	Verbal and nonverbal intelligence
Wechsler Individual Achievement Test (WIAT; Wechsler 1992)	6–16	Academic achievement in reading, mathematics, language, and writing (use ability-achievement discrepancy analysis between WISC-III and WIAT)
Wide Range Achievement Test, 3rd Edition (WRAT-3), Level 2 (Wilkinson 1993)	12–75	Spelling, arithmetic, reading
Boder Test of Reading-Spelling Patterns (Boder and Jarrico 1982)	All	Reading disabilities
Scholastic Abilities Test for Adults (SATA; Bryant et al. 1991)	16-0—79-11	Aptitude and achievement (relative strengths and weaknesses) (mostly untimed) (use aptitude-achievement discrepancy analysis)
Raven's Progressive Matrices and Coloured Progressive Matrices (Raven 1938, 1947)	6–Adult	Reasoning (untimed, nonverbal, nonmotor test) (used as nonverbal assessment of intelligence)
Symbol Digit Modalities Test (SDMT; A. Smith 1991)	8–78	Reading readiness; reading difficulties predicted and identified early

(continued)

Table 5–2. Neuropsychological assessments for validation and discrimination of reading disorder in children, adolescents, and adults *(continued)*

Test	Normed for ages	Functions assessed
Woodcock Reading Mastery Test—Revised Subtests: Visual-Auditory Learning Word Attack (Woodcock 1987)	5–75+	Visual-auditory associations that simulate the learning-to-read process; decoding skills without contextual clues
Goldman-Fristoe-Woodcock Test of Auditory Discrimination (Goldman et al. 1974)	3–0—Adult	Auditory discrimination of words
Test of Language Development—Primary, 3rd Edition (TOLD-P:3) (relevant subtests) (Newcomer and Hammill 1998)	4–0—8–11	Auditory discrimination and memory, receptive and expressive language, oral/pointing responses
Test of Adolescent Language—3 (TOAL-3) (relevant subtests) (Hammill et al. 1998)	11–0—17–5	Receptive and expressive language, oral/written responses
Boston Naming Test (BNT; Kaplan et al. 1983)	5–5—10–5; 18–59	Mild word retrieval deficits
Gray Oral Reading Test, 3rd Edition (GORT-3; Wiederholt and Bryant 1992)	7–0—18–11	Oral reading rate/ accuracy, oral reading comprehension, oral reading miscues
Token Test for Children (DiSimoni and Vignolo 1962)	3–0—12–0	Receptive auditory syntax, following verbal instructions
Developmental Test of Visual-Motor Integration (Beery and Buktenica 1989)	2—14–11 (retains validity for older age groups and adults)	Visual-motor integration (copying of geometric line drawings)

(continued)

Table 5–2.   Neuropsychological assessments for validation and discrimination of reading disorder in children, adolescents, and adults *(continued)*

Test	Normed for ages	Functions assessed
Rey-Osterrieth Complex Figure (copy, immediate and delayed memory) (Rey 1941; Osterrieth 1944)	6–85	Visuospatial constructional ability and visual memory
Hooper Visual Organization Test (HVOT; Hooper 1958)	25–69	Visual-conceptual integration, nonmotor
Wide Range Assessment of Memory and Learning (WRAML; Sheslow and Adams 1990) • Picture Memory • Design Memory • Verbal Learning • Story Memory	5–0—17–11	Visual and verbal memory; immediate and delayed recall
Trail Making Test A and B (Reitan 1969b)	8–79	Speed for visual search, attention, mental flexibility, and motor function
Motor-Free Visual Perception Test (Colarusso and Hammill 1996)	4–8 (retains validity with older children)	Visual perception without motor component; five visual-perceptual areas
Dyslexia Screening Instrument (Coon et al. 1994)	6–21	Reading and writing problems associated with dyslexia (based on classroom teachers' observations/rating)

An alternative method to remediate deficit areas is "teaching to strengths," in which intact areas of cognitive functioning are focal points of remediation. This modality permits the development of compensatory strategies. The "whole word" teaching method (Stauffer 1970), use of flash card drills, a method that breaks words into visual chunks (i.e., root, prefix, suffix) (Chall 1967), and fingertip number writing (Reitan 1969a) have been used to develop compensatory strategies, as long as visual and tactile sensory perception abilities are intact. In children whose visuospatial deficits are identified as an underlying basis of their dyslexia, integrated phonics programs such as the Science Research Associates (SRA) basic reading program are recommended. Interesting new research has shown a method of modifying acoustic signals and temporal processing associated with receptive language that may mediate underlying phonological processing deficits in reading disorder (Tallal et al. 1996). Receptive phonology, morphology, and syntax significantly improved in children (age 5–10 years) with language-learning impairment after use of this training method (see Tallal et al. 1996).

In summary, comprehensive neuropsychological evaluations are critical to assess areas of cognitive strengths and weaknesses in individuals with reading disorders. Identifying and mediating early developmental precursors to a reading disorder further enhance the possibility of a child's potential for some recovery or compensation. Moreover, early intervention may help minimize the emotional overlay that often accompanies dyslexia. Use of compensatory devices (e.g., word processing/ handheld "spell check") is recommended to circumvent spelling difficulties, because spelling deficits are more refractory to interventions (Pennington 1991a). Additional compensatory mechanisms, such as the use of tape recorders, oral examinations, and extended test-taking time, may be helpful. Acoustically modified speech training may prove useful in enhancing language comprehension. Adolescents and adults with dyslexia may benefit from remedial strategies that focus on enhancement of study skills, reading comprehension, and reading time management. Nonstandard test administration (e.g., extended time) and reduction of course load will assist individuals with slower reading skills (Denckla 1993).

Pharmacological treatment.   Pharmacological treatment of dyslexia has gained some support. Literature suggests that psychostimulant medications, such as methylphenidate (Ritalin), may be useful in treating dyslexia with comorbid hyperactivity and attentional problems. Word recognition was enhanced in groups of hyperactive children with dyslexia, believed to be associated with improvement in attention, recall, and verbal retrieval (Kupietz et al. 1988; Richardson et al. 1988). Piracetam, a drug structurally related to γ-aminobutyric acid (GABA) and vasopressin, was somewhat effective in laboratory measures and in clinical trials. Verbal learning, short-term memory, single word reading, and reading rate were enhanced in dyslexic boys in 12 double-blind, placebo-controlled studies (see Rapoport 1987). One study, however, found no significant improvement in dyslexic children receiving piracetam relative to placebo (Ackerman et al. 1991). An integration of pharmacotherapy and cognitive remediation may be most effective in treating dyslexia.

Mathematics Disorder

Diagnostic Criteria and Definition

Mathematics disorder is characterized by mathematical skills that are substantially underdeveloped relative to that which is expected given one's chronological age, measured intelligence, and age-appropriate education, as measured by standardized assessments (American Psychiatric Association 1994).

A variety of mathematical skills may be impaired in mathematics disorder, including linguistic, perceptual, attentional, and mathematical abilities. Linguistic impairment may manifest in difficulty comprehending or expressing mathematical concepts, terms, or operations and/or coding mathematical symbols from text. Perceptual deficits are evidenced by difficulty recognizing mathematical signs and symbols as well as grouping objects. Impairment associated with attention includes carelessness in copying numbers, attending to the type of operational signs, and remembering to "carry over." Deficits in mathematical skills themselves include counting objects, adhering to sequential processes in mathematical operations, and learning multiplication tables (American Psychiatric Association 1994).

Symptoms associated with mathematics disorder have also been described as *developmental dyscalculia*. Shalev and Gross-Tsur (1993, p. 134) stated that "Developmental Dyscalculia (DDC) is defined as marked impairment of arithmetic skills in an otherwise healthy child . . . , refractory to special educational interventions." They also stated, quite significantly, that "evaluation by a multidisciplinary team, . . . [for potentially dyscalculic children is] strongly recommended, because achievement in mathematics is very sensitive to a variety of factors, foremost among them neurological conditions" (Shalev and Gross-Tsur 1993, p. 134). Furthermore, "complex cognitive skills, such as calculating, language, and reading, call for the integrated activity of many brain systems, so these children often have a disorder affecting more than one function" (Shalev and Gross-Tsur 1993, p. 134).

Subtypes. There is some debate as to the appropriate categorizing of developmental dyscalculia. According to S. Hughes et al. (1994):

◆ Badian denotes four subtypes: 1) spatial, 2) anarithmetria, 3) attentional-sequential, and 4) alexia and agraphia for numbers.
◆ Sharma and Loveless describe six subtypes: 1) verbal, 2) practognostic, 3) lexical, 4) graphic, 5) ideognostic, and 6) operational.
◆ Hooper and Willis suggest that empirical support is insufficient to validate subtyping.

Comorbidity. Reading disorder, disorder of written expression, and ADHD frequently co-occur with mathematics disorder.

Prevalence

Prevalence estimates are as high as 1% of school-age children and one in every five cases of learning disorder that does not co-occur with other disorders. These are rough estimates, however, because of the limited number of studies in this area (American Psychiatric Association 1994). Developmental dyscalculia does not seem to occur more frequently in boys than girls (Russell and Ginsburg 1984; Shalev et al. 1988), as do developmental dyslexia and ADHD. However, prevalence is increased in girls who have epilepsy, sex chromosome anomalies, and fragile X (Pennington 1991b).

Pathology and Neuropsychological Function

As cited in C. Hughes et al. (1994), Cohn attributed developmental dyscalculia to "lesions in widely disparate regions of the brain, including regions outside the visual system" (Hughes et al. 1994, p. 64). Hecaen, based on Luria, claimed that spatial dyscalculia is due to right-hemispheric lesions, whereas arithmetical dyscalculia is due to left-hemispheric lesions (Hughes et al. 1994).

Links between developmental dyscalculia and right-cerebral-hemisphere dysfunction. According to N. Gordon (1992, p. 459), subject to the relation between spatial and mathematical abilities, errors can result from the "inability to point accurately to objects being counted." Furthermore, "speech articulation, and the acquisition of reasonably neat writing" also may be affected (N. Gordon 1992, p. 460). He noted that "children with treated phenylketonuria tend to show deficits in conceptual and visual spatial skills, . . . [and in a study by Berry et al.] had no apparent reading and spelling disability, but their arithmetic scores were significantly low" (N. Gordon 1992, p. 460). Also, "the results of psychometric tests in Turner's syndrome show that affected girls do relatively well on verbal tests, but poorly on performance and numerical ones. It is suggested that in this syndrome, there is involvement of the right parietal lobe, possibly related to the basic chromosome defects" (Gordon 1992, p. 460).

With regard to social behavior, Gordon cited Weintraub and Mesulam (1983), who described right-cerebral-hemisphere dysfunction, in which "affected children suffer from emotional and interpersonal difficulties, shyness, visuospatial disturbances and problems with mathematics, . . . poor eye contact, absence of gesture, lack of speech prosody, . . . [low] social maturity, . . . difficulty understanding the affective state of others, and . . . a poor comprehension of non-verbal communication" (N. Gordon 1992, p. 461). There may also be "right-left confusion, poor sense of direction, and difficulty with tasks such as riding a bicycle" (N. Gordon 1992, p. 461).

O'Hare et al. (1991, p. 360) also discussed right-hemisphere dysfunction and stated that

> These dyscalculic children characteristically have a profound inability to conceptualize number quantity, but their symbol recognition and production is preserved . . . they may have associated features such as left-limb atrophy, incoordination of the left hand, constructional dyspraxia, poor development of visual spatial and visual motor skills, sensory inattention, absence of stereoscopic vision, and dysprosodia.

Links between developmental dyscalculia and left-cerebral-hemisphere dysfunction.

> These dyscalculic children [with left-hemispheric lesions] . . . characteristically are unable to recognize and produce number and operator symbols. They have number quantity concept, but mental arithmetic is disturbed by poor sequencing skills and reduced short-term auditory memory, associated with damage to the left temporal-parietal region. They may also have features . . . of . . . Gerstmann syndrome, which includes spelling dysgraphia, right-left disorientation and finger agnosia, . . . (O'Hare et al. 1991, pp. 358, 360)

as well as dyslexia, associated with deficits in the left superior angular gyrus and the posterior supramarginal gyrus (Roeltgen et al. 1983b).

However, it has also been shown that the dyscalculia associated with Gerstmann's syndrome is not specific to the type of dyscalculic deficits associated with right-hemispheric dysfunction (Critchley 1953; Kinsbourne and Warrington 1963).

Developmental Course

Table 5–3 describes the normal developmental course of arithmetic skill acquisition.

Mathematics disorder is considered when arithmetic skill acquisition substantially deviates from the normal course of development (see Table 5–3) in relation to the diagnostic criteria indicated above. Although symptoms of the disorder may manifest during kindergarten or first grade, the disorder is not usually diagnosed until at least the end of first grade when formal mathematical instruction and assessments have begun. Recognition of this disorder may be even more difficult in children with high IQs, in which case mathematics disorder may only become apparent in the later grades.

Prognosis depends on the nature of spared function in relation to the specific deficit profile, because dyscalculia rarely occurs in isolation. The prognosis is poor for dyscalculia associated with right-hemisphere dysfunction, and it frequently persists into adulthood (O'Hare et al. 1991). Moreover, although language skills are often intact, social, conceptual, visuospatial, visuoconstructional, and neuromotor deficits often accompany right-hemispheric dyscalculia, further complicating development and adult functioning. This clinical profile mimics the symptom cluster associated with nonverbal learning disability, which has core symptoms

Table 5–3. Course of arithmetic skill development

Operation	Task	Age
Counting	Active counting of objects	Preschool
Quantity: counting objects in linear array	4 objects	3.5–4 years
	15 objects	5 years
Number and operator symbol recognition and production	Correctly writes 3-digit number	8 years
Calculation	Simple addition/subtraction without concrete materials	7+ years
	Multiply single written integer	10.5+ years
	Division	13+ years

of dyscalculia, socioemotional difficulties, communication problems, Verbal Scale IQ higher than Performance Scale IQ, visuospatial deficits, and increased left-sided soft neurological signs (Gross-Tsur et al. 1995). In contrast, dyscalculia associated with left-hemispheric dysfunction often results in dyslexia, Performance Scale IQ higher than Verbal Scale IQ, and right-sided soft neurological signs but no visuospatial problems. Interestingly, one study found that although impairment in either hemisphere has a profound effect on mathematical skill development (arithmetic scores >2 SD below the mean), left-hemisphere dysfunction was associated with an even greater level of impairment (>3 SD below the mean) in select areas (Shalev et al. 1995). Thus, specific mathematical deficits associated with left-hemispheric dysfunction may be more severe than those associated with right-hemispheric dysfunction. However, in conjunction with comorbid problems associated with left-hemispheric dyscalculia, the effect on overall level of functioning may be more discrete relative to that in right-hemispheric dyscalculia.

Neuropsychological Patterns and Assessments

Initial identification of possible developmental dyscalculia was determined by a cutoff score at the fifth percentile on a battery of arithmetic tests given to 200 nonimpaired children in grades 3–6. Shalev et al. (1993) noted that low scores correlated well with teachers' assessments of students' arithmetic skills but not reading ability. The "inability to recognize number symbols; mirror writing; failure to recognize the basic mathematical operations or use of operator or separator symbols; inability to recall tables and 'carry' numbers in multiplication; and failure to maintain the proper order of numbers in calculation" are often found among children with developmental dyscalculia (Gordon 1992, p. 462).

Treatment

Nonpharmacological treatment. For right-hemisphere dysfunction, computer software that provides language support for mathematical skills may be of use (O'Hare et al. 1991). Other aids include use of Cuisenaire rods, use of graph paper for column alignment, acquisition of the ability to estimate answers before calculation, and use of a calculator to check answers (Pennington 1991a).

For left-hemisphere dysfunction, software that uses color to identify symbols is recommended (O'Hare et al. 1991), as well as step-by-step formulas for solving multistep problems (Pennington 1991a).

Pharmacological treatment. No specific pharmacological treatment for mathematics disorder has been identified at this time. However, case studies reflect how treatment of comorbid conditions may affect improvement in mathematics disorder. For example, Shalev and Gross-Tsur (1993) described two children with known learning disorders who were not progressing in mathematics despite extensive remediation and were, therefore, examined by a multidisciplinary team. One 8½-year-old girl had normal reading and writing skills but problems with arithmetic. She was given a diagnosis of attention deficit disorder without hyperactivity. After treatment with Ritalin, she made slow but steady progress in arithmetic. Another 8½-year-old girl had short staring spells several times a day for more than 3 years, severe arithmetic difficulties, and minor problems in reading and writing. She was given a diagnosis of petit mal seizures. After treatment with valproic acid, her academic skills improved rapidly.

Disorder of Written Expression

Diagnostic Criteria and Definition

Disorder of written expression, also referred to as *dysgraphia,* is characterized by writing skills that are substantially underdeveloped relative to that which is expected given one's chronological age, measured intelligence, and age-appropriate education (American Psychiatric Association 1994). Writing skills are evaluated by either standardized or functional assessments. More specifically, evidence of punctuation and grammatical errors, multiple spelling errors, poorly organized paragraphs, and substantially impaired handwriting is often observed in written text. Other learning disabilities such as reading and mathematics disorders often accompany disorder of written expression, along with other language and perceptual motor deficits (American Psychiatric Association 1994).

Prevalence

The prevalence of disorder of written expression is unknown because deficits associated with this disorder are more generally clustered into overall categories of learning disabilities in much of the literature (American Psychiatric Association 1994).

Pathology and Neuropsychological Function

Linguistic and motor functions are two major components associated with the development of writing skills. The linguistic component includes the ability to choose correct letter and word meanings (i.e., spelling and semantics). The motor component includes neuropsychological functions that are involved in motor output necessary for producing the correct form for spelling and semantics. The following section provides an overview of these basic components involved in the multiplex of possible neurological functions that may be impaired in writing disorders associated with agraphia (see Roeltgen 1985 for a comprehensive review). Investigations of dysgraphia and developmental dysgraphia are frequently based on very small samples or single-case studies and are sparsely listed in the literature.

Linguistic components and disorders associated with written expression. Writing disorders involving linguistic components include the following:

◆ *Lexical agraphia.* The lexical approach to spelling and writing is the "whole word" approach.

> The lexical strategy is necessary for spelling familiar orthographically irregular words (words that cannot be spelled utilizing direct sound-to-letter correspondence rules, e.g., "comb") and ambiguous words (words with sounds that may be represented by multiple letters or letter clusters, e.g., "phone"). The lexical system can also be used for spelling familiar orthographically regular words (words with direct sound-to-letter correspondence, e.g., "animal") that the phonological system can also handle. (Roeltgen 1985, pp. 79–80)

Individuals with lexical agraphia misspell words that are accurate phonologically (e.g., "pikcher" for "picture") and have difficulty with irregular and ambiguous words. The ability to spell regular words and nonwords is intact. Neuroanatomical substrates of lexical agraphia may include impairment in the junction of the posterior angular gyrus and the parieto-occipital lobule, as evidenced by computed tomography (CT) scans of four patients with lexical agraphia (Roeltgen 1985).

◆ *Phonological agraphia.* The phonological approach involves phonological decoding of speech sounds (phonemes) that are subsequently transformed into letters (phoneme-grapheme conversion). This approach is used when "spelling unfamiliar orthographically regular words and pronounceable nonwords (e.g., 'flig')" (Roeltgen 1985, p. 82). Individuals with phonological agraphia have difficulty spelling nonwords, but the capacity to write regular and irregular words is preserved. Spelling errors reflect visual similarity rather than phonological accuracy (Roeltgen 1985). Neuroanatomical correlates of phonological agraphia include the supramarginal gyrus and/or the insula medial to it (Roeltgen et al. 1983a; Shallice 1981).

◆ *Semantic-related agraphias.* Interaction between lexical and phonological strategy allows an individual to process the meaning of words. Semantic-related writing disorders have been subtyped into three categories: 1) semantic agraphia, 2) phonological agraphia and Wernicke's aphasia, and 3) lexical agraphia with semantic paragraphia (see Roeltgen 1985, pp. 84–85, for a review).

Motor components and disorders associated with written expression. An integration of motor and visuospatial skills is involved in writing letters. Four subtypes of agraphia related to motor components of written expression have been described (see Roeltgen 1985, pp. 86–88, for full review) and include the following:

◆ *Apraxic agraphia.* Apraxic agraphia refers to impaired ability to hold a writing instrument correctly and to use fine motor movements associated with letter formation. Impairment in the hemisphere opposite the dominant hand is usually associated with the apraxia (Roeltgen 1985).

◆ *Agraphia without apraxia.* This disorder is characterized by impaired letter formation, with otherwise intact practic function and oral spelling ability. Deficits in letter formation occur during spontaneous writing and writing to dictation (Roeltgen 1985). Parietal-lobe impairment is believed to be associated with this disorder (Roeltgen and Heilman 1983).

◆ *Visuospatial agraphia.* Letter and word formation requires an integration of visuospatial skills and graphomotor output. Impairment in this process may result in visuospatial agraphia. Manifestations of this disorder include "1) reiteration of strokes; 2) inability to write on a straight line; and 3) insertion of blank spaces between graphemes" (Roeltgen 1985, p. 87). Nondominant parietal-lobe lesions have been associated with this disorder. Problems in handwriting and mathematics often overlap and may be related to an underlying impairment in spatial function. In what has been referred to as right-hemisphere learning disorder, problems in mathematics, handwriting, and art are often observed. Within this disorder, handwriting may be slow and labored. Pencil grip may be awkward and tight, so that heavy, dark strokes may appear, with spatial disorganization of letters to one another, lines on the page, and placement within the page appearing variable/displaced (left margins may be shifted to the right) (Pennington 1991a). Comorbid problems may include impaired social cognition, attention, and conceptual skills. Children may become oppositional toward completing homework assignments and written work in school. Spelling problems also may be observed. The greater the requirement for written output, the more likely that problems and resistance will surface (Levine et al. 1981). These problems may initially manifest in the form of depression, social withdrawal, oppositional behavior, or motivational difficulties. Girls with a specific genetic disorder, Turner's syndrome, often have problems in handwriting and math (Money 1973; Pennington et al. 1985).

◆ *Unilateral (callosal) agraphia.* Unilateral agraphia may occur when interhemispheric communication between the left hemisphere's spelling and graphemic systems and the right hemisphere's motor system nondominant hand control is disrupted. The manifestation of this disorder is illegible writing. Oral spelling and reading are usually intact (Roeltgen 1985). Impairment of the genu of corpus callosum has been hypothesized as a neuroanatomical substrate associated with this disorder (Watson and Heilman 1983).

Developmental Course

Early signs of deficits in written expression may be observed in first grade, manifested by difficulty in writing (e.g., poor copying ability, extremely poor handwriting, and difficulty remembering letter sequences in familiar words). The disorder may not be diagnosed until children have formal written instruction, usually during second grade (American Psychiatric Association 1994). Because of the paucity of information in the literature regarding this disorder developmentally, its progression into adolescence and adulthood is unclear.

Developmental dysgraphia. Developmental dysgraphia is characterized by an impaired ability to progress from an alphabetical stage to an orthographical stage of reading development (Frith 1985). The alphabetical stage begins when children learn to connect speech sounds to individual written letters and later use these abilities to read and spell familiar and unfamiliar words. The orthographical stage begins when children recognize and spell familiar words from a lexical basis only, without phonological input (Frith 1985; Seymour and MacGregor 1984).

In a study of two adolescent boys (ages 14 and 16) with developmental dysgraphia, spelling errors were correlated with level of orthographical ambiguity and with word frequency (Thomas-Anterion et al. 1994). These types of deficits are typically found in acquired dysgraphia. The spelling of ambiguous irregular words during writing appeared more difficult than their recognition during reading, implying that the phonological system was more intact than the lexical system. Long-term recall (20-minute delay) of irregular words was impaired, whereas short-term and working memory were intact. One of the two adolescents learned 20 irregular words via selective reminding of errors. These authors posited that the angular gyrus is a neuroanatomical correlate of developmental dysgraphia as has been proposed in adult acquired lexical agraphia.

Thus, as in other learning disorders, the specific impairment associated with dysgraphia may vary depending on the underlying deficit, genesis of the deficit (i.e., developmental or acquired), patient's age, exposure to skill development, and psychosocial factors.

Neuropsychological Patterns and Assessments

Far fewer standardized tests are available to assess disorders of written expression compared with other learning disorders. For elementary-school-age children, the extent and nature of the writing disorder must be assessed both formally and informally. A three-part writing test was initially developed to evaluate writing disorders (Chedru and Geschwind 1972). The test includes 1) writing to command (spontaneous), 2) writing to dictation, and 3) copying. Clinicians have used this general model consistently to help diagnose and identify specific deficits associated with this disorder. Writing to command includes asking the individual to write about a familiar topic or to write a story based on a picture. A writing sample based on a picture can be compared with a sample written at a different time to analyze content and form. Writing to dictation (words/sentences) allows the clinician to examine specific features that may be associated with the manifest deficit, such as difficulty with the length, commonality, regularity, and/or abstractability of a word. Further, mode of expression may be varied (i.e., type, spell orally, spell from blocks) to determine whether the impairment is related to a selective writing process or whether it is associated with a more global linguistic impairment. A copying task may vary in length of stimuli presented.

Standardized tests that will help identify specific deficits associated with writing disorders include the

◆ Test of Language Development—Primary, 3rd Edition (TOLD—P:3): ages 4–0 to 8–11 years
◆ Test of Adolescent Language—3 (TOAL—3; Hammill et al. 1998): ages 12–0 to 24–11 years
◆ Test of Written Language—3 (TOWL—3): ages 7.6–17.11 years

In addition, specific tests that assess phonological ability, letter recognition, reading, and spelling are essential (see Table 5–2). Moreover, assessments should include tests of visuospatial, visuoperceptual, and constructional abilities; ideomotor praxis (i.e., selection, sequencing, spatial orientation of gestural movements); and basic motor and sensory functions to determine whether impairment in any of these areas exists and thus interferes with the capacity for written expression.

These neuropsychological and neurological assessments may help classify the type of dysgraphia and may also help identify underlying symptoms associated with the specific variant of the disorder. Remedial efforts can then be directed.

Treatment

Writing depends on an integration of multiple neuropsychological functions; thus, remediation of writing disorders also depends on the specific cognitive profile associated with the disorder. Unfortunately, very little research has been conducted in this area. The literature is speckled with case studies of individuals with developmental or acquired dysgraphia, in which individually tailored remedial programs for specific deficit profiles are described. Remedial approaches may involve either retraining select deficits or teaching compensatory mechanisms to minimize the effects of a writing disorder. Treatment of a handwriting problem may include teaching a child to type on a word processor, allowing additional time to complete written assignments in school, and if deficits are severe enough, undergoing occupational therapy (Pennington 1991a).

◈ PERVASIVE DEVELOPMENTAL DISORDERS

"Pervasive Developmental Disorders are characterized by severe and pervasive impairment in several areas of development: reciprocal social interaction skills, communication skills, or the presence of stereotyped behavior, interests, and activities" (American Psychiatric Association 1994, p. 65) relative to one's developmental level or mental age. Specific disorders include autistic disorder, Asperger's disorder, Rett's disorder, and childhood disintegrative disorder. Delays and deviations in development associated with these disorders may be recognized as early as infancy. They may become more obvious as a deviation, instead of a delay, in development, as children progress through their first few years. Other conditions may accompany these disorders, including mental retardation and/or "medical conditions (e.g., chromosomal abnormalities, congenital infections, structural abnormalities of the central nervous system)" (American Psychiatric Association 1994, pp. 65–66).

Diagnostic boundaries among the pervasive developmental disorders are not always clearly defined. Although some distinctions are based on factors such as onset of the disorder following a normal developmental period (e.g., Rett's disorder, childhood disintegrative disorder), or lack of significant language delays (e.g., Asperger's disorder), other characteristics are nonspecific. As such, deficits in social interaction and communication characterize the various pervasive developmental disorders. Deficits in neuromotor development are part of the pervasive developmental disorder profile. Continued investigations will further validate convergent and divergent factors associated with specific pervasive developmental disorders via phenomenological, neurobiological, and neuropsychological assessments.

In the following section, we discuss autism and Asperger's disorder. Rett's disorder and childhood disintegrative disorder are not discussed because they are less common and are not seen as frequently as autism and Asperger's disorder in general practice.

Autistic Disorder

Diagnostic Criteria and Definition

Autistic disorder is characterized by "markedly abnormal or impaired development in social interaction and communication and a markedly restricted repertoire of activity and interests" (American Psychiatric Association 1994, p. 66). Delays or deficits in social interaction, in use of language in social communication, or in symbolic or imaginative play occur prior to age 3 years (American Psychiatric Association 1994).

This behavioral triad has been consistently linked to autistic disorder. More specifically, impairment in social interaction includes

1. Lack of eye contact
2. Poor or absent attachments
3. Impairment in imitation
4. Aloofness or indifference toward others
5. Lack of empathy
6. Lack of comfort-seeking from others

Disturbances in speech and communication include

1. Mute, delayed, or abnormal speech
2. Monotonous or peculiar vocal intonation and prosody
3. Lack of gestural communication
4. Echolalia
5. Concrete thinking
6. Deficits in pragmatic communication
7. Impairment in semantic development
8. Failure to use language for social interaction

Inflexible patterns of behavior include

1. Preoccupation with stereotyped and restricted interests and activities
2. Rituals
3. Repetitive mannerisms (e.g., hand flapping, spinning)
4. Interest in nonfunctional aspects of objects (e.g., taste or feel)
5. Deficits in play skills and imaginative play (e.g., taking toys apart; lining up)
6. Bizarre affective responses to change (e.g., in routine, in the environment; new situations)

Additionally, aggressive behavior is often part of the autistic profile and may be directed toward the self or others. Additional behavioral symptoms include hyperactivity, impulsivity, inattention, abnormalities in eating and sleeping patterns, hypersensitivity to certain sounds (e.g., vacuum cleaner) or touch, hyposensitivity to pain, and abnormalities in mood and affect (American Psychiatric Association 1994).

It is unlikely that autism is a single neurological disorder. The etiology, symptoms, and course associated with this disorder may vary from one affected individual to the next.

Associated disorders. Other disorders associated with autism include Rett's disorder (in girls) (Tridon et al. 1989; Witt-Engerstrom and Gillberg 1987), rubella embryopathy (Wing 1989), and seizure disorders (Olsson et al. 1988; Rutter 1970). Other medical conditions that have been described in autism include congenital infections, such as cytomegalovirus infection, syphilis, toxoplasmosis, varicella, and rubeola, and postnatal central nervous system (CNS) infections, including herpes encephalitis and mumps. Furthermore, prenatal abnormalities, including midtrimester uterine bleeding, parental exposure to chemical toxins, histories of infertility and spontaneous abortions, and parental thyroid disorders (which have been linked to immune disorders in some autistic patients), have been associated with autism (Pomeroy 1990).

Prevalence

Prevalence estimates of autistic disorder range from 2 to 5 cases per 10,000 individuals. Autistic disorder male-to-female ratios range from 2:1 in a French study (Cialdella and Mamelle 1989) and 2.9:1 in a Swedish study (Steffenburg and Gillberg 1986) to 4–5:1 in the United States (American Psychiatric Association 1994). Although autistic disorder occurs less frequently in females, the severity level of mental retardation is increased relative to males. Prevalence estimates of epilepsy in autistic children range from 5% (Bryson et al. 1988; Cialdella and Mammelle 1989) to 14% (Steffenburg and Gillberg 1986) and to 25% in adolescence and in early adulthood (Gillberg and Steffenberg 1987).

Etiology

Evidence suggests that autism is a familial, heritable, and genetically heterogeneous disorder. Furthermore, the interaction between environmental and genetic factors may compound the risk for development of this disorder.

Autism is estimated to be familial at the rate of 3% (Rutter et al. 1990b; for a review, see Smalley et al. 1988). As such, the prevalence of autism in siblings of autistic patients is approximately 50–100 times that in the general population. Heritability of autism has been supported by many twin studies. However, many of these studies had methodological limitations, such as ascertainment biases, which result in the reporting of inflated concordance rates in monozygotic and dizygotic twins (up to 90% for monozygotic and 25% for dizygotic twins). One study that avoided these limitations, based on 21 pairs of twins, reported a 36% concordance rate of autism in monozygotic twins and 0% concordance in dizygotic twins (Folstein and Rutter 1977). When these twins were combined with a new sample of twins, the reexamined data suggested that in the combined sample, 60% of monozygotic pairs and 0% of dizygotic pairs were concordant for autism (Bailey et al. 1995). Concordance rates for cognitive and language deficits in the original study of monozygotic pairs (82%) and dizygotic pairs (10%) were also reported (Folstein and Rutter 1977). Twin studies have also provided evidence to support the gene-environment interaction effect in the development of autism. Rates of perinatal problems were higher in the autistic probands in monozygotic pairs who were discordant for autism but concordant for language or cognitive disorders (Folstein and Rutter 1977) and, as adults, social impairment (Rutter et al. 1990b). These studies suggest that although genetics may play an important role in the development of social, language-related, and cognitive factors associated with autism, the interaction between genetic predisposition and early environmental insult may have a large effect on the development of autism.

Genetic studies of autism have provided some evidence for possible genetic subtyping, including "multifactorial inheritance, autosomal recessive inheritance, X-linked inheritance, and nonfamilial chromosomal anomalies" (Pennington 1991b, p. 137). Preliminary evidence of linkage and association between the serotonin transporter gene and autism has been implicated (Cook et al. 1997) because potent serotonin reuptake inhibitors have been effective in reducing repetitive behaviors in individuals with autistic disorder (McDougle et al. 1996). Pennington (1991b) suggested three articles for a full review of the genetics of autism (see Folstein and Rutter 1988; Rutter et al. 1990b; Smalley et al. 1988).

Genetic disorders associated with autism include fragile X syndrome (August and Lockhart 1984; Brown et al. 1982, 1986; Gillberg 1983; Hagerman et al. 1986; Le Couteur 1988); phenylketonuria (PKU) (Hackney et al. 1968); and two neurocutaneous disorders, tuberous sclerosis (A. Hunt and Dennis 1987; Mansheim 1979) and neurofibromatosis (Gaffney et al. 1988; Gillberg and Forsell 1984).

Pathology and Neuropsychological Function

Autism is a complex developmental disorder. Literature on the neuropathology of autism is vast and often contradictory. Although clinical manifestations of autism may cluster into core components, symptomatology varies among individuals with this disorder. Moreover, multiple underlying neuropathological mechanisms appear to be associated with autism. Considering the heterogeneity that exists among individuals with autism, conflicting results in studies of autism are not unexpected. Furthermore, treatment requires appropriate delineation of behavioral and/or neurobiological profiles associated with each autistic individual.

Neuroanatomy and neuroimaging. Postmortem brain studies and neuroimaging studies have provided evidence of neuroanatomical abnormalities in autism. Structural and cellular abnormalities have been found in the hippocampus, amygdala, and cerebellum (Bauman and Kemper 1985), including loss of Purkinje's cells, which provide the sole output of the cerebellar cortex (Bauman and Kemper 1985; Ritvo et al. 1986a). These abnormalities have been associated with deficits in socioemotional skills, sensory processing, and motor planning.

Neuroimaging, such as MRI, studies have implicated hypoplasia (i.e., defective or incomplete development) of the cerebellar vermal lobules (Courchesne et al. 1988; Hashimoto et al. 1995) and brain stem (Gaffney et al. 1988; Hashimoto et al. 1995). However, findings of reductions in cerebellar volume and vermis size were not always replicated (Kleiman et al. 1992), especially when age, IQ, and brain cross-sectional area in the midsagittal plane were controlled for in the analyses (Holttum et al. 1992; Piven et al. 1992). These results suggest the possibility of nonspecific findings in mental retardation or other developmental disorders rather than specific findings in autism (Peterson 1995). Other positive MRI findings include widening of the fourth ventricle (Gaffney et al. 1988), parietal-lobe impairment (Egaas et al. 1995; Saitoh et al. 1995), and a significantly smaller right-sided anterior cingulate gyrus in autistic patients relative to control subjects (Buchsbaum and Haznedar 1995). Anterior cingulate gyrus impairment has implications for the affective and socioemotional deficits in autism (for a review of magnetic resonance and autopsy studies in autism, see Courchesne 1995; Courchesne et al. 1994a; and Gillberg 1990). Moreover, total brain enlargement has been found, which is believed to be associated with significantly greater brain tissue volume and greater lateral ventricle volume in male autistic subjects relative to matched nonautistic control subjects (Piven et al. 1995).

Single photon emission computed tomography (SPECT) studies also have had mixed findings. In one study, brain metabolic dysfunction of cortical areas was found (Minshew 1994), whereas in another study, findings were negative (Zilbovicius et al. 1992).

Findings from PET studies have been mixed. One study yielded significantly decreased metabolism in the thalamus and increased metabolism in the cerebral peduncles in a group of patients with autistic and Asperger's disorder relative to control subjects (Buchsbaum and Haznedar 1995). In addition, metabolism was decreased in the anterior cingulate gyrus in the subgroup of autistic patients. These studies have implications for the impairment in affiliative behavior, attention, and information processing that has been found in autism. Abnormalities have also been found in the interactions between frontal or parietal lobes and the neostriatum and thalamus (Siegel et al. 1992), areas believed to be involved in directed attention (Mesulam 1981, 1983). Other studies have shown normal regional glucose metabolic rates (DeVolder et al. 1987; Jacobsen et al. 1988).

Differences in findings may be accounted for by differences in methodologies, such as the use of cortical activation procedures during PET. For example, the use of cortical activation procedures yielded very significant differences in regional metabolic rates in a group of autistic adults relative to nonautistic control subjects who were restudied (Buchsbaum et al. 1992), compared with earlier findings of the same group without the use of these activation procedures (Chris-Heh et al. 1989). Differences in findings also may be accounted for by sample selection. Schifter et al. (1994) found metabolic abnormalities in reduced [18F]fluorodeoxyglucose (FDG) uptake primarily in parietal, occipital, and temporal areas in autistic patients who had coexisting seizure disorders. Thus, it is important to note methodological similarities and differences when reviewing PET findings in autism.

In summary, although findings have been mixed, both structural and functional neuroimaging findings suggest that abnormalities are present in autistic individuals, especially in the brain stem, cerebellar, limbic, and frontal-lobe areas. As brain banks develop and become more accessible to researchers, and as brain imaging techniques become more sophisticated, research findings should become more precise, consistent, and reliable. An integration of the findings from these studies with the results of neurochemical, neurophysiological, and neuropsychological assessments will provide further insights into effective treatment of the various components of autism.

Neurophysiology. Event-related brain potentials (ERPs), electroencephalography (EEG), evoked potentials (EPs), and oculomotor function have been studied in patients with autism. ERP studies have reported small P3 waves in individuals with autism (Courchesne et al. 1985; Dawson et al. 1988; Lincoln et al. 1993). These studies support the impairment in selective attention in autistic individuals. Electroencephalographic patterns generally have been bilateral or a combination of localized and diffuse abnormalities. EP studies have reported extended reaction times in brain-stem auditory EPs, which may be related to the hypotonia sometimes observed in autistic children (Pomeroy 1990). Saccadic eye movement abnormalities have also been found in autistic patients (Rosenhall et al. 1988). Thus, neurophysiological findings provide further evidence of abnormalities in autism.

Neurochemistry. Neurochemical investigations in autism have been conducted to identify the underlying pathophysiology associated with its core components. Results from these studies have provided insight toward the development of new and effective pharmacological treatments (for a review, see Cook 1990; Gillberg 1990; Wing 1988). Neurochemical research has focused primarily on the study of monoamines and peptides.

Serotonin. Studies of the serotonergic system in autistic individuals are important because serotonin (5-HT) has been linked to the associated compulsive symptoms, including restricted interests, rigidity, need for sameness, and stereotypic and repetitive behavior. However, it is important to keep in mind that serotonergic dysfunction is associated with most disorders and, as such, is nonspecific to the pathophysiology of autism.

Blood, urine, and cerebrospinal fluid (CSF) samples of autistic patients that have been examined showed increased levels of whole-blood and platelet-bound serotonin. Hyperserotonemia, as evidenced in whole blood and platelets, has been documented in several studies of autism (Campbell et al. 1974; Hanley et al. 1977; Leboyer et al. 1994; Ritvo et al. 1970; Schain and Freedman 1961). However, this finding also has been documented in other disorders, including severe mental retardation (Hanley et al. 1977; Partington et al. 1973), chronic schizophrenia (Freedman et al. 1981), Huntington's disease (Belendiuk et al. 1981), and motor neuron disease (Belendiuk et al. 1980). It is important to note that whole-blood serotonin (Cook et al. 1990) and platelet serotonin (Kuperman et al. 1987) were not correlated with IQ in autistic children. Thus, associated mental retardation may not account for the hyperserotonemia in autism.

The mechanisms associated with hyperserotonemia are not well understood. Examinations of measures of uptake and excretion of serotonin have not clarified this finding. Moreover, the relation between serotonin blood levels and brain functioning is unclear. Conflicting reports have emerged regarding the roles of platelet serotonin receptors and serotonin receptor functioning in autism, whereby both increased (Katsui et al. 1986) and normal (Langer et al. 1981) platelet serotonin uptake were found in autistic children. Similarly, both decreased (McBride et al. 1989b) and normal (B. D. Perry et al. 1989) maximal binding capacity (B_{max}) of platelet 5-HT$_2$ binding were found in male autistic adults and children or adolescents, respectively, with no significant correlations between whole-blood serotonin and 5-HT$_2$ receptor binding site B_{max}.

Urinary indolamine data have also showed conflicting results. Urinary excretion of the serotonin metabolite 5-hydroxyindoleacetic acid (5-HIAA) was increased in a subgroup of hyperserotonemic autistic children (Minderaa et al. 1987), although no overall between-group differences were found when autistic patients were compared with control subjects. Interestingly, differences in whole-blood serotonin levels between groups were significant, which did not correlate with urinary 5-HIAA excretion. In contrast, urinary serotonin excretion was decreased in a group of autistic patients compared with nonautistic control subjects, and a subgroup of hyperserotonemic autistic patients had blunted levels relative to the control subjects (G. M. Anderson et al. 1989). Thus, these contradictory findings make it difficult to understand the possible relation between serotonin turnover and hyperserotonemia.

Studies have not identified increased levels of CSF 5-HIAA in autistic children relative to other patient control groups (D. J. Cohen et al. 1974, 1977; Gillberg et al. 1983a, 1983b; Leckman et al. 1980). CSF 5-HIAA levels in subgroups of hyperserotonemic autistic children have not been examined, and, moreover, the relation between CSF 5-HIAA levels and whole-blood serotonin has not been established. In summary, the relation between CSF 5-HIAA and serotonin dysfunction in autism has not been established.

Neurochemical challenge procedures provide indirect information about steady state and dynamic function of the central serotonin system via baseline and stimulated hormonal levels (e.g., prolactin, cortisol). Although no differences in baseline prolactin levels were found between groups of unmedicated autistic adolescents and adults relative to nonautistic control subjects (McBride et al. 1989a; Minderaa et al. 1989), after a single-dose administration of oral fenfluramine (a serotonin releasing agent and reuptake blocker), prolactin levels were blunted in the autistic patients (McBride et al. 1989a, 1989b). However, a blunted prolactin response to a serotonergic agent in a challenge setting is not unique to autistic patients; this type of response also has been documented in other groups of psychiatric patients, including those with OCD (Hollander et al. 1992), mood disorder (Coccaro et al. 1989; Siever et al. 1984), and impulsive-aggressive behavior (Coccaro et al. 1989). Furthermore, compulsive, depressive, and impulsive-aggressive behaviors are common in autistic patients. Alternatively, the serotonergic dysregulation found in autistic patients may reflect mediation via neurotransmitter system interactions, such as dopaminergic-serotonergic interactions (Cook 1990), that may or may not be specific to autism.

Norepinephrine and epinephrine. Studies of norepinephrine and epinephrine function may provide insight into problems associated with attention and arousal (impulsive, aggressive, self-injurious behavior) in autism, although the role appears to be limited. Although plasma norepinephrine and epinephrine levels were increased in autistic patients in several studies, some methodological limitations may have confounded findings (Cook et al. 1990; Lake et al. 1977; Launay et al. 1987; Leboyer et al. 1994; Leventhal et al. 1990). In platelet norepinephrine and epinephrine studies, both decreased levels (Launay et al. 1987) and normal uptake (Sankar 1970) were found in autistic patients. Similarly, levels of urinary norepinephrine and epinephrine (Young et al. 1978) and 3-methoxy-4-hydroxy-phenylglycol (MHPG) (Young et al. 1979) were decreased, and levels of urinary norepinephrine and epinephrine and MHPG excretion were normal (Launay et al. 1987). CSF findings showed no significant difference in CSF MHPG levels between autistic and control subjects (Gillberg et al. 1983b). In summary, the only consistent finding among neurobiological studies reported in the literature of norepinephrine and epinephrine function in autism was an increase in plasma norepinephrine and epinephrine, and these studies are not without methodological limitations.

Dopamine. The dopaminergic system has been associated with speech and communication skills and information-processing skills (i.e., use of cognitive strategies for efficient organization of information). These areas of cognitive functioning are impaired in autism. Increased dopamine levels have been associated with increased motoric and ticlike behavior, whereas decreased dopamine levels have been linked to decreased communication and information processing (functional deficits of autism).

Similar to other studies of neurotransmitter function in autism, dopaminergic function has been investigated via plasma, platelet, urine, and CSF studies. Studies have shown both elevated (Israngkun et al. 1986) and nonelevated levels of plasma dopamine (Launay et al. 1987) and its principal metabolite, plasma homovanillic acid (HVA) (Minderaa et al. 1989). Consistent with platelet norepinephrine and epinephrine findings, platelet dopamine levels were decreased in autistic subjects relative to control subjects (Launay et al. 1987). Urine dopamine studies have yielded mixed results: urinary HVA levels were elevated in groups of medicated autistic subjects (Garnier et al. 1986; Lelord et al. 1981), and urinary HVA excretion was nonelevated in unmedicated autistic subjects relative to nonautistic control subjects (Minderaa et al. 1989). Moreover, no difference in urinary dopamine concentration was found in autistic children relative to control subjects (Launay et al. 1987). Of note, blunted basal urinary HVA levels were found in children who responded to fenfluramine treatment relative to those who did not (Barthelemy et al. 1989). CSF HVA levels were elevated in autistic children (Gillberg et al. 1983b) relative to control subjects. This finding, along with the finding of decreased platelet dopamine in autistic patients, may be associated with dopamine D_2-receptor antagonist treatment efficacy (Cook 1990).

Thus, although impaired dopaminergic function has been shown, inconsistent findings have emerged with regard to its contribution to the pathogenesis of autism.

Peptides.   Opiate activity has been investigated in autism because behaviors associated with a dysregulated opiate system (i.e., self-injurious behavior, decreased pain sensitivity, stereotypies, attentional dysfunction, and social withdrawal) also have been associated with autism. Levels of CSF endorphin fraction II (Gillberg et al. 1985) and CSF β-endorphin (D. L. Ross et al. 1987) have been elevated in autistic children compared with control subjects. Abnormalities associated with the reduction of striatal β-endorphin content, which otherwise occurs through maturation, have been thought to contribute to the development of autistic disorder (D. L. Ross et al. 1987). Blood levels of endorphin H have been significantly decreased in autistic and schizophrenic subjects relative to control subjects (Weizman et al. 1984). In a replication study, median N-terminally directed β-endorphin immunoreactivity was slightly decreased in autistic children (boys and girls) and higher in children (girls) with Rett's disorder, whereas median C-terminally directed β-endorphin immunoreactivity was elevated in both samples (substantially more elevated in the autistic children) compared with nonimpaired control subjects (Leboyer et al. 1994). The authors report that this difference may suggest abnormalities in processing the pro-opiomelanocortin gene in autism.

In preclinical studies, oxytocin (the 9-amino acid peptide) induced affiliative and prosocial behavior in animals (Insel 1992), whereas administration of oxytocin antagonists resulted in social avoidance in certain animals. Interestingly, in another preclinical study, retention of a learned response was decreased either before treatment (1 hour prior) or after treatment (immediately following administration) with oxytocin (Bohus et al. 1978). This finding suggests that in rats, oxytocin administration may be related to attenuation of consolidation processes and retrieval processes, respectively. These studies provide direction for hypothesis-generating clinical research.

In summary, contradictory findings and methodological limitations are associated with much of the research on the neuropathology of autism. The most consistent findings suggest that patients with autism have abnormalities within the brain stem, cerebellum, midbrain, and frontal lobe. Although serotonergic and peptide function have been most vigorously researched and implicated in the neuropathology of autism, other neurotransmitter and peptide abnormalities have been implicated. Further research is needed to elucidate the underlying pathophysiology and the interrelationships among various neurobiological systems that may be associated with the development, behavioral manifestations, and treatment of autism.

Neuropsychological Patterns and Assessments

Investigations of neuropsychological function in autism have yielded findings that are consistent with neurological abnormalities found in the brain stem, cerebellum, midbrain, and frontal lobe. The range of neuropsychological deficits associated with the neuropathology reflects the complexity of and the interactions among the neuroanatomical, neurophysiological, and neurochemical abnormalities that have been linked to this disorder (for a review, see Huebner 1992). Neuropsychological deficits associated with autism include impairment in general intellectual ability (Bartak and Rutter 1976; Hoffman and Prior 1982); language capacities, especially verbal comprehension (Lincoln et al. 1988); attentional set-shifting (Courchesne et al. 1994b; C. Hughes et al. 1994); abstract problem-solving; cognitive flexibility (Rumsey and Hamburger 1988); socioemotional abilities (Fein et al. 1990); visual memory (Ameli et al. 1988); and motor planning (V. Jones and Prior 1985). Cognitive sparing of perceptual-motor function and rote memory have been demonstrated (Asarnow et al. 1987; Lincoln et al. 1988; Prior and Hoffman 1990).

More specifically, a large proportion (70%–80%) of children with autism are mentally deficient (Young et al. 1989). Although estimates of the male-to-female ratio range from 4:1 (Gillberg 1988) to 5:1 (Rapin 1988), the level of intellectual impairment has been estimated to be much greater in females than in males. Approximately 85% of females had IQ scores below 50 compared with 33% of males (DeLong and Dwyer 1988). Autistic patients performed significantly better on Wechsler Adult Intelligence Scale—Revised (Wechsler 1981; WAIS-R) performance subtests than on verbal subtests, especially verbal comprehension subtests (Asarnow et al. 1987; Lincoln et al. 1988; Smalley and Asarnow 1990), which suggests left-hemispheric dysfunction (Dawson et al. 1983; Hoffman and Prior 1982). However, not all studies showed significant language deficits in autism (Rumsey and Hamburger 1988). Impaired verbal and nonverbal problem-solving, especially related to social and conceptual reasoning, lends support to frontal-lobe-subcortical dysfunction (Prior and Hoffman 1990; Rumsey and Hamburger 1988).

Autistic children also have socioemotional deficits. In one study, autistic children had difficulty recognizing emotional gestures, context, vocalization, and tone (Hobson 1986). Two schools of thought exist regarding the basis for socioemotional impairment in autism. One line of thinking characterizes social aloofness as a primary element of autism that contributes to impaired cognitive development (Fein et al. 1986). A second perspective suggests that autistic children have a fundamental cognitive disorder characterized by impairment in the development of a theory of mind (Baron-Cohen 1991; Leslie and Frith 1990), that is, the ability to incorporate another person's beliefs or knowledge. Autistic children had difficulty in perceiving a situation from another individual's perspective or in alternative ways (i.e., metarepresentation), including role-playing and imaginative play, predicting another person's behavior, and exhibiting empathy (Baron-Cohen 1991; Leslie and Frith 1990).

Moreover, these children had language deficits related to a theory of mind. Thus, socioemotional deficits that manifest may be a function of cognitive impairment in autism.

Attention deficits have been evidenced by excessive attention to detail (Fein et al. 1990) and impaired ability to shift attention rapidly and accurately between auditory and visual stimuli (Courchesne et al. 1994b). These authors suggested that the findings correspond to an association between capacity to shift attention and cerebellar abnormalities (Courchesne et al. 1994b). Moreover, attentional deficits associated with abnormal cerebellar development may contribute to impaired cognitive and social development (Botez et al. 1985; Courchesne et al. 1994b; Hamilton et al. 1983). Alternatively, deficits in attentional set-shifting and planning have been associated with executive function and frontal-lobe activity in autistic adolescents (C. Hughes et al. 1994).

Autistic patients had deficits in visual memory recognition for meaningless material, thought to reflect impairment in cognitive flexibility and poor generalization of task learning and, thus, compromised frontal-lobe function (Ameli et al. 1988). This proposal contrasts the idea that memory impairment in autism may be mediated by hippocampal-amygdala function related to behavioral rigidity and socioemotional deficits.

Motor and visuomotor deficits in autistic patients generally have been thought to reflect difficulties with cognitive flexibility. In one study, among a group of autistic children, dyspraxia (e.g., difficulty imitating arm and hand gestures) and neurological soft signs (e.g., choreiform movements, coordination and balance difficulties, tactile stimulation discrimination difficulty, thumb-finger touching difficulty, impaired speech-sound production) (V. Jones and Prior 1985) were found, thought to be associated with impairment in play and functional skill development.

In summary, neuropsychological deficits in autism include cognitive deficits such as compromised IQ, impaired verbal and nonverbal reasoning and abstract thinking, inferential thinking, and a lack of metarepresentation. Socioemotional deficits have been associated with impaired social reasoning, empathy, and adaptability; theory of mind; and deficits in socially laden language. Attention and memory deficits include excessive attentional detailing, poor attentional regulation, perseveration, and lack of memory for nonmeaningful visual information. Motor impairment includes poor motor and visuomotor coordination, neurological soft signs, and dyspraxia. With this complex array of impairment, it is not surprising that individuals with autism frequently have great difficulty navigating through daily life.

Neuropsychological assessment of children with autism should begin with diagnostic inventories/interviews; tests of general intelligence, adaptive functioning, academic achievement, and specific neuropsychological functions; and a neurological soft sign examination. Diagnostic inventories, after assessment on the basis of DSM-IV (American Psychiatric Association 1994) criteria, include the Autism Diagnostic Interview-R (ADI-R; Rutter et al. 1990a), a semistructured psychiatric interview of the patient's primary caregiver or family member (1–2 hours); the Autism Diagnostic Observation Schedule (ADOS; Lord et al. 1989), a clinician behavioral observation of autistic individuals (half-hour), or the Pre-Linguistic Autism Diagnostic Observation Schedule (PL-ADOS; DiLavore et al. 1995); and the Child Autism Rating Scale (CARS; Schopler et al. 1988), a dimensional 15-scale instrument (half-hour).

Tests of general intellectual functioning include the Wechsler Intelligence Scale for Children, Third Edition (WISC-III; Wechsler 1991), the Leiter International Performance Scale (Leiter 1969), and the Raven's Coloured Progressive Matrices (Raven 1947). Adaptive functioning can be assessed with the Vineland Adaptive Behavior Scales (Sparrow et al. 1984). Achievement tests include the Wechsler Individual Achievement Test (Psychological Corporation 1992) and the Wide Range Achievement Test, 3rd Edition (Wilkinson 1993). Discrepancies between intellectual and academic functioning, as well as between intellectual and adaptive functioning, will identify specific learning disabilities or mental retardation.

Language tests include the TOLD—P:3 (Newcomer and Hammill 1998), verbal fluency tests such as animal naming and the Benton Verbal Fluency Test (Benton and Hamsher 1983), the Peabody Picture Vocabulary Test—Revised (PPVT-R; Dunn and Dunn 1981), and the Test of Linguistic Competency (TLC; Wiig and Secord 1988) to test figurative language skills.

Learning and memory tests include the Wide Range Assessment of Memory and Learning (WRAML; Sheslow and Adams 1990) and the Buschke Selective Reminding Test (Buschke 1973). Tests of attention and executive function include target detection tests, continuous performance tests (e.g., Vigil Computerized Test 1993), the Trail Making Test (Reitan 1969a), the Matching Familiar Figures Test (MFFT; Kagan et al. 1964), the Wisconsin Card Sorting Test (WCST; Heaton 1981), the Stroop Color and Word Test (Golden 1978; Stroop 1935), and the Rey-

Osterrieth Complex Figure (Osterrieth 1944; Rey 1941) (copy, immediate, and delayed memory).

Visual and sensory perception may be assessed by the Money's Road Map Test of Direction Sense (Money et al. 1965), the Numberless Clocks/Draw-a-Clock (Mattis 1988), the Motor-Free Visual Perception Test (Colarusso and Hammill 1996), and a clinical examination that evaluates visual fields and double simultaneous stimulation, stereognosis, graphesthesia, and finger agnosia.

Motor and graphomotor function may be evaluated by the Purdue Pegboard Test (Tiffin 1968; Tiffin and Asher 1948), the Grooved Pegboard, the Denckla Motor Performance Battery: revised PANESS (Denckla 1985), the Developmental Test of Visual-Motor Integration (VMI; Beery and Buktenica 1989), and the Alternating Writing Sequence (Mattis 1988).

Assessments of facial recognition, emotional labeling, and empathy include the Benton Facial Recognition Test (Benton et al. 1994), the Pictures of Facial Affect test (Ekman and Friesen 1976), and the Rosenzweig Picture Frustration Test (Rosenzweig 1978).

Treatment

Nonpharmacological treatment. Nonpharmacological treatment of autism includes megavitamin treatment, physical and sensory stimulation, vigorous aerobic exercise, dietary intervention, and facilitated communication. However, the usefulness and generalizability of these therapies are limited because scientific validity and reliability are lacking. Intensive behavioral and educational programming, including parental training, has been used to treat autism in preschool children (Lovaas 1987). A "squeeze machine" (Grandin and Scariano 1986) and holding techniques (Zappella 1990) have been used to create an intensive pressure around the body to help calm and organize an autistic child's behavior when he or she is overaroused or in a rage. Social skills training groups also have been conducted, during which the focus is on skill development in pretending and perceiving emotions and social responses. Exaggeration of facial expression may enhance learning of associated emotional labels. Play therapy that permits the autistic child to initiate activities and to have choices has been found to decrease social avoidance (Koegel et al. 1987).

Pharmacological treatment. Based on evidence that implicates serotonin dysfunction, pharmacological agents that affect the serotonin system have been investigated. Treatment studies with lysergic acid diethylamide (LSD) (Bender et al. 1963; Freedman et al. 1962), imipramine (Campbell et al. 1971), lithium (Campbell et al. 1972), 5-hydroxytryptophan (5-HTP) (Sverd et al. 1978), buspirone (Realmuto et al. 1989), and risperidone (Purdon et al. 1994) have been conducted in children and adults with autism. These studies were open, uncontrolled treatment trials with small and sometimes diagnostically mixed patient samples and mixed results. Treatment with serotonin reuptake inhibitors has resulted in somewhat more consistent findings, such that fluvoxamine (McDougle et al. 1990, 1996), fluoxetine (Mehlinger et al. 1990), and sertraline (McDougle et al. 1998) treatment yielded positive findings, whereas clomipramine yielded both positive (C. T. Gordon et al. 1992) and negative findings (Sanchez et al. 1996). Fenfluramine, a serotonin releaser and reuptake inhibitor, also yielded mixed findings regarding treatment efficacy (Campbell 1988; E. Geller et al. 1982; Ritvo et al. 1986b).

In an open treatment study of eight autistic adults (Ratey et al. 1987a, 1987b), treatment with β-blockers (propranolol or nadolol), which block norepinephrine receptors and reduce overall norepinephrine transmission, led to a reduction in aggressive, impulsive, and self-injurious behavior, and socialization and speech also improved. Of note, many of these patients were also receiving neuroleptic or mood-stabilizing drugs. A reduction in chronic hyperarousal was thought to be associated with symptom improvement. In a double-blind, placebo-controlled crossover study, an α_2 noradrenergic receptor antagonist, clonidine, moderately decreased hyperactivity and irritability in eight autistic boys according to parent and teacher ratings (Jaselskis et al. 1992). Clinician ratings, however, showed no difference.

Dopamine antagonists have been found to reduce hyperactivity, stereotypies, and speech and communication impairment in autistic children, as has been observed in several double-blind, placebo-controlled treatment studies with haloperidol (L. T. Anderson et al. 1989; Campbell et al. 1978; Naruse et al. 1982; R. Perry et al. 1989), pimozide (Naruse et al. 1982), and trifluoperazine (Fish et al. 1966). These findings were independent of sedative effects of these medications. The undesirable side effects of neuroleptics limit their use. Treatment with dopamine agonists has yielded mixed findings. Decreased withdrawal, communication deficits, stereotypies, and idiosyncratic responses to the environment were found in an open trial of bromocriptine, but treatment with L-dopa has not been effective (Campbell et al. 1976; Ritvo et al. 1971). Amphetamines, indirect dopamine agonists, exacerbated stereotypies and hyperactivity in some autistic children (Campbell et al. 1972).

Opioid receptor antagonists, such as naltrexone, have been used to treat particular core symptoms in autistic patients. Increased prosocial behavior (Campbell et al. 1989; Herman et al. 1993; Kolmen et al. 1995) and decreased stereotypies (Campbell et al. 1989; Herman et al. 1993; Leboyer et al. 1992), hyperactivity, inattention (Campbell et al. 1989; Kolmen et al. 1995; Leboyer et al. 1992), and self-injurious behavior (Herman 1990; Leboyer et al. 1992) were found after treatment with naltrexone, although self-injurious behavior did not decline in all studies (Willemsen-Swinkels et al. 1995).

Asperger's Disorder

Diagnostic Criteria and Definition

Asperger's disorder is characterized by "severe and sustained impairment in social interaction . . . and the development of restricted, repetitive patterns of behavior, interests, and activities" (American Psychiatric Association 1994, p. 75) that cause significant impairment in daily living, such as in social and occupational functioning. There are no clinically significant delays in language, cognitive, age-appropriate self-help skill, and adaptive behavior development (except for social impairment) as is often observed in autism (American Psychiatric Association 1994). In one study, no significant differences were found between individuals with Asperger's disorder and individuals with autistic disorder on measures of nonverbal communication, nonverbal cognition, and motor development (Szatmari et al. 1995).

Impairment in social interaction may be reflected by limited and/or inappropriate use of nonverbal communication skills used to facilitate social behavior, such as eye-to-eye gaze, facial expression, posturing, and gesturing. Facial expression may be limited, except with strong emotions such as anger or misery. Vocal intonation tends to be monotonous or exaggerated. Gestures may be limited or exaggerated, clumsy, or inappropriate to speech content. Comprehension of others' gestures or expressions may be poor. Subtle verbal jokes may not be understood. Social impairment may also manifest in limited development of age-appropriate peer relationships, a lack of shared interests or pleasures with others, and a lack of socioemotional reciprocity (American Psychiatric Association 1994). Individuals with Asperger's disorder have difficulty comprehending and using rules governing social behavior, which consequently appears naive and peculiar.

Restricted and repetitive interests may manifest in preoccupation with a behavior, activity, or interest in which the intensity or focus is beyond the normal range. Further, these characteristics may be observed in nonfunctional, rigid patterns of behavior; stereotyped and repetitive motor movements (e.g., hand flapping); or preoccupation with parts of objects (American Psychiatric Association 1994).

Developmental delays in Asperger's disorder may be observed in the acquisition of motor milestones. Motor clumsiness may develop, and posture and gait may appear odd. Difficulty with games involving motor skills may be apparent, and writing and drawing skills may be impaired.

Speech content is impoverished and is often heavily attached to minute details or lengthy discourse on favorite subjects. Thought processes are usually confined to a narrow, literal, but logical sequence of reasoning. Pronouns may not be used correctly, with substitutions of second or third person for first-person forms. Specific learning problems affecting arithmetic, reading, and writing skills may develop. Despite these difficulties, excellent rote memory often develops, and full command of grammar is usually acquired.

Psychological difficulties may manifest in the form of adjustment problems, especially during adolescence. At this time, patients may develop varying degrees of anxiety and depression in relation to the awareness of their differences from others.

Although Asperger's disorder has been categorized in DSM-IV as a pervasive developmental disorder, debate continues as to whether it truly represents a qualitatively distinct diagnostic entity or is a less severe form of autism. Furthermore, the phenomenological and neuropsychological profile of Asperger's disorder also parallels learning disorders such as nonverbal learning disabilities syndrome (Rourke 1989), developmental learning disability of the right hemispheres (Denckla 1983; Voeller 1986), and semantic-pragmatic disorder (Bishop 1989). Neuropsychological deficits found in these disorders include visuospatial, graphomotor, complex motor, organizational, and sequential difficulties, similar to those found in Asperger's disorder. Moreover, social interaction deficits associated with these learning disorders parallel those found in Asperger's disorder and include difficulty recognizing faces and facial expressions, difficulty recognizing rhythm and intonation in speech and gesture, difficulty with speech pragmatics, misinterpretation of tactile stimulation (e.g., a handshake) in social situations, and difficulty understanding cause-and-effect relationships (Brumback et al. 1996).

More specifically, Rourke (1988) described neuropsychological, academic, and socioemotional and adaptive deficits associated with non-verbal learning disability. Neuropsychological deficits have been characterized by impaired

◆ Tactile perception, especially left-sided
◆ Visual discrimination and recognition of visual detail and relationships
◆ Psychomotor coordination, especially left-sided
◆ Integration of novel material
◆ Attention and memory for nonverbal, complex material, especially visual or tactile
◆ Exploratory behavior
◆ Concept formation and problem-solving
◆ Articulation, speech prosody, and linguistic pragmatics

Areas of academic difficulty include

◆ Graphomotor skills (difficulty with printing and writing)
◆ Reading comprehension
◆ Mechanical arithmetic and mathematical reasoning
◆ Academic subjects that require problem-solving and concept formation (e.g., science)

Socioemotional difficulties include

◆ Acclimation to new situations
◆ Social perception, judgment, and interactions, with withdrawal and isolation throughout course
◆ Psychiatric disorders such as anxiety and depression
◆ Hyperactivity, especially during childhood (for a full review, see Rourke 1988)

As is evident, the phenomenological and neuropsychological profile of a nonverbal learning disability mimics the Asperger's disorder profile. Thus, neuropsychological and neurobiological research may help to provide insights into the categorical exclusivity given to Asperger's disorder in DSM-IV.

Prevalence

No large-scale epidemiological study has been conducted, so prevalence rates of Asperger's disorder are unknown. One British study suggested a conservative estimate of 1.7 per 10,000 based on a clinically referred sample of physically and mentally disabled children in London (Wing 1981). Another study reported estimates from a nonretarded sample in the range of 10–26 per 10,000 (Gillberg and Gillberg 1989). Sex ratio estimates from these studies suggest a male-to-female ratio ranging from 4:1 to 9:1.

Etiology

Although little is known about the familial and environmental factors associated with Asperger's disorder, some evidence of familiality has been reported (Burgoine and Wing 1983; Gillberg and Gillberg 1989; Gillberg et al. 1987; Wing 1981). As observed in autism (DeLong and Dwyer 1988), a strong family history of bipolar illness was found in one case study of Asperger's syndrome (Gillberg 1985). Of note, Asperger's disorder was more common among relatives of nonretarded autistic probands than among retarded autistic probands, whereas the rate of bipolar disorder did not differ significantly between these groups (Pennington 1991a).

Environmental factors may be linked to the development of Asperger's disorder. In one study, about half of the patient sample had pre-, peri-, or postnatal complications (Wing 1981). Similarly, in another study, perinatal and neonatal histories included hemorrhage, obstructed labor with ruptured membranes, and anoxia in 12 boys later given the diagnosis of Asperger's disorder (Rickarby et al. 1991).

Extensive research is needed to identify further the familial, genetic, and environmental factors associated with Asperger's disorder.

Pathology and Neuropsychological Function

Very little is known about the underlying pathophysiology of Asperger's disorder. As reported in single case studies, abnormal left-hemispheric (El Badri and Lewis 1993; P. B. Jones and Kerwin 1990) and cerebellar (El Badri and Lewis 1993) function and agenesis or partial agenesis of the corpus callosum (David et al. 1993) were found in patients with Asperger's disorder.

In another study, patients with Tourette's disorder and comorbid Asperger's disorder (Tourette's with Asperger's disorder) and patients with Tourette's disorder without comorbid Asperger's disorder (Tourette's without Asperger's disorder) underwent MRI procedures. Five of seven Tourette's with Asperger's disorder patients and one of nine

Tourette's without Asperger's disorder patients had abnormal MRI scans (Berthier et al. 1993). In the Tourette's with Asperger's disorder group, anomalies included 1) abnormalities in the right central perisylvian area; 2) incomplete formation of the posterior-inferior frontal gyrus, inferior precentral gyrus, and anterior portion of the superior temporal gyrus, resulting in widening of the sylvian fissure and partial exposure of the insular cortex; 3) hypoplasia of the right temporo-occipital cortex; 4) small gyri in the posterior parietal lobes; and 5) moderate enlargement of the right lateral ventricle. The Tourette's with Asperger's disorder patients had significantly more schizoid traits, unsociability, emotional detachment, abnormalities in nonverbal expression, and neurological soft signs than the Tourette's without Asperger's disorder patients. Further, neuropsychological tests yielded poorer performance on tests of motor functioning, cognitive flexibility, and spatial orientation. Thus, this study implicates structural brain abnormalities, CNS dysfunction, and associated impairment in cognitive flexibility, spatial orientation, and motor function in Asperger's disorder.

In Asperger's disorder, cortical anomalies have been viewed as developmental and have been linked to abnormalities in neuronal migration, which occurs before the end of month 5 of gestation (Berthier et al. 1990; Piven et al. 1990). Brain imaging studies have identified areas of polymicrogyria in the cerebral cortex of patients with Asperger's disorder (Berthier et al. 1990), which suggests neurodevelopmental cortical anomalies in Asperger's disorder. Moreover, the localization and overall appearance of the MRI abnormalities were consistent with neuropathological studies of polymicrogyria (Becker et al. 1989; M. D. Cohen et al. 1989), offering additional evidence for neurodevelopmental abnormalities in Asperger's disorder.

Developmental Course

Onset (or recognition of the onset) of symptoms in Asperger's disorder appears somewhat later in life than the onset of autism. This delay in recognition may be related to the relatively spared language and cognitive abilities in Asperger's disorder (Klin 1994). Asperger's disorder is considered a lifelong disorder, and the full impact may not be realized until adolescence or young adulthood. During this period, development of social relationships is critical. Awareness of atypical development in this arena may precipitate anxiety, mood disorders, and suicidal behavior (Wing 1981). Prognosis may be affected by the occurrence of comorbid illness.

Neuropsychological Patterns and Assessments

Neuropsychological studies in Asperger's disorder have yielded mixed findings with regard to cognitive functioning. Both similarities and differences have been found between individuals with Asperger's disorder and individuals with high-functioning autism. These two diagnostic groups have been discriminated by differences in clinical features, including social responsiveness, imaginative play, and types of restricted interests or preoccupations, and may be associated more with level of severity than with etiological differences (Szatmari et al. 1989a; Wing 1981). Distinguishing cognitive functions associated with Asperger's disorder and high-functioning autism has been more controversial and inconsistent. Differences in sample selection, based on the lack of standard diagnostic criteria prior to DSM-IV, have contributed to these inconsistencies and have made it difficult to compare studies. For example, in one study, patients with Asperger's disorder and autism (IQ > 85) showed significant impairment on both verbal and performance measures on the Wechsler Intelligence Scales relative to an outpatient control group (Szatmari et al. 1990). Language comprehension, facial recognition, and motor coordination were substantially impaired in both groups compared with the control group. Variation in the pattern of deficits in patients with Asperger's disorder and high-functioning autism was thought to be associated with developmental level rather than absolute differences in cognitive function. In another study, executive function was impaired among individuals with high-functioning autism and Asperger's disorder and those with high-functioning autism without Asperger's disorder. However, only the high-functioning autism without Asperger's disorder group had difficulty on theory of mind tasks (Ozonoff et al. 1991).

In contrast, other investigations have yielded divergent findings between individuals with Asperger's disorder and individuals with high-functioning autism. Discrepancies in Verbal Scale IQ and Performance Scale IQ have been found. Verbal Scale IQ has been found to be greater than Performance Scale IQ in Asperger's disorder and Performance Scale IQ greater than Verbal Scale IQ in high-functioning autism (Dawson et al. 1983; Gillberg 1989; Klin et al. 1995; Lincoln et al. 1988; Volkmar et al. 1994; Wing 1981). Individuals with Asperger's disorder may have a higher Full Scale and Verbal Scale IQ than those with high-functioning autism (Ramberg et al. 1996).

More recently, studies have found a Verbal Scale IQ greater than Performance Scale IQ in Asperger's disorder but no IQ discrepancy in high-functioning autism (Klin et al. 1995; Minshew 1992; Volkmar et al. 1994). Moreover, individuals with Asperger's disorder, compared with high-functioning autistic patients, had greater deficits in 1) gross and fine motor skills, 2) visuomotor integration, 3) visuospatial perception, 4) visual memory, and 5) nonverbal concept formation. By contrast, those with high-functioning autism, relative to patients with Asperger's disorder, had increased deficits in 1) auditory perception, 2) verbal memory, 3) articulation, 4) vocabulary, and 5) verbal output. No significant between-group differences were found in the frequency of deficits in novel and rote material, verbal content and concept formation, prosody, pragmatics, word decoding, reading/comprehension, arithmetic, social competence, and emotional material. Language comprehension may not discriminate between the two groups once the effects of IQ have been accounted for (Ramberg et al. 1996).

Following diagnostic assessments based on DSM-IV criteria and the ADI-R, neuropsychological assessment should be comprehensive and include tests of general intellectual and adaptive functioning, academic achievement, communication skills, and discrete neuropsychological and psychological functions. Tests of general intelligence include the WISC-III, the WAIS-R, and Raven's Progressive Matrices, with specific emphasis on problem-solving, concept formation, and visual-perceptual skills. Adaptive functioning tests should focus on social development and the level of self-sufficiency in daily living. Academic achievement should be compared with IQ levels to diagnose specific learning disabilities. Communication skills assessments should include tests of articulation, tone, and pitch. The clinician should also administer receptive and expressive language assessments of syntactic, semantic, figurative, and pragmatic language skills. Nonverbal communication skills (e.g., gaze and gesturing) and the nature, content, and coherence of verbal production should be examined. Additional neuropsychological assessments should include examination of executive functions, verbal and nonverbal concept formation, visual memory, visual-perceptual skills, visuomotor integration, motor function, and emotional labeling. (See subsection "Neuropsychological Patterns and Assessments" in the "Autism" section earlier in this chapter for specific instruments.)

Psychological assessments should include 1) observation of social and affective presentation and interaction, 2) metarepresentation, 3) identification of restricted interests and use of leisure time, 4) development of peer relationships, 5) response to unfamiliar situations, 6) use of compensatory adaptive strategies, and 7) mood and anxiety symptoms and disorders.

Treatment

Remediation and treatment may vary according to the particular cluster of neurocognitive deficits and comorbid disorders in the individual.

Nonpharmacological treatment. Instruction in the use of compensatory mechanisms may help the patient circumvent impaired areas. Skill development should be taught in a straightforward and rote manner, with sequential, parts-to-whole verbal instruction (Klin 1994). Development of problem-solving skills, especially in novel and social situations, is critical. Social skills groups should focus on development of comprehending and expressing nonverbal behavior with regard to social interaction. This type of treatment requires direct and explicit instruction; practice in a structured setting; and support, reassurance, and feedback in noncontrolled daily living situations (Foss 1991).

Pharmacological treatment. Pharmacological treatment of symptom clusters in Asperger's disorder may mirror treatment of the same in autism. In addition, serotonin reuptake inhibitors (e.g., clomipramine) and selective serotonin reuptake inhibitors (SSRIs) (e.g., fluvoxamine, fluoxetine, sertraline) may be used to treat comorbid depression and OCD, and antianxiety agents, such as buspirone or clonazepam, may be used to reduce comorbid anxiety. Note that because patients with Asperger's disorder have difficulty identifying and verbalizing emotions, they may have difficulty recognizing and describing their mood and anxiety symptoms. Therefore, the treating clinician must carefully monitor the potential development of these conditions. (For treatment of socioemotional impairment and the compulsive, restricted, stereotyped behaviors, refer to the references cited in the "Pharmacological Treatment" subsection in the "Autism" section earlier in this chapter.)

◆ ATTENTION-DEFICIT/ HYPERACTIVITY DISORDER

Diagnostic Criteria and Definition

ADHD is associated with the core symptoms of attentional dysfunction, defective response inhibition or impulsivity, and motor restlessness or hyperactivity. Symptoms must begin before age 7 years, are maladaptive, and are inconsistent with the individual's developmental level (American Psychiatric Association 1994). DSM-IV diagnostic criteria require that ADHD-related behaviors exist in at least two different settings (e.g., home, school), cause significant impairment, and not be better accounted for by another disorder.

Inattention symptoms include difficulty 1) attending to detail, 2) sustaining attention, 3) following instructions and tasks to completion, 4) organizing, and 5) keeping objects necessary to perform tasks. *Hyperactivity* symptoms include 1) fidgeting, 2) difficulty staying in a seat, 3) being restless, 4) running or climbing (if age inappropriate), 5) difficulty playing quietly, 6) behaving as if "driven by a motor," and 7) talking excessively. *Impulsivity* symptoms include 1) blurting out responses before questions are completely asked, 2) difficulty awaiting one's turn, and 3) interrupting or intruding on others (e.g., bursting into activities or conversation).

ADHD may be diagnosed when 1) both inattention and hyperactivity-impulsivity are primarily present; 2) inattention is the primary feature, and hyperactivity or impulsivity symptoms have not been evident for the past 6 months; or 3) hyperactivity-impulsivity is predominant, and inattention symptoms have not been evident for the past 6 months (American Psychiatric Association 1994).

Comorbidity

Biederman et al. (1991c) reported comorbidity rates for clinically referred patients with ADHD: 30%–50% for conduct/oppositional defiant disorder, 15%–75% for mood disorders, 10%–92% for learning disabilities, and 25% for anxiety disorders. ADHD is more common in first-degree biological relatives of child probands with ADHD than in non-ADHD control probands (Faraone et al. 1997). In addition, the prevalence of mood, anxiety, learning, and substance disorders and antisocial personality disorder is greater in first-degree biological relatives of ADHD probands than in non-ADHD control probands (Biederman et al. 1991a, 1991b). Such comorbidity and associated social and academic difficulties suggest a heterogeneous disorder and contribute to clinical complexity, which significantly influences conceptions of etiology, prognosis, and treatment.

Prevalence

The estimated prevalence of ADHD varies widely as a function of whether DSM-III, DSM-III-R (American Psychiatric Association 1980, 1987), or DSM-IV diagnostic criteria were used. Prevalence estimates also vary depending on the populations sampled and whether attention deficit disorder (ADD) without hyperactivity was included. ADD without hyperactivity is approximately half as prevalent as strictly defined ADHD. Nationwide prevalence estimates of ADHD in school-age children are 3%–5% (American Psychiatric Association 1987, 1994). Prevalence data for adolescence and adulthood are limited.

Pathology and Neuropsychological Function

In addition to inattention, distractibility, restlessness, and motor activity, a host of physical, cognitive, academic, behavior, and social problems occur in children with ADHD. Minor physical anomalies (Fogel et al. 1985); neurological soft signs, such as impaired fine motor coordination, balance difficulties, and clumsiness; and frontal-lobe deficits on neuropsychological tests have been found in ADHD. These findings implicate CNS mechanisms in the development of ADHD symptoms (Anastopoulos and Barkley 1988; Chelune et al. 1986; Lou et al. 1984). However, the pathophysiology of ADHD is not well understood. Therefore, the clinician should evaluate the functional neuropsychiatric status of the child's CNS, because it pertains, in part, to neuropsychological competencies.

The right cerebral hemisphere plays a role in vigilance (Weinberg and Harper 1993), maintenance of attention, processing of visuospatial information, and expression and interpretation of emotional stimuli (Flor-Henry 1979; Heilman et al. 1985; Mesulam 1981; E. D. Ross 1981). Voeller (1987) found that 93% of children with right-hemisphere deficits had ADD with or without hyperactivity. Brumback and Staton (1982) also suggested the relation between right-hemisphere involvement, ADHD, and depression; they postulated that ADHD results from anatomical dysfunction—either cortical damage or delayed cortical maturation of the right cerebral hemisphere. Voeller and Heilman (1988) added that ADHD may result from either right-hemisphere dysfunction or dysfunction of related brain stem and diencephalic structures subserving attentional functions. Heilman et al. (1991) found that this theory was consistent with the speculation that behavioral abnormalities in ADHD reflect functional impairment of frontal striatal systems with which the right, nondominant hemisphere has preferential involvement. Moreover, MRI findings of low brain volumes in the corpus callosum regions and significantly smaller mean right caudate volume in ADHD than in control boys (Castellanos et al. 1994) likewise support developmental abnormalities of frontal striatal circuits in ADHD. Further corroboration is found in the neuropsychological literature on deficient "frontal-lobe functioning" in children and adolescents with ADHD (Grodzinsky and Diamond 1992).

Developmental Course

Excessive motor activity is typically first identified when the children are toddlers. The disorder usually is first diagnosed during grade school, when behavior is disruptive in the classroom, and remains stable through early adolescence. In most cases, symptoms diminish in late adolescence and adulthood; a minority of individuals have full symptomatology into adulthood. Follow-up studies of childhood-onset ADHD provide the most reliable source of information about adult residua. Milder behavioral problems and ADHD symptoms persist in an estimated 50%–65% of young adults. Comorbid adult disorders include antisocial personality disorder and substance abuse, particularly alcohol abuse. Lower educational and socioeconomic status was found, with academic failures significantly noted in adulthood more often than in control subjects or in comparison with their own siblings (for a full review, see Weiss and Hechtman 1986). Furthermore, adults with ADHD are less able to work independently, less persistent in completing tasks, and less likely to maintain stable relationships with supervisors than are adults without ADHD (Gittelman et al. 1985; Weiss and Hechtman 1986). Intelligence, absence of aggressivity, and family environment contribute to better outcome. Nevertheless, academic problems provide the greatest risk for consequent vocational underachievement, regardless of intelligence and emotional stability. Because adults are expected to operate with well-developed executive functions (e.g., attention, inhibition, organization, goal-setting and maintenance), deficits in these capacities create havoc in academic, vocational, and interpersonal functioning (Kane et al. 1990; Weiss and Hechtman 1986).

Neuropsychological Patterns and Assessments

Neuropsychological evaluation should not be used to diagnose ADHD nor should it be used alone to establish prognosis and plan treatment. Observational and informant adjunctive instruments in addition to clinical interviews with the child or adolescent and parents are required to obtain a full behavioral profile of the child or adolescent. Parent rating scales include the Conners Parent Rating Scale—Revised (CPRS-R; Goyette et al. 1978) and the Child Behavior Checklist (CBCL; Achenbach and Edelbrock 1983). Teacher rating scales include the Conners Teacher Rating Scale—Revised (CTRS-R; Goyette et al. 1978) and the Child Behavior Checklist—Teacher Report Form (CBCL-TRF; Edelbrock and Achenbach 1986). (For a full review of such ADHD patient and informant rating scales, see Barkley 1990.)

Neuropsychological evaluation provides the opportunity to assess, in the controlled environment of the test situation, ADHD components of rule-governed behavior, executive processes, inattention, and behavioral inhibition in comparison to data from normative samples. However, no sine qua non neuropsychological evaluation or test pattern characterizes the child or adolescent with ADHD. Therefore, the examination of qualitative as well as quantitative aspects of the child's performance is crucial in the evaluation. Aspects such as problem-solving style, task approach and preferences, planning and strategy implementation, set-shifting, and particularly compensatory mechanisms all constitute qualitative task performance variables that provide significant information about academic planning and remediation for the child or adolescent with ADHD. Other extratest variables for consideration include the relative contribution of medication to task performance and psychological variables such as motivation, esteem, and attributions made for success and failure.

Hallmark neuropsychological features of ADHD are intertest and intratest "scatter," or variability, in which the child fails simple items and responds correctly to more difficult items. This outcome is accounted for by waxing and waning attention. In addition, Zentall (1986) claimed that variability is likewise dependent on the test stimulus in ADHD; for example, performance is poorer when tasks are overly familiar. Finally, task difficulty or variability may result if tasks are not only familiar but also perceived as rote or boring, such as memorizing definitions for vocabulary words, historical dates and events, or multiplication tables. The clinician should ascertain whether difficulties on such tasks result from inattention or boredom or from specific learning disabilities, such as auditory recall or visuoperceptual deficits. Because approximately 25% of children with ADHD have some type of learning disability, neuropsychological assessment may include a "second-level" (Barkley 1990) evaluation in which more specific information is required about ability and risk for such learning disability.

Neuropsychological evaluation of ADHD first must include solid measures of baseline cognitive and intellectual functioning, such as the WISC-III. Typical neuropsychological evaluations have included vigilance tasks such as the continuous performance tasks (CPTs). CPTs are used to assess attention and routinely distinguish children with ADHD from children without ADHD (Horn et al. 1989; Seidel and Joschko 1990). Omission scores on the CPT are believed to measure inattention (Aman and Turbott 1986). The CPT has many variations, including visual and auditory versions, such as the Conners Computerized Continuous Performance Test (Conners 1994), the Vigil Continuous Performance Test (1993), and the Test of Variables of Attention (TOVA; Greenberg and Waldman 1993). The most widely adopted CPT in clinical practice is the Gordon Diagnostic System (Gordon 1983). Several pencil-and-paper CPT versions have been used in the absence of computerized CPTs (e.g., the Children's Checking Test [CCT]) and often have been termed *cancellation tasks* (Margolis 1972).

Time estimation tests also have been conducted to distinguish children with and without ADHD (Barkley et al. 1997). Children with ADHD were less accurate than control subjects at most durations of temporal reproductions and were affected by distraction. Time estimation improved after administration of methylphenidate.

One of the earliest and most commonly used measures of impulsivity is the MFFT. The differential reinforcement of low rate behavior is another impulsivity task that significantly differentiates children with ADHD from children without ADHD (McClure and Gordon 1984). Delay of gratification paradigms have been increasingly used as tests of impulsivity (Rapport et al. 1986), in which ADHD subjects select immediate over delayed reward tasks (Schweitzer and Sulzer 1995).

The neuropsychological evaluation also should include tasks of neuropsychiatric status, including coordination, involuntary movements, sensory and visuospatial functioning, and laterality (such as an examination for neurological soft signs) (Denckla 1985). Because a review of neuropsychological studies suggested that children with ADHD and ADD without hyperactivity may differ electrophysiologically and that children with ADD without hyperactivity may have automaticity impairments similar to those in children with learning disabilities (Goodyear et al. 1992), automaticity should be evaluated by the Rapid Automatized Naming Test (RAN) or similar tasks. Distractibility may be assessed by the Stroop Color and Word Test. Immediate visual recall may be assessed by the Benton Visual Retention Test—Revised (BVRT-R; Benton 1974) and visual organization by the Rey-Osterrieth Complex Figure. Immediate and delayed visual and verbal learning and memory can be evaluated by the WRAML, and verbal learning also may be evaluated by the Rey Auditory-Verbal Learning Test (RVLT; Rey 1964) and the California Verbal Learning Test—Children's Version (CVLT-C; Delis et al. 1994). Anticipation and planning may be assessed by the Porteus Maze Test (Porteus 1933, 1942) and the maze test of the WISC-III. The assessment of motor skills is an important part of the neuropsychological test battery because up to 52% of children with ADHD in comparison to up to 35% of children without ADHD are characterized as having poor motor coordination (Szatmari et al. 1989b), in particular, fine motor coordination (Shaywitz and Shaywitz 1984). Motor function is assessed by tasks such as the Purdue Pegboard Test (Tiffin 1968; Tiffin and Asher 1948), the Kaufman Assessment Battery for Children (K-ABC; Kaufman and Kaufman 1983; Hand Movement subtest; adapted from Luria 1980), the Go–No-Go Test, and the Finger Tapping Test (Reitan 1969b). Many of the above-mentioned tasks simultaneously evaluate frontal and executive functions.

Finally, to evaluate the symptom of hyperactivity in laboratory settings, an actometer is typically attached to the wrist or ankle to measure activity levels of children with ADHD and has differentiated children with ADHD from children without ADHD (Luk 1985; Tryon 1984). Moreover, the actometer may be used during attentional and selected neuropsychological tests.

Most of the traditional neuropsychological and analogue behavior instruments have been criticized as having only moderate generalizability to real-life situations in children with ADHD (Barkley 1990). Moreover, many measures lack adequate psychometric properties, including normative data, reliability, and validity, and provide inadequate information about sensitivity, specificity, and, particularly, prediction of pharmacological and nonpharmacological treatment response. One solution proposed by Atkins et al. (1985) is to use direct observations of ADHD symptoms in their natural settings; for example, incorporating academic performance measures, direct classroom and desk organization, and playroom and clinic observations into a scorable, psychometrically sound test battery (Abikoff et al. 1977; Milich et al. 1982). When this method is not feasible, analogue laboratory and clinic measures, CPT, and CCT-type tasks, in combination with parent and teacher ratings, are the next best methodology.

Treatment

Nonpharmacological Treatment

Psychosocial treatments, behavior therapy (Northup et al. 1995; Waldrop 1994), school-based interventions (Blackman et al. 1991; Bloomquist et al. 1991), individual and group parent training for families (Newby et al. 1991; Pisterman et al. 1992), and other multimodal treatments (Ialongo et al. 1993) have been claimed to be effective for childhood and adolescent ADHD.

Pharmacological Treatment

CNS psychostimulant medication is the most common treatment of ADHD in children. Research has clearly shown the efficacy of pharmacotherapy in the short-term enhancement of the core behavioral, academic, and social symptoms of ADHD in most children. The most commonly prescribed medications are methylphenidate, dextroamphetamine, and pemoline. (For a full review of the pharmacology, neurobiology, and prevalence of use of psychostimulants in ADHD, see Wilens and Biederman 1992.)

Although psychostimulants may normalize aggressive behavior and other indexes of sociality, they are not intended as sole treatments of ADHD. Psychostimulants instead maximize the benefits of concurrent treatments, such as behavior modification and academic tutoring (Barkley 1990). Moreover, few well-controlled studies indicate that short-term benefits of psychostimulants improve the long-term neuropsychological (Risser and Bowers 1993) and general prognosis of children with ADHD who receive treatment. Other claims of pharmacological treatment efficacy of ADHD in children have been made for tricyclic antidepressants such as desipramine (Gualtieri et al. 1991) and nortriptyline, other antidepressants such as bupropion (Barrickman et al. 1995), noradrenergic agonists such as clonidine and guanfacine (R. D. Hunt et al. 1995), SSRIs such as fluoxetine (Barrickman et al. 1991), the noradrenergic-serotonergic medication venlafaxine (Pleak and Gormly

1995), and the reversible monoamine oxidase inhibitor moclobemide (Trott et al. 1992). Finally, combined pharmacotherapy for ADHD patients with psychiatric comorbidity, treatment refractoriness, and moderate benefits from single medications has been proposed (Wilens et al. 1995). Typical pharmacological treatment combinations are fluoxetine and methylphenidate (Bussing and Levin 1993; Gammon and Brown 1993).

A National Institute of Mental Health (NIMH) collaborative multisite multimodal treatment study of children with ADHD has been conducted. A conclusion drawn from this study was that despite decades of ADHD treatment, clinicians are unable to predict the circumstances and/or child characteristics that would differentially benefit from specific treatments or treatment combinations. Moreover, the effect of specific treatments on specific domains of functioning and treatment length and the underlying process of change have not been determined (Richters et al. 1995).

Finally, combined pharmacological and nonpharmacological treatment of ADHD may be viewed as providing cooperative, additive benefits in comparison to any single treatment alone (DuPaul and Barkley 1993; Engeland 1993).

◈   **OTHER CHILDHOOD NEUROPSYCHIATRIC DISORDERS**

Obsessive-Compulsive Disorder

Over the past decade, evidence has accrued to suggest that OCD involves neuropsychiatric (Hollander et al. 1990), neuropsychological (Aronowitz et al. 1994), and neuroanatomical (Laplane et al. 1989) specific and nonspecific dysfunction in children, adolescents (Rapoport et al. 1981), and adults. Thus, OCD is justified as a childhood disorder with neuropsychiatric and neuropsychological findings sufficiently significant to warrant further investigation, ultimately leading to increased understanding of the pathophysiology of the disorder. We thus discuss OCD as a prototype of other childhood neuropsychiatric disorders, such as Tourette's disorder and other tic disorders, which are beyond the scope of this review.

Diagnostic Criteria and Definition

OCD is relatively common in the general population, with onset typically in adolescence or early adulthood. However, onset also has frequently been reported in childhood. The individual must have either obsessions or compulsions to receive the diagnosis of OCD (American Psychiatric Association 1994) (see O'Donnell and Calev, Chapter 4, in this volume for a review of diagnostic criteria). Although Criterion B of the DSM-IV diagnostic criteria stipulates that at some point during the disorder, the person realizes that the obsessive thoughts and/or compulsive behaviors are excessive or irrational, this condition does not apply to children because they may lack sufficient cognitive awareness to make this judgment.

Obsessions are distracting, thereby frequently resulting in inefficient performance on cognitive tasks that require concentration, such as reading or mathematical computations. Obsessions and compulsions can displace useful thoughts and behaviors and may severely disrupt academic, social, and occupational functioning. Finally, mild to extensive avoidance of situations provoking obsessions or compulsions results in significantly restricted overall functioning and lifestyle and may result in the patient being housebound.

Comorbidity. Hypochondriasis is frequently associated with OCD. Concerns may lead to repeated visits to physicians to seek reassurance. Children who have subjective feelings of illness may seek reassurance about health from parents and caregivers. Guilt, pathological responsibility, and sleep disturbances may be present. Patients with OCD may use excessive amounts of alcohol and substances such as sedatives, hypnotics, or anxiolytic medications in attempts to self-medicate debilitating anxiety and guilt in adolescence and continuing into adulthood. Furthermore, a high rate of morbidity and dysfunction such as depression, eating disorders, other anxiety disorders, tic disorders, and disorders involving lack of empathy (e.g., autistic disorder) have been reported (Rapoport et al. 1993; Thomsen 1994).

Prevalence

OCD is much more common in children and adolescents than was previously thought and may have an onset as young as age 2 years (Rapoport et al. 1993), with a 2% lifetime prevalence (McGough et al. 1993) and chronic course (Swedo et al. 1992b). The most prevalent obsessions in children and adolescents include fear of harm, illness and death, and contamination, as well as obsessions with numbers. These obsessions are often associated with the compulsions of washing, checking, repeating, counting, and symmetry (G. B. Adams et al. 1994).

Etiology

Concordance rates for OCD in monozygotic twins are higher than those in dizygotic twins, and the rate of OCD in first-degree biological relatives of OCD and Tourette's disorder probands is higher than that in the general population. Moreover, in a pilot study (Aronowitz et al. 1992), we found that the first-degree relatives of OCD probands with many neurological soft signs (four or more soft signs) had a significantly higher rate of OCD and broadly defined OCD—both DSM-III-R OCD and obsessions and compulsions that did not meet disorder impairment criteria—in comparison with the first-degree relatives of OCD probands with few neurological soft signs (one or no soft signs). The latter group had increased rates of generalized anxiety disorder. This finding suggested that diagnostic heterogeneity may be stratified along neuropsychiatric and familial lines in OCD. One homogeneous subgroup may be characterized by neurological deficits and high familial aggregation of OCD or obsessive-compulsive symptoms and the other by a lack of neurological findings and high familial aggregation of generalized anxiety disorder.

Pathology and Neuropsychological Function

Neuropsychological studies of OCD generally agree on localization of dysfunction—that is, prefrontal and frontal regions, limbic system, and basal ganglia (Alarcon et al. 1994; Otto 1992). However, they disagree as to hemisphere and frontal-lobe side of impairment, other brain area involvement, pathophysiological connections, and developmental phase effects. (For neuropsychological manifestations of OCD in adults, see Chapter 4.)

Childhood OCD has been associated with high degrees of neuropsychological (Rapoport et al. 1993; Thomsen 1994), neurological (Thomsen 1994), and neurotransmitter dysfunction (Oades et al. 1994). Swedo et al. (1992a) examined selected CSF peptides and monoamine metabolites in 43 children and adolescents with OCD. Results suggested that subgroups had primary hypothalamic-neurohypophysial dysfunction that resulted in perseverative OCD behavior. Other authors (Allen et al. 1995) have implicated an autoimmune subtype of pediatric OCD and a generalized CNS syndrome by the investigation of antineuronal antibodies (Kiessling et al. 1994). Oades et al. (1994) found that young OCD patients had increased serotonergic activity and unusual arousal with high adrenergic, serotonergic, and HVA levels in comparison with controls.

Neuropsychological investigations of childhood and adolescent OCD are scant. Behar et al. (1984) and Cox et al. (1989) have conducted most work in this area. Neuropsychological functions assessed in children and adolescents with OCD included attention, verbal and visual learning and memory, visuospatial orientation and judgment, and auditory and visual-perceptual processes. The structures examined were frontal, parietal, right parietal, and caudate, and laterality was assessed. Cox et al. (1989) found that children and adolescents with OCD were impaired on a selected subset of neuropsychological tests, implicating frontal lobe–basal ganglia structures.

Developmental Course

OCD onset is typically gradual, but acute onset is not uncommon and may result from stressful or traumatic life events. OCD is usually characterized by a chronic waxing and waning course, with symptomatic exacerbation during stress. After repeated failures to resist obsessions and/or compulsions, individuals may ultimately yield to almost all of them, cease to experience desire for resistance, and incorporate obsessions and/or compulsions into their routines, which may further exacerbate the clinical course of the disorder and lead to a vicious cycle.

Neuropsychological Patterns and Assessments

Typical neuropsychological tests administered to children with OCD are the WISC-III or selected subtests intended as a baseline measure of cognitive functioning. The Money's Road Map of Direction Sense and the Stylus Maze Learning Test both assess anticipation, planning, and visuospatial ability. Mental flexibility in shifting of cognitive set may be assessed with the WCST or its variants adapted for children. Psychomotor speed has been evaluated with the Digit Symbol subtest of the WISC-III. Memory and constructional abilities have been assessed with the Rey-Osterrieth Complex Figure. Verbal learning and recognition may be examined with the Rey Auditory-Verbal Learning Test, and other memory skills may be assessed with the WRAML. Outcome measures used in children include the NIMH Clinician's Global Impression Obsessive-Compulsive Disorders Scale (CGI-OCD), the Children's Yale-Brown Obsessive-Compulsive Scale (CY-BOCS) (March et al. 1994), and the Leyton Obsessional Inventory—Child Version (Berg et al. 1986; Cooper 1970).

Treatment

Nonpharmacological treatment. Cognitive-behavior therapy has been the main nonpharmacological treatment used in children and adolescents with OCD. Graded exposure and response prevention are the core components of this treatment. Of the 32 investigations identified in the literature, which are largely case studies, all but 1 showed some benefit of cognitive-behavioral interventions in childhood and adolescent OCD.

Other adjunctive treatments for children include relaxation, coping, and anxiety management training. Environmental manipulation, including family treatment (Piacentini et al. 1994), and OCD-related family interventions, such as familial cessation of reassurance and participation in OCD rituals, may attenuate avoidance, which is a serious complication of OCD.

The use of multiple simultaneous long-term treatments has improved the outcome for child and adolescent OCD. In addition, a great deal of clinical and newly emergent empirical evidence suggests that the combination of cognitive-behavior therapy and pharmacotherapy is effective in the treatment of child and adolescent OCD (Fisman and Walsh 1994). However, treatment difficulties include poor patient and family compliance and inconsistently applied treatment. Poorly operationalized techniques make comparative assessment of efficacy difficult between studies.

Pharmacological treatment. Pharmacological treatment of OCD has been widely available since the tricyclic antidepressant clomipramine was found to be superior to placebo in the treatment of OCD. In addition, the most successful pharmacotherapy for OCD in adults and children has been with antidepressants with potent serotonin reuptake inhibition properties (Montgomery 1993; Piacentini et al. 1992), such as clomipramine and fluoxetine. Fluoxetine provided moderate to marked reduction in OCD symptoms in 74% of pediatric psychopharmacology clinic children and adolescents at average follow-up of 19 months (D. A. Geller et al. 1995) and in comparison to placebo in a double-blind crossover trial (Riddle et al. 1992). The SSRI fluvoxamine likewise provided benefit for children (Riddle et al. 1996) and adolescents (Apter et al. 1994; Riddle et al. 1996) with OCD. Clonazepam augmentation of fluoxetine for severe, refractory childhood OCD has been reported as beneficial (H. L. Leonard et al. 1994).

Possible gastrointestinal, autonomic, hepatic, and cardiac problems accompanying clomipramine treatment should be considered in the clinical management of child and adolescent OCD (Scahill and Lynch 1995). Moreover, the long-term efficacy of antiobsessional agents such as fluoxetine and other SSRIs has not been systematically studied in young children. Decisions to use medication ultimately require careful examination of child and adolescent overall development and determination of the presence and severity of OCD symptoms.

Questions pertaining to childhood OCD concern the continuity of OCD with normal development, the nature of the relation between OCD and other psychiatric comorbidity, an etiology focused on neurobiological determinants, and long-term prognosis.

Conclusion

In this chapter, we have reviewed some of the prominent childhood mental disorders from a neuropsychological perspective. We highlighted convergent and divergent findings based on phenomenological, neurobiological, and neuropsychological factors in learning disorders (reading disorder, mathematics disorder, disorder of written expression), pervasive developmental disorders (autism and Asperger's disorder), ADHD, and OCD. For many of these disorders, the lack of systematic studies makes it difficult to assess the validity of the specificity of diagnostic criteria, neurobiological markers, and neuropsychological deficits. Researchers need to understand better what role shared characteristics, abnormalities, and spared functions play in each disorder, as well as to clarify further what other factors differentiate one disorder from another. Moreover, these disorders must be better understood from a developmental perspective so that researchers may address identification of risk, prevention strategies, and methods of treatment and remediation. Table 5–4 summarizes the most salient neuropsychological, neuroanatomical, and neurobiological findings in the disorders highlighted in this chapter.

Large controlled studies need to be conducted across all areas of research described in this chapter and in several settings to compare

Table 5–4. Cognitive deficits and neuroanatomical/neurobiological findings in childhood mental disorders

Disorder	Cognitive deficits	Neuroanatomical/ Neurobiological impairment
Learning disorders		
Reading disorder	Phonological processing	• Left-hemisphere planum temporale
	Onset of speech acquisition	
	Articulation	
	Naming	
	Word finding	
	Letter transposition	
	Verbal sequencing	
	Visuospatial processing	
	Word recognition	
	Reading comprehension	
	Spelling accuracy/fluency	
	Verbal short-term memory	
Mathematics disorder	Conceptualization of number quantity	• Right-hemisphere dysfunction
	Left-limb atrophy	• Left-hemisphere temporal-parietal dysfunction
	Incoordination of left hand	
	Constructional apraxia	
	Visuospatial processing	
	Visuomotor skills	

(continued)

Sensory inattention

Absence of stereoscopic vision

Dysprosodia

Poor eye contact

Absence of gesture

Poor comprehension of nonverbal communication

Understanding affective states of others

Recognition/production of number/operator symbols difficulties

Poor sequencing skills

Reduced short-term auditory memory

• Angular gyrus

Disorder of written expression

Difficulty copying words/sentences

Extremely poor handwriting

Letter sequencing difficulty

Nonword reading impairment

Spelling of ambiguous, irregular words during writing

Long-term recall of irregular words

Difficulty writing to dictation

Spontaneous writing

Table 5–4. Cognitive deficits and neuroanatomical/neurobiological findings in childhood mental disorders (*continued*)

Disorder	Cognitive deficits	Neuroanatomical/Neurobiological impairment
Pervasive developmental disorders		
Autism	General intellectual ability Sensory processing Metarepresentation Selective attention Attention set-shifting Verbal comprehension Inferential thinking Abstract problem-solving Cognitive flexibility Visual memory Visuomotor Motor planning Soft neurological signs Affiliative behavior Social reasoning/empathy Adaptability	• Hippocampus • Amygdala • Brain stem • Cerebellar vermal lobules • Anterior cingulate gyrus • Parietal-lobe impairment • Fourth ventricle widening • Abnormalities in the interactions between frontal or parietal lobes and neostriatum and thalamus • Decreased anterior cingulate gyrus metabolism • Small P3 waves • Saccadic eye movement abnormalities • Serotonergic dysfunction • Endorphin abnormalities
Asperger's disorder	Cognitive flexibility Language comprehension	• Cerebellar abnormalities • Agenesis of corpus callosum

Disorder	Neuropsychological functions	Brain abnormalities
	Nonverbal concept formation Visuospatial perception Visual memory Visuomotor integration Spatial orientation Facial recognition Gross and fine motor skills	• Right central perisylvian abnormalities • Sylvian fissure widening • Hypoplasia of right temporo-occipital cortex • Small posterior parietal lobe gyri • Moderate enlargement of right lateral ventricle • Polymicrogyria—cerebral cortex
Other disorders Attention-deficit/ hyperactivity disorder	Attention Organization/planning Motor coordination Balance Clumsiness Impulsivity Verbal/visual learning and memory	• Low brain volume in corpus callosum • Small right caudate volume • Noradrenergic/serotonergic dysfunction
Obsessive-compulsive disorder	Cognitive flexibility Verbal/visual learning and memory Visuospatial Psychomotor speed	• Hypothalamic-hypophysial abnormalities • Serotonergic/noradrenergic dysfunction • Prefrontal/frontal, limbic, and basal ganglia abnormalities

Note. LH = left hemisphere; RH = right hemisphere.

results among samples drawn from a range of clinical, academic, and community settings. Standardized diagnostic and assessment instruments also need to be developed.

◈ REFERENCES

Abikoff H, Gittelman-Klein R, Klein D: Validation of a classroom observation code for hyperactive children. J Consult Clin Psychol 45:772–783, 1977

Achenbach TM, Edelbrock CS: Manual for the Child Behavior Checklist and Revised Child Behavior Profile. Burlington, University of Vermont, Department of Psychiatry, 1983

Ackerman PT, Dykman RA, Holloway C, et al: A trial of piracetam in two subgroups of students with dyslexia enrolled in summer tutoring. Journal of Learning Disabilities 24:542–549, 1991

Adams GB, Waas GA, March JS, et al: Obsessive compulsive disorder in children and adolescents: the role of the school psychologist in identification, assessment, and treatment. School Psychology Quarterly 9:274–294, 1994

Adams MJ: Learning to Read. Cambridge, MA, MIT Press, 1990

Alarcon RD, Libb JW, Boll T: Neuropsychological testing in obsessive-compulsive disorder: a clinical review. J Neuropsychiatry Clin Neurosci 6:217–228, 1994

Allen AJ, Leonard HL, Swedo SE: Case study: a new infection-triggered, autoimmune subtype of pediatric OCD and Tourette's syndrome. J Am Acad Child Adolesc Psychiatry 34:307–311, 1995

Aman MG, Turbott SH: Incidental learning, distraction and sustained attention in hyperactive and control subjects. J Abnorm Child Psychol 14:441–455, 1986

Ameli R, Courchesne E, Lincoln A, et al: Visual memory processes in high-functioning individuals with autism. J Autism Dev Disord 18:601–615, 1988

American Psychiatric Association: Diagnostic and Statistical Manual of Mental Disorders, 3rd Edition. Washington, DC, American Psychiatric Association, 1980

American Psychiatric Association: Diagnostic and Statistical Manual of Mental Disorders, 3rd Edition, Revised. Washington, DC, American Psychiatric Association, 1987

American Psychiatric Association: Diagnostic and Statistical Manual of Mental Disorders, 4th Edition. Washington, DC, American Psychiatric Association, 1994, pp 37–78

Anastopoulos AD, Barkley RA: Biological factors in attention deficit-hyperactivity disorder. Behavior Therapy 11:47–53, 1988

Anderson GM, Minderaa RB, Cho SC, et al: The issue of hyperserotonemia and platelet serotonin exposure: a preliminary study. J Autism Dev Disord 19: 349–351, 1989

Anderson LT, Campbell M, Adams P, et al: The effects of haloperidol on discrimination learning and behavioral symptoms in autistic children. J Autism Dev Disord 19:227–239, 1989

Apter A, Ratzoni G, King RA, et al: Fluvoxamine open-label treatment of adolescent inpatients with obsessive-compulsive disorder or depression. J Am Acad Child Adolesc Psychiatry 33:342–348, 1994

Arnold LE: Learning disorders, in Psychiatric Disorders in Children and Adolescents. Edited by Garfinkel BD, Carlson GA, Weller EB. Philadelphia, PA, WB Saunders, 1990, pp 237–256

Aronowitz BR, Hollander E, Mannuzza S, et al: Soft signs and familial transmission of obsessive-compulsive disorder. Young Investigators New Research Poster presented at the 145th annual meeting of the American Psychiatric Association, Washington, DC, May 2–7, 1992

Aronowitz BR, Hollander E, Rosen W, et al: Neuropsychology of obsessive-compulsive disorder: preliminary findings. Neuropsychiatry Neuropsychol Behav Neurol 7:81–86, 1994

Asarnow RF, Tanguay PE, Bott L, et al: Patterns of intellectual functioning in non-retarded autistic and schizophrenia children. J Child Psychol Psychiatry 28:273–280, 1987

Atkins MS, Pelham WE, Licht JH: A comparison of objective classroom measures and teacher ratings of attention deficit disorder. J Abnorm Child Psychol 13: 155–167, 1985

August GJ, Lockhart LH: Familial autism and the fragile X chromosome. J Autism Dev Disord 14:197–204, 1984

Badian NA: Reading disability in an epidemiological context: incidence and environmental correlates. Journal of Learning Disabilities 17:129–136, 1984

Badian N, McAnulty GB, Duffy FH, et al: Prediction of dyslexia in kindergarten boys. Annals of Dyslexia 40:152–169, 1990

Bailey A, LeCouteur A, Gottesman I, et al: Autism as a strongly genetic disorder: evidence from a British twin study. Psychol Med 25:63–77, 1995

Barkley RA: Attention Deficit Hyperactivity Disorder: A Handbook for Diagnosis and Treatment. New York, Guilford, 1990

Barkley RA, Koplowitz S, Anderson T: Sense of time in children with ADHD: effects of duration, distraction, and stimulant medication. Journal of International Neuropsychological Society 3:359–369, 1997

Baron-Cohen S: The development of a theory of mind in autism: deviance and delay? Psychiatr Clin North Am 14:33–51, 1991

Barrickman LL, Noyes R, Kuperman S, et al: Treatment of ADHD with fluoxetine: a preliminary trial. J Am Acad Child Adolesc Psychiatry 30:762–767, 1991

Barrickman LL, Perry PJ, Allen AJ, et al: Bupropion versus methylphenidate in the treatment of attention-deficit hyperactivity disorder. J Am Acad Child Adolesc Psychiatry 34:649–657, 1995

Bartak L, Rutter M: Differences between mentally retarded and normally intelligent autistic children. Journal of Autism and Childhood Schizophrenia 6: 109–122, 1976

Barthelemy C, Bruneau N, Jouve J, et al: Urinary dopamine metabolites as indicators of responsiveness to fenfluramine treatment in children with autistic behavior. J Autism Dev Disord 19:241–254, 1989

Bauman M, Kemper TL: Histoanatomic observations of the brain in early infantile autism. Neurology 35:866–874, 1985

Becker PS, Dixon AM, Troncoso JC: Bilateral opercular polymicrogyria. Ann Neurol 25:90–92, 1989

Beery KE, Buktenica NA: Developmental Test of Visual-Motor Integration—3rd Revision. Los Angeles, CA, Western Psychological Services, 1989

Behar D, Rapoport JL, Berg CJ, et al: Computerized tomography and neuropsychological test measures in adolescents with obsessive compulsive disorder. Am J Psychiatry 141:363–369, 1984

Belendiuk K, Belendiuk GW, Freedman DX: Blood monoamine metabolism in Huntington's disease. Arch Gen Psychiatry 37:325–332, 1980

Belendiuk K, Belendiuk GW, Freedman DX, et al: Neurotransmitter abnormalities in patients with motor neuron disease. Arch Neurol 38:415–417, 1981

Bender L, Faretra G, Cobrinik L: LSD and UML treatment of hospitalized disturbed children, in Recent Advances in Biological Psychiatry, Vol 5. Edited by Wortis J. New York, Plenum, 1963, pp 84–92

Benton AL: Revised Visual Retention Test—4th Edition. San Antonio, TX, Psychological Corporation, 1974

Benton AL, Hamsher K: Multilingual Aphasia Examination (Word Fluency Subtest). Iowa City, IA, AJA Associates, 1983

Benton AL, Hamsher K deS, Varney NR, et al: Benton Facial Recognition Test, in Contributions to Neuropsychological Assessment: A Clinical Manual, 2nd Edition. Edited by Benton AL, Sivan AB, Hamsher K, et al. New York, Oxford University Press, 1994

Berg CZ, Rapoport JL, Flament M: The Leyton Obsessional Inventory—Child Version. J Am Acad Child Adolesc Psychiatry 25:84–91, 1986

Berthier ML, Starkstein SE, Leiguarda R: Developmental cortical anomalies in Asperger's syndrome; neuroradiological findings in two patients. J Neuropsychiatry Clin Neurosci 2:197–201, 1990

Berthier ML, Bayes A, Tolosa E: Magnetic resonance imaging in patients with concurrent Tourette's disorder and Asperger's syndrome. J Am Acad Child Adolesc Psychiatry 32:633–639, 1993

Biederman J, Faraone SV, Keenan K, et al: Evidence of familial association between attention deficit disorder and major affective disorders. Arch Gen Psychiatry 48:633–642, 1991a

Biederman J, Faraone SV, Keenen K, et al: Familial association between attention deficit disorder and anxiety disorder. Am J Psychiatry 148:251–256, 1991b

Biederman J, Newcorn J, Sprich S: Comorbidity of attention deficit hyperactivity disorder with conduct, depressive, anxiety and other disorders. Am J Psychiatry 148:564–577, 1991c

Bigler ED: On the neuropsychology of suicide. Journal of Learning Disabilities 22:180–185, 1989

Bishop DVM: Autism, Asperger's syndrome and semantic-pragmatic disorder: where are the boundaries? British Journal of Disorders of Communication 24:107–121, 1989

Blackman JA, Westervelt VD, Stevenson R, et al: Management of preschool children with attention deficit-hyperactivity disorder. Topics in Early Childhood Special Education 11:91–104, 1991

Bloomquist ML, August GJ, Ostrander R: Effects of a school-based cognitive-behavioral intervention for ADHD children. J Abnorm Child Psychol 19:591–605, 1991

Boder E, Jarrico S: Boder Test of Reading-Spelling Patterns. San Antonio, TX, Psychological Corporation, 1982

Bohus B, Kovacs G, deWied D: Oxytocin, vasopressin, and memory: opposite effects on consolidation and retrieval processes. Brain Res 157:414–417, 1978

Botez MI, Gravel J, Attig E, et al: Reversible chronic cerebellar ataxia after phenytoin intoxication: possible role of cerebellum in cognitive thought. Neurology 35:1152–1157, 1985

Brown WT, Jenkins EC, Friedman E, et al: Autism is associated with the fragile-X syndrome. J Autism Dev Disord 12:303–308, 1982

Brown WT, Jenkins EC, Cohen IL, et al: Fragile X and autism: a multicenter survey. Am J Med Genet 23:341–352, 1986

Brumback RA, Staton RD: An hypothesis regarding the commonality of right hemisphere involvement in learning disability attentional disorder, and childhood major depressive disorder. Percept Mot Skills 55:1091–1097, 1982

Brumback RA, Harper CR, Weinberg WA: Nonverbal learning disabilities, Asperger's syndrome, pervasive developmental disorder—should we care? J Child Neurol 11:427–429, 1996

Bryant BR, Patton JR, Dunn C: Scholastic Abilities Test for Adults. Austin, TX, Pro-Ed, 1991

Bryson SE, Clark BS, Smith IM: First report of a Canadian epidemiological study of autistic syndromes. J Child Psychol Psychiatry 29:433–445, 1988

Buchsbaum M, Haznedar M: Functional imaging with PET in autism. Presented at the symposium, "New Insights in the Diagnosis, Neurobiology, Genetics and Treatment of Autism." Mount Sinai School of Medicine, New York, NY, November 1995

Buchsbaum MS, Siegel BU, Wu JC, et al: Brief report: attention performance in autism and regional brain metabolic rate assessed by positron emission tomography. J Autism Dev Disord 22:115–125, 1992

Burgoine E, Wing L: Identical triplets with Asperger's syndrome. Br J Psychiatry 143:261–265, 1983

Buschke H: Selective reminding for analysis of memory and learning. Journal of Verbal Learning and Verbal Behavior 12:543–550, 1973

Bussing R, Levin GM: Methamphetamine and fluoxetine treatment of a child with attention-deficit hyperactivity disorder and obsessive-compulsive disorder. J Child Adololesc Psychopharmacol 3:53–58, 1993

Campbell M: Fenfluramine treatment of autism. J Child Psychol Psychiatry 29: 1–10, 1988

Campbell M, Fish B, Shapiro T, et al: Imipramine in preschool autistic and schizophrenic children. Journal of Autism and Childhood Schizophrenia 1: 267–282, 1971

Campbell M, Fish B, Korein J, et al: Lithium and chlorpromazine: a controlled crossover study of hyperactive severely disturbed young children. Journal of Autism and Childhood Schizophrenia 2:343–358, 1972

Campbell M, Freidman E, DeVito E, et al: Blood serotonin in psychotic and brain damaged children. Journal of Autism and Childhood Schizophrenia 4:33–41, 1974

Campbell M, Small AM, Collins PJ, et al: Levodopa and levoamphetamine: a crossover study in young schizophrenic children. Curr Ther Res 19:70–86, 1976

Campbell M, Anderson LT, Meier M, et al: A comparison of haloperidol and behavior therapy and their interaction in autistic children. Journal of the American Academy of Child Psychiatry 17:640–655, 1978

Campbell M, Small AM, Anderson LT, et al: A double-blind and placebo controlled study of naltrexone in autistic children, in Proceedings of the American Academy of Child and Adolescent Psychiatry, Washington, DC, American Academy of Child and Adolescent Psychiatry, 1989, pp 66–67

Castellanos FX, Giedd JN, Eckburg P, et al: Quantitative morphology of the caudate nucleus in attention deficit hyperactivity disorder. Am J Psychiatry 151:1791–1796, 1994

Chall JS: Learning to Read: The Great Debate. New York, McGraw-Hill, 1967

Chedru F, Geschwind N: Writing disturbances in acute confusional states. Neuropsychologia 10:343–353, 1972

Chelune GJ, Ferguson W, Koon R, et al: Frontal lobe disinhibition in attention deficit disorder. Child Psychiatry Hum Dev 16:221–234, 1986

Chris-Heh CW, Smith R, Wu J, et al: Positron emission tomography of the cerebellum in autism. Am J Psychiatry 146:242–245, 1989

Cialdella P, Mamelle N: An epidemiological study of infantile autism in a French department (Rhone): a research note. J Child Psychol Psychiatry 30:165–175, 1989

Clark DB: Dyslexia: Theory and Practice of Remedial Instruction. Parkton, MD, York Press, 1988

Coccaro E, Siever LJ, Klar HM, et al: Serotonergic studies in patients with affective and personality disorders: correlates with suicidal and impulsive aggressive behavior. Arch Gen Psychiatry 46:587–599, 1989

Cohen DJ, Shaywitz BA, Johnson WT, et al: Biogenic amines in autistic and atypical children: cerebrospinal fluid measures of homovanillic acid and 5-hydroxyindoleacetic acid. Arch Gen Psychiatry 31:845–853, 1974

Cohen DJ, Caparulo BK, Shaywitz GA, et al: Dopamine and serotonin metabolism in neuropsychiatrically disturbed children. Arch Gen Psychiatry 34:545–550, 1977

Cohen MD, Campbell R, Yaghmai F: Neuropathological abnormalities in developmental dysphasia. Ann Neurol 25:567–570, 1989

Colarusso RP, Hammill DD: Motor-Free Visual Perception Test. Novato, CA, Academic Therapy Publications, 1996

Conners CK: Conners' Continuous Performance Test: Computer Program, Version 3.0 (CPT). San Antonio, TX, Psychological Corporation, 1994

Cook EH: Autism: review of neurochemical investigation. Synapse 6:292–308, 1990

Cook EH, Leventhal BL, Heller W, et al: Autistic children and their first-degree relatives: relationships between serotonin and norepinephrine levels and intelligence. J Neuropsychiatry Clin Neurosci 2:268–274, 1990

Cook E, Lord C, Courchesne R, et al: Preliminary evidence of linkage and association between HTT and autistic disorder (abstract). Biol Psychiatry 41: 1S–120S, 1997

Coon KB, Polk MJ, McCoy Waguespack M: Dyslexia Screening Instrument. San Antonio, TX, Psychological Corporation, 1994

Cooper JL: The Leyton Obsessional Inventory. Psychol Med 1:48–64, 1970

Courchesne E: New evidence of cerebellar and brainstem hypoplasia in autistic infants, children and adolescents: the MR imaging study by Hashimoto and colleagues. J Autism Dev Disord 25:19–22, 1995

Courchesne E, Lincoln AJ, Kilman BA, et al: Event-related brain potential correlates of the processing of novel visual and auditory information in autism. J Autism Dev Disord 15:55–76, 1985

Courchesne E, Yeung-Courchene R, Press GA, et al: Hypoplasia of cerebellar vermal lobules VI and VII in autism. N Engl J Med 318:1349–1354, 1988

Courchesne E, Townsend J, Saitoh O: The brain in infantile autism: posterior fossa structures are abnormal. Neurology 44:214–223, 1994a

Courchesne E, Townsend J, Akshoomoff NA, et al: Impairment in shifting attention in autistic and cerebellar patients. Behav Neurosci 108:848–865, 1994b

Cox CS, Fedio P, Rapoport JL: Neuropsychological testing of obsessive-compulsive adolescents, in Obsessive-Compulsive Disorder in Children and Adolescents. Edited by Rapoport JL. Washington, DC, American Psychiatric Press, 1989, pp 73–85

Critchley M: The Parietal Lobes. London, Arnold, 1953

David AS, Wacharasindhu A, Lishman WA: Severe psychiatric disturbance and abnormalities of the corpus callosum: review and case series. J Neurol Neurosurg Psychiatry 56:85–93, 1993

Dawson G, Warrenburg S, Fuller P: Hemispheric functioning and motor imitation in autistic persons. Brain Cogn 2:346–354, 1983

Dawson G, Finley C, Phillips S, et al: Reduced P3 amplitude of the event-related brain potential: its relationship to language ability in autism. J Autism Dev Disord 18:493–504, 1988

DeFries JC: Gender ratios in reading-disabled children and their affected relatives: a commentary. Journal of Learning Disabilities 22:544–555, 1989

DeFries JC, Fulker DW, LaBuda MC: Reading disability in twins: evidence for a genetic etiology. Nature 329:537–539, 1987

Delis DC, Kramer JH, Kaplan E, et al: California Verbal Learning Test—Children's Version. San Antonio, TX, Psychological Corporation, 1994

DeLong RG, Dwyer JT: Correlation of family history with specific autistic subgroups: Asperger's syndrome and bipolar affective disease. J Autism Dev Disord 18:593–600, 1988

Denckla MB: The neuropsychology of social-emotional learning disabilities. Arch Neurol 40:461–462, 1983

Denckla MB: Revised PANESS. Psychopharmacol Bull 21:773–800, 1985

Denckla MB: The child with developmental disabilities grown up: adult residua of childhood disorders. Neurol Clin 11:105–125, 1993

DeRenzi E, Lucchelli F: Developmental dysmnesia in a poor reader. Brain 13:1337–1345, 1990

DeVolder A, Bol A, Michel C, et al: Brain glucose metabolism in children with autistic syndrome: positron emission tomography analysis. Brain Development 9:581–587, 1987

DiLavore PC, Lord C, Rutter M: The Pre-Linguistic Autism Diagnostic Observation Schedule. J Autism Dev Disord 25:355–379, 1995

DiSimoni E, Vignolo L: The Token Test: a sensitive test to detect receptive disturbances in aphasics. Brain 85:665–678, 1962

Duffy FH, McAnulty G: Neuropsychological heterogeneity and the definition of dyslexia: preliminary evidence for plasticity. Neuropsychologia 28:555–571, 1990

Dunn D, Dunn L: Peabody Picture Vocabulary Test—Revised. Circle Pines, MN, American Guidance Services, 1981

DuPaul GJ, Barkley RA: Behavioral contributions to pharmacotherapy: the utility of behavioral methodology in medication treatment of children with attention deficit hyperactivity disorder. Behav Ther 24:47–65, 1993

Edelbrock CS, Achenbach TA: The teacher version of the Child Behavior Profile, I: boys aged 6–11. J Consult Clin Psychol 52:207–217, 1986

Egaas B, Courchesne E, Saitoh O: Reduced size of the corpus callosum in autism. Arch Neurol 52:794–801, 1995

Eisenberg L: Definitions of dyslexia: their consequences for research and policy, in Dyslexia. Edited by Benton AL, Pearl D. New York, Oxford University Press, 1978, pp 29–42

Ekman P, Friesen WV: Pictures of Facial Affect Manual. San Francisco, CA, Human Interaction Laboratory: University of California Medical Center, 1976

El Badri SM, Lewis M: Left hemisphere and cerebellar damage in Asperger's syndrome. Irish Journal of Psychological Medicine 10:22–23, 1993

Eliason MJ, Richman LC: Behavior and attention in LD children. Learning Disability Quarterly 11:360–369, 1988

Engeland HV: Pharmacotherapy and behavior therapy: competition or cooperation? Acta Paedopsychiatrica 56:123–127, 1993

Faraone SV, Biederman J, Jetton JG, et al: Attention deficit disorder and conduct disorder: longitudinal evidence for a familial subtype. Psychol Med 27: 291–300, 1997

Fein D, Pennington B, Markowitz P, et al: Toward a neuropsychological model of infantile autism: are the social deficits primary? Journal of the American Academy of Child Psychiatry 25:198–212, 1986

Fein D, Lucci D, Waterhouse L: Brief report: fragmented drawings in autistic children. J Autism Dev Disord 20:263–268, 1990

Felton RH, Naylor CE, Wood FB: Neuropsychological profile of adult dyslexics. Brain Lang 39:485–497, 1990

Finucci JM, Guthrie JT, Childs AL, et al: The genetics of specific reading disability. Annual Review of Human Genetics 40:1–23, 1976

Fish B, Shapiro T, Campbell M: Long-term prognosis and the response of schizophrenic children to drug therapy: a controlled study of trifluoperazine. Am J Psychiatry 123:32–39, 1966

Fisman SN, Walsh L: Obsessive-compulsive disorder and fear of AIDS contamination in childhood. J Am Acad Child Adolesc Psychiatry 33:349–353, 1994

Flor-Henry P: On certain aspects of localization of the cerebral systems regulating and determining emotion. Biol Psychiatry 14:677–698, 1979

Flowers DL, Wood FB, Naylor CE: Regional cerebral bloodflow correlates of language processes in reading disability. Arch Neurol 48:637–643, 1991

Fogel CA, Mednick SA, Michelson N: Hyperactive behavior and minor physical anomalies. Acta Psychiatr Scand 72:551–556, 1985

Folstein S, Rutter M: Infantile autism: a genetic study of 21 twin pairs. J Child Psychol Psychiatry 18:297–321, 1977

Folstein SE, Rutter ML: Autism: familial aggregation and genetic implications. J Autism Dev Disord 18:3–30, 1988

Foss JM: Nonverbal learning disabilities and remedial interventions. Annals of Dyslexia 41:128–140, 1991

Freedman AM, Ebin EV, Wilson EA: Autistic schizophrenic children: an experiment in the use of d-lysergic acid diethylamide (LSD-25). Arch Gen Psychiatry 6:203–213, 1962

Freedman DX, Belendiuk K, Belendiuk GW, et al: Blood tryptophan metabolism in chronic schizophrenics. Arch Gen Psychiatry 38:655–659, 1981

Frith U: Beneath the surface of developmental dyslexia, in Surface Dyslexia. Edited by Patterson K, Marshall JC, Coltheart M. Hove, England, Lawrence Erlbaum Associates, 1985

Gaffney GR, Kuperman S, Tsai LY, et al: Morphological evidence for brainstem involvement in infantile autism. Biol Psychiatry 24:578–586, 1988

Galaburda AM: Neurology of developmental dyslexia. Curr Opin Neurobiol 3: 237–242, 1993

Galaburda AM, Kemper TL: Cytoarchitectonic abnormalities in developmental dyslexia: a case study. Ann Neurol 6:94–100, 1979

Galaburda AM, Sherman GF, Rosen GD, et al: Developmental dyslexia: four consecutive patients with cortical anomalies. Ann Neurol 18:222–232, 1985

Galaburda AM, Menard MT, Rosen GD: Evidence for aberrant auditory anatomy in developmental dyslexia. Proc Natl Acad Sci U S A 91:8010–8013, 1994

Gammon GD, Brown TE: Fluoxetine and methylphenidate in combination for treatment of attention deficit disorder and comorbid depressive disorder. J Child Adolesc Psychopharmacol 3:1–10, 1993

Garnier C, Comoy E, Barthelemy C, et al: Dopamine-beta-hydroxylase (DBH) and homovanillic acid (HVA) in autistic children. J Autism Dev Disord 16:23–29, 1986

Geller DA, Biederman J, Reed ED, et al: Similarities in response to fluoxetine in the treatment of children and adolescents with obsessive-compulsive disorder. J Am Acad Child Adolesc Psychiatry 43:36–44, 1995

Geller E, Ritvo ER, Freeman BJ, et al: Preliminary observations on the effect of fenfluramine on blood serotonin and symptoms in three autistic boys. N Engl J Med 307:165–169, 1982

Gillberg C: Identical triplets with infantile autism and the fragile X syndrome. Br J Psychiatry 143:256–260, 1983

Gillberg C: Asperger's syndrome and recurrent psychosis: a case study. J Autism Dev Disord 15:389–397, 1985

Gillberg C: Annotation: the neurobiology of infantile autism. J Child Psychol Psychiatry 29:257–266, 1988

Gillberg C: Asperger's syndrome in 23 Swedish children. Dev Med Child Neurol 31:520–531, 1989

Gillberg C: Autism and pervasive developmental disorders. J Child Psychol Psychiatry 31:99–119, 1990

Gillberg C, Forsell C: Childhood psychosis and neurofibromatosis—more than a coincidence. J Autism Dev Disord 14:1–9, 1984

Gillberg C, Gillberg C: Asperger syndrome—some epidemiological considerations: a research note. J Child Psychol Psychiatry 30:631–638, 1989

Gillberg C, Steffenburg S: Outcome and prognostic factors in infantile autism and similar conditions. J Autism Dev Disord 17:271–285, 1987

Gillberg C, Rosenhall U, Johansson E: Auditory brainstem responses in childhood psychosis. J Autism Dev Disord 13:181–194, 1983a

Gillberg C, Svennerholm L, Hamilton-Hellberg C: Childhood psychosis and monoamine metabolites in spinal fluid. J Autism Dev Disord 13:383–396, 1983b

Gillberg C, Terenius L, Lonnerholm G: Endorphin activity in childhood psychosis. Arch Gen Psychiatry 42:780–783, 1985

Gillberg C, Steffenburg S, Jakobson G: Neurological findings in 20 relatively gifted children with Kanner type autism or Asperger syndrome. Dev Med Child Neurol 29:641–649, 1987

Gittelman R, Mannuzza S, Shenker R, et al: Hyperactive boys almost grown up. Arch Gen Psychiatry 42:937–947, 1985

Golden JC: Stroop Color and Word Test: A Manual for Clinical and Experimental Uses. Los Angeles, CA, Western Psychological Services, 1978

Goldman R, Fristoe M, Woodcock RW: Goldman-Fristoe Woodcock Test of Auditory Discrimination. Circle Pines, MN, American Guidance Service, 1974

Goldman SM: Language in the preschool child: development and assessment, in Handbook of Clinical Assessment of Children and Adolescents, Vols 1 and 2. Edited by Kestenbaum CJ, Williams DT. New York, University Press, 1988, pp 259–295

Goodyear P, Hynd GW, Furman U: Attention-deficit disorder with (ADD/H) and without (ADD/WO) hyperactivity: behavioral and neuropsychological differentiation. J Clin Child Psychol 21:273–305, 1992

Gordon CT, Rapoport JL, Hamburger SD, et al: Differential response of seven subjects with autistic disorder to clomipramine and desipramine. Am J Psychiatry 149:363–366, 1992

Gordon M: The Gordon Diagnostic System. DeWitt, NY, Gordon Systems, 1983

Gordon N: Children with developmental dyscalculia. Dev Med Child Neurol 34:459–463, 1992

Goyette CH, Conners CK, Ulrich RF: Normative data on Revised Conners Parent and Teacher Rating Scales. J Abnorm Child Psychol 6:221–236, 1978

Grandin T, Scariano MM: Emergence Labeled Autistic. Novato, CA, Arena Press, 1986

Greenberg LM, Waldman ID: Developmental normative data on the Test of Variables of Attention (T.O.V.A.). J Am Acad Child Adolesc Psychiatry 34:1019–1030, 1993

Gregg N, Hoy C: Identifying the learning disabled. Journal of College Admission 129:30–34, 1990

Gregg N, Hoy C, King M, et al: The MMPI-2 profile of adults with learning disabilities in university and rehabilitation settings. Journal of Learning Disabilities 25:386–395, 1992

Gresham FM, Reschly DJ: Social skill deficits and low peer acceptance of mainstreamed learning disabled children. Learning Disability Quarterly 9: 23–32, 1986

Grodzinsky GM, Diamond R: Frontal lobe functioning in boys with attention-deficit hyperactivity disorder. Developmental Neuropsychology 8:427–445, 1992

Gross-Glenn K, Duara R, Barker WW, et al: Positron emission tomographic studies during serial word-reading by normal and dyslexic adults. J Clin Exp Neuropsychol 13:531–544, 1991

Gross-Tsur V, Shalev RS, Manor O, et al: Developmental right-hemisphere syndrome: clinical spectrum of the nonverbal learning disability. Journal of Learning Disabilities 28:80–86, 1995

Gualtieri CT, Keenen PA, Chandler M: Clinical and neuropsychological effects of desipramine in children with attention deficit hyperactivity disorder. J Clin Psychopharmacol 11:155–159, 1991

Hackney IM, Hanley WB, Davidson W, et al: Phenylketonuria: mental development, behaviour, and termination of the low phenylalanine diet. J Pediatr 72:646–655, 1968

Hagerman RJ, Chudley AE, Knoll JH, et al: Autism in fragile X females. Am J Med Genet 23:375–380, 1986

Hagman JO, Wood F, Buchsbaum MS, et al: Cerebral brain metabolism in adult dyslexic subjects assessed with positron emission tomography during performance of an auditory task. Arch Neurol 49:734–739, 1992

Hamilton NG, Frick RB, Takahashi T, et al: Psychiatric symptoms and cerebellar pathology. Am J Psychiatry 140:1322–1326, 1983

Hammill DD, Brown VL, Larsen SC, et al: Test of Adolescent Language—3rd Edition. Austin, TX, Pro-Ed, 1998

Hanley HG, Stahl SM, Freedman DX: Hyperserotonemia and amine metabolites in autistic and retarded children. Arch Gen Psychiatry 34:521–531, 1977

Hashimoto T, Tayama M, Murakawa K, et al: Development of the brainstem and cerebellum in autistic patients. J Autism Dev Disord 25:1–18, 1995

Heaton RK: Wisconsin Card Sorting Test Manaul. Odessa, FL, Psychological Assessment Resources, 1981

Heilman KM, Bowers D, Valenstein E: Emotional disorders associated with neurological diseases, in Neuropsychology. Edited by Heilman KM, Valenstein E. New York, Oxford University Press, 1985, pp 377–402

Heilman KM, Voeller KS, Nadeau SE: A possible pathophysiologic substrate of attention deficit hyperactivity disorder. J Child Neurol 6:576–581, 1991

Herman BH: A possible role of proopiomelanocortin peptides in self-injurious behavior. Prog Neuropsychopharmacol Biol Psychiatry 14 (suppl):S109–S139, 1990

Herman BH, Asleson G, Lukens E, et al: Acute and chronic naltrexone decreases the hyperactivity of autism. Society for Neuroscience Abstracts 19:1785, 1993

Hobson RP: The autistic child's appraisal of expressions of emotion. J Child Psychol Psychiatry 27:321–342, 1986

Hoffman WL, Prior MR: Neuropsychological dimensions of autism in children. Journal of Clinical Neuropsychology 4:27–41, 1982

Hollander E, Schiffman E, Cohen B, et al: Signs of central nervous system dysfunction in obsessive compulsive disorder. Arch Gen Psychiatry 47:27–32, 1990

Hollander E, DeCaria CM, Nitescu A, et al: Serotonergic function in obsessive-compulsive disorder: behavioral and neuroendocrine responses to oral m-chlorophenylpiperazine and fenfluramine in patients and healthy volunteers. Arch Gen Psychiatry 49:21–28, 1992

Holttum JR, Minshew NJ, Sanders RS, et al: Magnetic resonance imaging of the posterior fossa in autism. Biol Psychiatry 32:1091–1101, 1992

Hooper HE: The Hooper Visual Organization Test Manual. Los Angeles, CA, Western Psychological Services, 1958

Horn WF, Wagner AE, Ialongo N: Sex differences in school-aged children with pervasive attention deficit hyperactivity disorder. J Abnorm Child Psychol 17:109–125, 1989

Huebner R: Autistic disorder: a neuropsychological enigma. Am J Occup Ther 46:487–501, 1992

Hughes C, Russell J, Robbins TW: Evidence for executive dysfunction in autism. Neuropsychologia 32:477–492, 1994

Hughes S, Kolsted RK, Briggs LD: Dyscalculia and mathematics achievement. Journal of Instructional Psychology 21:64–67, 1994

Hunt A, Dennis J: Psychiatric disorder among children with tuberous sclerosis. Dev Med Child Neurol 29:190–198, 1987

Hunt RD, Arnsten AFT, Asbell MD: An open trial of guanfacine in the treatment of attention-deficit hyperactivity disorder. J Am Acad Child Adolesc Psychiatry 34:50–54, 1995

Hynd GW, Cohen MJ: Dyslexia, Neuropsychological Theory, Research, and Clinical Differentiation. New York, Grune & Stratton, 1983

Hynd GW, Semrud-Clikeman M, Lorys AR, et al: Brain morphology in developmental dyslexia and attention deficit disorder/hyperactivity. Arch Neurol 47:919–926, 1990

Ialongo NS, Horn WF, Pascoe JM, et al: The effects of a multimodal intervention with attention-deficit-hyperactivity-disorder children: a 9-month follow-up. J Am Acad Child Adolesc Psychiatry 32:182–189, 1993

Insel T: Oxytocin: a neuropeptide for affiliation—evidence from behavioral, receptor autoradiographic, and comparative studies. Psychoneuroendocrinology 17:3–33, 1992

Israngkun PP, Newman HAI, Patel ST: Potential biochemical markers for infantile autism. Neurochemistry Pathology 5:51–70, 1986

Jacobsen R, LeCouteur A, Howlin P, et al: Selective subcortical abnormalities in autism. Psychol Med 18:39–48, 1988

Jaselskis CA, Cook EH, Fletcher KE, et al: Clonidine treatment of hyperactive and impulsive children with autism disorder. J Clin Psychopharmacol 12: 322–327, 1992

Johnson DJ, Blalock J: Adults With Learning Disabilities. Orlando, FL, Grune & Stratton, 1987

Jones PB, Kerwin RW: Left temporal lobe damage in Asperger's syndrome. Br J Psychiatry 156:570–572, 1990

Jones V, Prior MR: Motor imitation abilities and neurological signs in autistic children. J Autism Dev Disord 15:37–46, 1985

Kagan J, Rosman B, Day D, et al: Information processing in the child: significance of analytic and reflective attitudes. Psychological Monographs 78: 578, 1964

Kane R, Mikalac C, Benjamin D, et al: Assessment and treatment of adults with attention-deficit hyperactivity disorder, in Attention Deficit Hyperactivity Disorder: A Handbook for Diagnosis and Treatment. Edited by Barkley RA. New York, Guilford, 1990, pp 613–654

Kaplan EF, Goodglass H, Weintraub S: The Boston Naming Test—2nd Edition. Philadelphia, PA, Lea & Febiger, 1983

Katsui T, Okuda M, Usuda S, et al: Kinetics of 3H-serotonin uptake by platelets in infantile autism and developmental language disorder (including five pairs of twins). J Autism Dev Disord 16:69–76, 1986

Kaufman AS, Kaufman NL: K-ABC: Kaufman Assessment Battery for Children. Circle Pines, MN, American Guidance Service, 1983

Kiessling LS, Marcotte AC, Culpepper L: Antineuronal antibodies: tics and obsessive-compulsive symptoms. J Dev Behav Pediatr 15:421–425, 1994

Kinsbourne M, Warrington EK: The developmental Gerstmann syndrome. Arch Neurol 8:490–501, 1963

Kleiman MD, Neff S, Rosman NP: The brain in infantile autism: are posterior fossa structures abnormal? Neurology 42:753–760, 1992

Klin A: Asperger syndrome. Child Adolesc Psychiatr Clin N Am 3:131–148, 1994

Klin A, Volkmar FR, Sparrow SS, et al: Validity and neuropsychological characterization of Asperger syndrome: convergence with nonverbal learning disabilities syndrome. J Child Psychol Psychiatry 36:1127–1140, 1995

Koegel RL, Dyer K, Bell LK: The influence of child-preferred activities on autistic children's social behavior. J Appl Behav Anal 20:243–252, 1987

Kolmen BK, Feldman HM, Handen BL, et al: Naltrexone in young autistic children: a double-blind, placebo-controlled crossover study. J Am Acad Child Adolesc Psychiatry 34:223–231, 1995

Kuperman S, Beeghly JHL, Burns TL, et al: Association of serotonin concentration to behavior and IQ in autistic children. J Autism Dev Disord 17:133–140, 1987

Kupietz SS, Winsberg BG, Richardson E, et al: Effects of methylphenidate dosage in hyperactive reading-disabled children, I: behavior and cognitive performance effects. J Am Acad Child Adolesc Psychiatry 27:70–77, 1988

Kurzweil SR: Developmental reading disorder: predictors of outcome in adolescents who receive early diagnosis and treatment. J Dev Behav Pediatr 13:399–404, 1992

Lake CR, Ziegler MG, Murphy DL: Increased norepinephrine levels and decreased dopamine-beta-hydroxylase activity in primary autism. Arch Gen Psychiatry 34:553–556, 1977

Langer SZ, Moret C, Raisman R, et al: High affinity binding of 3H-imipramine in brain and platelets and its relevance to affective disorders. Life Sci 29:211–220, 1981

Laplane D, Levasseur M, Pillon B, et al: Obsessive-compulsive and other behavioral changes with bilateral basal ganglia lesions: a neuropsychological, magnetic resonance imaging and positron tomography study. Brain 112:699–725, 1989

Larsen JP, Hoien T, Lundberg I, et al: MRI evaluation of the size and symmetry of the planum temporale in adolescents with developmental dyslexia. Brain Lang 39:289–301, 1990

Launay J, Bursztejn C, Ferrari P, et al: Catecholamines metabolism in infantile autism: a controlled study of 22 autistic children. J Autism Dev Disord 17:333–347, 1987

Leboyer M, Bouvard MP, Launay JM, et al: Brief report: a double blind study of naltrexone in infantile autism. J Autism Dev Disord 22:309–319, 1992

Leboyer M, Bouvard MP, Recasens C, et al: Difference between plasma N- and C-terminally directed B-endorphin immunoreactivity in infantile autism. Am J Psychiatry 151:1797–1801, 1994

Leckman JF, Cohen DJ, Shaywitz BA, et al: CSF monoamine metabolites in child and adult psychiatric patients: a developmental perspective. Arch Gen Psychiatry 37:677–681, 1980

Le Couteur A: The role of genetics in the aetiology of autism, including findings on the links with the fragile-X syndrome, in Aspects of Autism: Biological Research: Proceedings of a Conference Held at the University of Kent, September 1987. Edited by Wing L. Oxford, England, Alden Press, 1988, pp 39–52

Leiter RG: Examiners Manual for the Leiter International Performance Scale. Chicago, IL, Stoelting, 1969

Lelord G, Muh JP, Barthelemy C, et al: Effects of pyridoxine and magnesium on autistic symptoms—initial observations. J Autism Dev Disord 11:219–230, 1981

Leonard CM, Voeller KK, Lombardino LJ, et al: Anomalous cerebral structure in dyslexia revealed with magnetic resonance imaging. Arch Neurol 50:461–469, 1993

Leonard HL, Topol D, Bukstein O, et al: Clonazepam as an augmenting agent in the treatment of childhood-onset obsessive-compulsive disorder. J Am Acad Child Adolesc Psychiatry 33:792–794, 1994

Leslie AM, Frith U: Prospects for a cognitive neuropsychology of autism: Hobson's choice. Psychol Rev 97:122–131, 1990

Leventhal BL, Cook EH, Morford M, et al: Relationships of whole blood serotonin and plasma norepinephrine within families of autistic children. J Autism Dev Disord 20:499–511, 1990

Levine MD, Obkerlaid F, Meltzer L: Developmental output failure. Pediatrics 67:18–25, 1981

Lewitter FI, DeFries JC, Elston RC: Genetic models of reading disability. Behav Genet 10:9–39, 1980

Lincoln AJ, Courchesne E, Kilman BA: A study of intellectual abilities in high-functioning people with autism. J Autism Dev Disord 18:505–524, 1988

Lincoln AJ, Courchesne E, Harms L, et al: Contextual probability evaluation in autistic, receptive developmental language disorder, and control children: event-related potential evidence. J Autism Dev Disord 23:37–58, 1993

Lord C, Rutter M, Goode S, et al: Autism diagnostic observation schedule: a standardized observation of communicative and social behavior. J Autism Dev Disord 19:185–212, 1989

Lord C, Rutter M, LeCouteur A: Autism Diagnostic Interview—Revised: a revised version of a diagnostic interview for caregivers of individuals with possible pervasive developmental disorders. J Autism Dev Disord 24:659–685, 1994

Lou JD, Henriksen L, Bruhn P: Focal cerebral hypoperfusion in children with dysphasia and/or attention deficit disorder. Arch Neurol 41:825–829, 1984

Lovaas OI: Behavioral treatment and normal education and intellectual function in young autistic children. J Consult Clin Psychol 55:3–9, 1987

Luk S: Direct observations studies of hyperactive behaviors. J Am Acad Child Psychiatry 24:338–344, 1985

Luria A: Higher Cortical Functions in Man, 2nd Edition. New York, Basic Books, 1980

Maclean M, Bryant P, Bradley L: Rhymes, nursery rhymes, and reading in early childhood. Merrill-Palmer Quarterly 33:255–282, 1987

Mansheim P: Tuberous sclerosis and autistic behavior. J Clin Psychiatry 40:92–98, 1979

March JS, Nulle K, Herbel B: Behavioral psychotherapy for children and adolescents with obsessive-compulsive disorder: an open trial of a new protocol-driven treatment package. J Am Acad Child Adolesc Psychiatry 33:333–341, 1994

Margolis JS: Academic correlates of sustained attention. Unpublished doctoral dissertation, University of California, Los Angeles, 1972

Mattis S: (Modified) Dementia Rating Scale (Alternating Writing Sequence; Numberless Clocks). Odessa, FL, Psychological Assessment Resources, 1988

Mattis S, French JH, Rapin I: Dyslexia in children and adults: three independent neuropsychological syndromes. Dev Med Child Neurol 17:150–163, 1975

McBride PA, Anderson GM, Hertzig ME, et al: Serotonergic responsivity in male young adults with autistic disorder. Arch Gen Psychiatry 46:205–212, 1989a

McBride PA, Anderson GM, Mann JJ: Serotonin-mediated responses in autism (abstract). Biol Psychiatry 25:183A, 1989b

McClure RD, Gordon M: Performance of disturbed hyperactive and nonhyperactive children on an objective measure of hyperactivity. J Abnorm Child Psychol 12:561–572, 1984

McConaughy SH, Ritter DR: Social competence and behavioral problems of learning disabled boys aged 6–11. Journal of Learning Disabilities 19:101–106, 1986

McDougle CJ, Price LH, Goodman WK: Fluvoxamine treatment of coincident autistic disorder and obsessive-compulsive disorder: a case report. J Autism Dev Disord 20:537–543, 1990

McDougle CJ, Naylor ST, Cohen DJ, et al: A double-blind, placebo-controlled study of fluvoxamine in adults with autistic disorder. Arch Gen Psychiatry 53:1001–1008, 1996

McDougle CJ, Brodkin ES, Naylor ST, et al: Sertraline in adults with pervasive developmental disorders: a prospective open-label investigation. J Clin Psychopharmacol 18:62–66, 1998

McGough JJ, Spoeier PL, Cantwell DP: Obsessive-compulsive disorder in childhood and adolescence. School Psychology Review 22:243–251, 1993

Mehlinger R, Scheftner WA, Poznanski E: Fluoxetine and autism (letter). J Am Acad Child Adolesc Psychiatry 29:985, 1990

Mesulam MM: A cortical network for directed attention and unilateral neglect. Ann Neurol 10:309–325, 1981

Mesulam MM: The functional anatomy and hemispheric specialization for directed attention: the role of the parietal lobe and its connectivity. Trends Neurosci 6:384–387, 1983

Milich R, Loney J, Landau S: The independent dimensions of hyperactivity and aggression: a validation with playroom observation data. J Abnorm Psychol 91:183–198, 1982

Minderaa RB, Anderson GM, Volkmar FR, et al: Urinary 5-hydroxyindoleacetic acid and whole blood serotonin and tryptophan in autistic and normal subjects. Biol Psychiatry 22:933–940, 1987

Minderaa RB, Anderson GM, Volkmar FR, et al: Neurochemical study of dopamine functioning in autistic and normal subjects. J Am Acad Child Adolesc Psychiatry 28:190–194, 1989

Minshew NJ: Neurological localization in autism, in High-Functioning Individuals With Autism. Edited by Schopler E, Mesibov GB. New York, Plenum, 1992, pp 65–90

Minshew NJ: In vivo brain chemistry of autism: magnetic resonance spectroscopy studies, in The Neurobiology of Autism. Edited by Bauman M, Kemper TL. Baltimore, MD, Johns Hopkins University Press, 1994, pp 66–85

Money J: Turner's syndrome and parietal lobe functions. Cortex 9:387–393, 1973

Money J, Alexander D, Walker HT: A Standardized Road Map Test of Direction Sense. Baltimore, MD, Johns Hopkins University Press, 1965

Montgomery SA: Obsessive compulsive disorder is not an anxiety disorder. Int Clin Psychopharmacol 8 (suppl 1):57–62, 1993

Naidoo S: Specific Dyslexia. London, Pitman, 1972

Naruse H, Nagahata M, Nakane Y, et al: A multi-center double-blind trial of pimozide (Orap), haloperidol and placebo in children with behavioral disorders, using crossover design. Acta Paedopsychiatrica 48:173–184, 1982

Newby RF, Fischer M, Roman MA: Parent training for families of children with ADHD. School Psychology Review 20:252–265, 1991

Newcomer PL, Hammill DD: Tests of Language Development—Primary: 3rd Edition. Austin, TX, Pro-Ed, 1998

Northup J, Jones K, Broussard C, et al: A preliminary comparison of reinforcer assessment methods for children with attention deficit hyperactivity disorder. J Appl Behav Anal 28:99–100, 1995

Oades RD, Ropcke B, Eggers C: Monoamine activity reflected in urine of young patients with obsessive-compulsive disorder, psychosis with and without reality distortion and healthy subjects: an explorative analysis. J Neural Transm Gen Sect 96:143–159, 1994

O'Hare AE, Brown JK, Aitken K: Dyscalculia in children. Dev Med Child Neurol 33:356–361, 1991

Olson RK, Wise B, Conners F, et al: Specific deficits in component reading and language skills: genetic and environmental influences. Journal of Learning Disabilities 22:339–348, 1989

Olsson I, Steffenburg S, Gillberg C: Epilepsy in autism and autistic-like conditions: a population-based study. Arch Neurol 45:666–668, 1988

Osterrieth PA: Le test de copie d'une figure complex: contribution a l'etude de la perception et de la memoire [The complex figure text: contribution to the study of perception and memory]. Arch de Psychologie 30:286–356, 1944

Otto MW: Normal and abnormal information processing: neuropsychological perspective on obsessive-compulsive disorder. Psychiatr Clin North Am 15:825–848, 1992

Ozonoff S, Rogers S, Pennington BF: Asperger's syndrome: evidence of an empirical distinction from high functioning autism. J Child Psychol Psychiatry 32:1107–1122, 1991

Partington MW, Tu JB, Wong CY: Blood serotonin levels in severe mental retardation. Dev Med Child Neurol 15:616–627, 1973

Pennington BF: Diagnosing Learning Disorders: A Neuropsychological Framework. New York, Guilford, 1991a, pp 45–81, 111–134

Pennington BF: Genetics of learning disabilities. Semin Neurol 11:28–34, 1991b

Pennington BF, Van Doorninck WJ, McCabe LL, et al: Neuropsychological deficits in early treated phenylketonurics. American Journal of Mental Deficiency 89:467–474, 1985

Pennington BF, Van Orden G, Smith SD, et al: Phonological processing skills and deficits in adult dyslexics. Child Dev 61:1753–1778, 1990

Pennington BF, Van Orden G, Kirson D, et al: What is the causal relation between verbal STM problems and dyslexia? in Phonological Processes in Literacy. Edited by Brady S, Shankweiler D. Hillsdale, NJ, Lawrence Erlbaum, 1991, pp 173–186

Perry BD, Cook EH, Leventhal BL, et al: Platelet 5-HT2 receptor binding sites in autistic children and their first-degree relatives, in Proceedings of the American Academy of Child and Adolescent Psychiatry. Washington, DC, American Academy of Child and Adolescent Psychiatry, 1989, pp 67–68

Perry R, Campbell M, Adams P, et al: Long-term efficacy of haloperidol in autistic children: continuous versus discontinuous drug administration. J Am Acad Child Adolesc Psychiatry 28:93–96, 1989

Peterson BS: Neuroimaging in child and adolescent neuropsychiatric disorders. J Am Acad Child Adolesc Psychiatry 34:1560–1576, 1995

Petraukas R, Rourke B: Identification of subgroups of retarded readers: a neuropsychological multivariate approach. Journal of Clinical Neuropsychology 1:17–37, 1979

Piacentini J, Jaffer M, Gitow A, et al: Psychopharmacologic treatment of child and adolescent obsessive compulsive disorder. Psychiatr Clin North Am 15: 87–107, 1992

Piacentini J, Gitow A, Jaffer M, et al: Outpatient behavioral treatment of child and adolescent obsessive-compulsive disorder. J Anxiety Disord 8:277–289, 1994

Pisterman S, Firestone P, McGrath P, et al: The role of parent training in treatment of preschoolers with ADHD. Am J Orthopsychiatry 62:397–408, 1992

Piven J, Starkstein S, Berthier ML: Temporal lobe atrophy versus open operculum in Asperger's syndrome. Br J Psychiatry 157:457–458, 1990

Piven J, Nehme E, Simon J, et al: Magnetic resonance imaging in autism: measurement of the cerebellum, pons, and fourth ventricle. Biol Psychiatry 31: 491–504, 1992

Piven J, Arndt S, Bailey J, et al: An MRI study of brain size in autism. Am J Psychiatry 152:1145–1149, 1995

Pleak RR, Gormly LJ: Effects of venlafaxine treatment for ADHD in a child (letter). Am J Psychiatry 152:1099, 1995

Pomeroy JC: Infantile autism and childhood psychosis, in Psychiatric Disorders in Children and Adolescents. Edited by Garfinkel BD, Carlson GA, Weller EB. Philadelphia, PA, WB Saunders, 1990, pp 271–290

Porteus SD: Qualitative performance in the Maze Test. Vineland, NJ, Smith Printing House, 1933

Porteus SD: The Maze Test and Mental Differences. Vineland, NJ, Smith Printing House, 1942

Prior MR, Hoffman W: Brief report: neuropsychological testing of autistic children through an exploration with frontal lobe tests. J Autism Dev Disord 20:581–590, 1990

Psychological Corporation: Wechsler Individual Achievement Test. San Antonio, TX, Psychological Corporation, 1992

Purdon SE, Lit W, Labelle A, et al: Risperidone in the treatment of pervasive developmental disorder. Can J Psychiatry 39:400–405, 1994

Ramberg C, Ehlers S, Nyden A, et al: Language and pragmatic functions in school-age children on the autism spectrum. Eur J Disord Comm 31:387–413, 1996

Rapin I: Disorders of higher cerebral function in preschool children, part two: autistic spectrum disorders. American Journal of Diseases of Children 142: 1178–1182, 1988

Rapoport JL: Pediatric psychopharmacology: the last decade, in Psychopharmacology: The Third Generation of Progress. Edited by Meltzer HY. New York, Raven, 1987, pp 1211–1214

Rapoport J, Elkins R, Langer DH, et al: Childhood obsessive-compulsive disorder. Am J Psychiatry 138:1545–1555, 1981

Rapoport JL, Leonard HL, Swedo SE, et al: Obsessive compulsive disorder in children and adolescents: issues in management. J Clin Psychiatry 54 (6, suppl): 27–29, 1993

Rapport MD, Tucker SB, DuPaul GJ, et al: Hyperactivity and frustration: the influence of control over and size of rewards in delaying gratification. J Abnorm Child Psychol 14:191–204, 1986

Ratey J, Bemporad J, Sorgi P, et al: Brief report: open trial effects of beta-blockers on speech and social behaviors in 8 autistic adults. J Autism Dev Disord 17:439–446, 1987a

Ratey J, Mikkelsen E, Sorgi P, et al: Autism: the treatment of aggressive behaviors. J Clin Psychopharmacol 7:35–41, 1987b

Raven JC: Progressive Matrices: A Perceptual Test of Intelligence. London, HK Lewis, 1938

Raven JC: Coloured Progressive Matrices Sets A, Ab, B. London, HK Lewis, 1947

Realmuto GM, August GJ, Garfinkel BD: Clinical effect of buspirone in autistic children. J Clin Psychopharmacol 9:122–125, 1989

Reitan RM: Halstead-Reitan Neuropsychological Test Battery for Children. Bloomington, Indiana University Press, 1969a

Reitan RM: Manual for Administration of Neuropsychological Test Batteries for Adults and Children. Indianapolis University Medical Center, unpublished manuscript, 1969b

Rey A: L'examen psychologique dans les cas d'encephalopathie tramatique [The psychological exam in the cases of traumatic encephalopathy]. Archives de Psychologie 28:286–340, 1941

Rey A: Rey Auditory-Verbal Learning Test. [L'examen clinique en psychologie.] Paris, Press Universaire de France, 1964

Richardson E, Kupietz SS, Winsberg BG, et al: Effects of methylphenidate dosage in hyperactive reading-disabled children, II: reading achievement. J Am Acad Child Adolesc Psychiatry 27:78–87, 1988

Richters JE, Arnold LE, Jensen PS, et al: NIMH collaborative multisite multimodal treatment study of children with ADHD, I: background and rationale. J Am Acad Child Adolesc Psychiatry 34:987–1000, 1995

Rickarby G, Carruthers A, Mitchell M: Brief report: biological factors associated with Asperger syndrome. J Autism Dev Disord 21:341–348, 1991

Riddle MA, Scahill L, King RA, et al: Double-blind, crossover trial of fluoxetine and placebo in children and adolescents with obsessive-compulsive disorder. J Am Acad Child Adolesc Psychiatry 31:1062–1069, 1992

Riddle MA, Landbloom R, Yaryura-Tobias J, et al: Fluvoxamine in the treatment of OCD in children and adolescents: a multicenter, double-blind, placebo-controlled trial. Presented at the annual meeting of the American Psychiatric Association, New York, NY, May 1996

Risser MG, Bowers TG: Cognitive and neuropsychological characteristics of attention deficit hyperactivity disorder children receiving stimulant medications. Percept Mot Skills 77:1023–1031, 1993

Ritvo ER, Yuwiler A, Geller E, et al: Increased blood serotonin and platelets in early infantile autism. Arch Gen Psychiatry 23:566–572, 1970

Ritvo ER, Yuwiler A, Geller E, et al: Effects of L-dopa in autism. Journal of Autism and Child Schizophrenia 1:190–205, 1971

Ritvo ER, Freeman BJ, Scheibel AB, et al: Lower Purkinje cell counts in the cerebella of four autistic subjects: initial findings. UCLA-NSAC Autopsy Research Report. Am J Psychiatry 143:862–866, 1986a

Ritvo ER, Freeman BJ, Yuwiler A, et al: Fenfluramine treatment of autism: UCLA collaborative study of 81 patients at nine medical centers. Psychopharmacol Bull 22:133–140, 1986b

Roeltgen D: Agraphia, in Clinical Neuropsychology, 2nd Edition. Edited by Heilman KM, Valenstein E. New York, Oxford University Press, 1985, pp 75–96

Roeltgen DP, Heilman KM: Apractic agraphia in a patient with normal praxis. Brain Lang 18:35–46, 1983

Roeltgen DP, Sevush S, Heilman KM: Phonological agraphia, writing by the lexical-semantic route. Neurology 33:755–765, 1983a

Roeltgen DP, Sevush S, Heilman K: Pure Gerstmann's syndrome from a focal lesion. Arch Neurol 40:46–47, 1983b

Rosenhall U, Johansson E, Gillberg C: Oculomotor findings in autistic children. J Laryngol Otol 102:435–439, 1988

Rosenthal J: Self-esteem in dyslexic children. Academic Therapy 9:27–39, 1973

Rosenzweig S: The Rosenzweig Picture-Frustration (P-F) Study Basic Manual. Odessa, FL, Psychological Corporation, 1978

Ross DL, Klykylo WM, Hitzemann R: Reduction of elevated CSF beta-endorphin by fenfluramine in infantile autism. Pediatr Neurol 3:83–86, 1987

Ross ED: The aprosodias: functional-anatomic organization of the affect components of language in the right hemisphere. Arch Neurol 38:561–569, 1981

Rourke BP: The syndrome of nonverbal learning disabilities: developmental manifestations in neurological disease, disorder, and dysfunction. The Clinical Neuropsychologist 2:293–330, 1988

Rourke B: Nonverbal Learning Disabilities: The Syndrome and the Model. New York, Guilford, 1989

Rumsey JM, Hamburger SD: Neuropsychological findings in high-functioning men with infantile autism, residual state. J Clin Exp Neuropsychol 10:201–221, 1988

Rumsey JM, Andreason P, Zametkin AJ, et al: Failure to activate the left temporoparietal cortex in dyslexia: an oxygen 15 positron emission tomographic study. Arch Neurol 49:527–534, 1992

Russell RL, Ginsburg HP: Cognitive analysis of children's mathematical difficulties. Cognition and Instruction 1:217–244, 1984

Rutter M: Autistic children: infancy to adulthood. Seminars in Psychiatry 2:435–450, 1970

Rutter M, Lord C, LeCateir A: Autism Diagnostic Interview-R Research, 1990a

Rutter M, MacDonald H, Le Couteur A, et al: Genetic factors in child psychiatric disorders—empirical findings. J Child Psychol Psychiatry 31:39–83, 1990b

Saitoh O, Courchesne E, Egaas B, et al: Cross-sectional area of posterior hippocampus in autistic patients with cerebellar and corpus callosum abnormalities. Neurology 45:317–324, 1995

Sanchez LE, Campbell M, Small AM, et al: A pilot study of clomipramine in young autistic children. J Am Acad Child Adolesc Psychiatry 35:537–544, 1996

Sankar DVS: Biogenic amine uptake by blood platelets and RBC in childhood schizophrenia. Acta Paedopsychiatrica 37:174–182, 1970

Scahill L, Lynch KA: Clomipramine and obsessive-compulsive disorder. Journal of Child and Adolescent Psychiatric Nursing 8:42–45, 1995

Schain RJ, Freedman DX: Studies on 5-hydroxyindole metabolism in autistic and other mentally retarded children. J Pediatr 58:315–320, 1961

Schifter T, Hoffman JM, Hatten HP, et al: Neuroimaging in infantile autism. J Child Neurol 9:155–161, 1994

Schopler E, Reichler R, Renner B: The Childhood Autism Rating Scale. Los Angeles, CA, Western Psychological Services, 1988

Schultz RT, Cho NK, Staib LH, et al: Brain morphology in normal and dyslexic children: the influence of sex and age. Ann Neurol 35:732–742, 1994

Schweitzer JB, Sulzer AB: Self-control in boys with attention deficit hyperactivity disorder: effects of added stimulation and time. J Child Psychol Psychiatry 36:671–686, 1995

Seidel WT, Joschko M: Evidence of difficulties in sustained attention in children with ADHD. J Abnorm Child Psychol 18:217–229, 1990

Seymour PK, MacGregor CJ: Developmental dyslexia: a cognitive experimental analysis of phonological, morphemic and visual impairments. Cognitive Neuropsychology 1:43–82, 1984

Shalev RS, Gross-Tsur V: Developmental dyscalculia and medical assessment. Journal of Learning Disabilities 26:134–137, 1993

Shalev RS, Weirtman R, Amir N: Developmental dyscalculia. Cortex 24:555–561, 1988

Shalev R, Manor O, Amir N, et al: The acquisition of arithmetic in normal children: assessment by a cognitive model of dyscalculia. Dev Med Child Neurol 35:593–601, 1993

Shalev RS, Manor O, Amir N, et al: Developmental dyscalculia and brain laterality. Cortex 31:357–365, 1995

Shallice T: Phonological agraphia and the lexical route in writing. Brain 104:412–429, 1981

Shaywitz SE, Shaywitz B: Diagnosis and management of attention deficit disorder: a pediatric perspective. Pediatr Clin North Am 31:429–457, 1984

Shaywitz SE, Shaywitz B, Fletcher JM, et al: Prevalence of reading disabilities in boys and girls: results of the Connecticut Longitudinal Study. JAMA 264:S998–S1002, 1990

Sheslow D, Adams W: Wide Range Assessment of Memory and Learning Administration Manual. San Antonio, TX, Psychological Corporation, 1990

Siegel BV, Asernow R, Tanguay P, et al: Regional cerebral glucose metabolism and attention in adults with a history of childhood autism. J Neuropsychiatry Clin Neurosci 4:406–414, 1992

Siever LJ, Murphy KL, Slater S, et al: Plasma prolactin changes following fenfluramine in depressed patients compared to controls: an evaluation of central serotonergic responsivity in depression. Life Sci 34:1029–1039, 1984

Simon-Soret C, Borenstein P: Essai de la bromocriptine dans le traitement de l'autisme infantile [Trial of bromocriptine in the treatment of child autism]. Presse Med 16:1286, 1987

Smalley SL, Asarnow RF: Brief report: cognitive subclinical markers in autism. J Autism Dev Disord 20:271–278, 1990

Smalley SL, Asarnow RF, Spence MA: Autism and genetics: a decade of research. Arch Gen Psychiatry 45:953–961, 1988

Smith A: Symbol Digit Modalities Test. Los Angeles, CA, Western Psychological Services, 1991

Smith SD, Kimberling WJ, Pennington BF, et al: Specific reading disability: identification of an inherited form through linkage and analysis. Science 219: 1345–1347, 1983

Smith SD, Pennington BF, Kimberling WJ, et al: Familial dyslexia: use of genetic linkage data to define subtypes. J Am Acad Child Adolesc Psychiatry 29: 204–213, 1990

Sparrow SS, Balla DA, Cicchetti DV: Vineland Adaptive Behavior Scales. Circle Pines, MN, American Guidance Service, 1984

Stauffer RG: The Language Experience Approach to the Teaching of Reading. New York, Harper & Row, 1970

Steffenburg S, Gillberg C: Autism and autistic-like conditions in Swedish rural and urban areas: a population study. Br J Psychiatry 149:81–87, 1986

Stone LW, La Greca AM: The social status of children with learning disabilities: a reexamination. Journal of Learning Disabilities 23:32–37, 1990

Stroop JR: Studies of interference in serial verbal reaction. J Exp Psychol 18: 643–662, 1935

Sverd J, Kupietz SS, Winsberg BG, et al: Effects of 1-5-hydroxytryptophan in autistic children. Journal of Autism and Child Schizophrenia 8:171–180, 1978

Swedo SE, Leonard HL, Kruesi MJ, et al: Cerebrospinal fluid neurochemistry in children and adolescents with obsessive-compulsive disorder. Arch Gen Psychiatry 49:29–36, 1992a

Swedo SE, Leonard HL, Rapoport JL: Childhood-onset obsessive-compulsive disorder. Psychiatr Clin North Am 15:767–775, 1992b

Szatmari P, Bartolucci G, Bremner R: Asperger's syndrome and autism: comparisons on early history and outcome. Dev Med Child Neurol 31:709–720, 1989a

Szatmari P, Offord DR, Boyle MH: Correlates, associated impairments and patterns of service utilization of children with attention deficit disorders: findings from the Ontario child health study. J Child Psychol Psychiatry 30:205–217, 1989b

Szatmari P, Tuff L, Finlayson A, et al: Asperger's syndrome and autism: neurocognitive aspects. J Am Acad Child Adolesc Psychiatry 29:130–136, 1990

Szatmari P, Archer L, Fisman S, et al: Asperger's syndrome and autism: differences in behavior, cognition, and adaptive functioning. J Am Acad Child Adolesc Psychiatry 34:1662–1671, 1995

Tallal P, Miller SL, Bedi G, et al: Language comprehension in language-learning impaired children improved with acoustically modified speech. Science 271:81–84, 1996

Thomas-Anterion C, Laurent B, Le Henaff H, et al: Trouble de l'apprentissage de l'orthographe: etude neuropsychologique de deux adolescents presentant une dysgraphie developpementale [Trouble in learning how to spell: neuropsychological study of two adolescents presenting developmental dysgraphia]. Rev Neurol (Paris) 150:827–834, 1994

Thomsen PH: Obsessive-compulsive disorder in children and adolescents: a review of the literature. Eur Child Adolesc Psychiatry 3:138–158, 1994

Tiffin J: Purdue Pegboard: Examiner Manual. Chicago, IL, Science Research Associates, 1968

Tiffin J, Asher EJ: The Purdue Pegboard: norms and studies of reliability and validity. J Appl Psychol 32:234–247, 1948

Tridon P, Schweitzer F, Six V: A propos du syndrome de Rett. Annales Medico Psychologiques 147:245–250, 1989

Trott GE, Friese HJ, Menzel M, et al: Use of moclobemide in children with attention deficit hyperactivity disorder. Psychopharmacology 106:134–136, 1992

Tryon WW: Principles and methods of mechanically measuring motor activity. Behavioral Assessment 6:129–140, 1984

Vellutino FR: Dyslexia: theory and research. Cambridge, MA, MIT Press, 1979

Vigil Continuous Performance Test: Software for the Assessment of Attention. Hollis, NH, For Thought, 1993

Voeller KK: Right-hemisphere deficit syndrome in children. Am J Psychiatry 143:1004–1009, 1986

Voeller KK: Right-hemisphere deficit syndrome in children. Annual Progress in Child Psychiatry and Child Development 381–393, 1987

Voeller KK, Heilman KM: Attention deficit disorder in children: a neglect syndrome? Neurology 38:806–808, 1988

Volger GP, DeFries JC, Decker SN: Family history as an indicator of risk for reading disability. Journal of Learning Disabilities 18:419–421, 1985

Volkmar FR, Klin A, Siegel B, et al: DSM-IV autism/pervasive developmental disorders field trial. Am J Psychiatry 151:579–592, 1994

Wagner RK, Torgesen JK: The nature of phonological processing and its causal role in the acquisition of reading skills. Psychol Bull 101:192–212, 1987

Waldrop RD: Selection of patients for management of attention deficit hyperactivity disorder in a private practice setting. Clin Pediatr 33:83–87, 1994

Wallach L, Wallach MA, Dozier MG, et al: Poor children learning to read do not have trouble with auditory discrimination but do have trouble with phoneme recognition. Journal of Educational Psychology 69:36–69, 1977

Watson RT, Heilman KM: Callosal apraxia. Brain 106:391–404, 1983

Wechsler D: Wechsler Adult Intelligence Scale—Revised. San Antonio, TX, Psychological Corporation, 1981

Wechsler D: Manual for the Wechsler Intelligence Scale for Children, Third Edition. San Antonio, TX, Psychological Corporation, 1991

Weinberg WA, Harper CR: Vigilance and its disorders. Neurol Clin 11:59–78, 1993

Weintraub S, Mesulam MM: Developmental learning disabilities of the right hemisphere: emotional, interpersonal, and cognitive components. Arch Neurol 40:463–468, 1983

Weiss G, Hechtman L: Hyperactive Children Grown Up. New York, Guilford, 1986

Weizman R, Weizman A, Tyano S: Humoral endorphin blood levels in autistic, schizophrenic and healthy subjects. Psychopharmacology 82:368–370, 1984

Wiederholt JL, Bryant BR: Gray Oral Reading Test—3rd Edition. Austin, TX, Pro-Ed, 1992

Wiig EH, Secord W: Test of Linguistic Competency—Expanded Edition. San Antonio, TX, Psychological Corporation, 1988

Wilens TE, Biederman J: The stimulants. Psychiatr Clin North Am 15:191–222, 1992

Wilens TE, Spencer T, Biederman J, et al: Combined pharmacotherapy: an emerging trend in pediatric psychopharmacology. J Am Acad Child Adolesc Psychiatry 34:110–112, 1995

Wilkinson GS: The Wide Range Achievement Test Administration Manual. Wilmington, DE, Wide Range, 1993

Willemsen-Swinkels SH, Buitelaar JK, Nijhof GJ, et al: Failure of naltrexone hydrochloride to reduce self-injurious and autistic behavior in mentally retarded adults: double-blind placebo-controlled studies. Arch Gen Psychiatry 52:766–773, 1995

Wing L: Asperger's syndrome: a clinical account. Psychol Med 11:115–130, 1981

Wing L (ed): Aspects of Autism: Biological Research. Oxford, England, Alden Press, 1988

Wing L: Diagnosis of autism, in Diagnosis and Treatment of Autism. Edited by Gillberg C. New York, Plenum, 1989, pp 5–23

Witt-Engerstrom I, Gillberg C: Autism and Rett syndrome: a preliminary epidemiological study of diagnostic overlap. J Autism Dev Disord 17:149–150, 1987

Woodcock RW: Woodcock Reading Mastery Test—Revised. Circle Pines, MN, American Guidance Services, 1987

Young JG, Cohen DJ, Brown S, et al: Decreased urinary free catecholamines in childhood autism. Journal of the American Academy of Child Psychiatry 17: 671–679, 1978

Young JG, Cohen DJ, Caparulo BK, et al: Decreased 24-hour urinary MHPG in childhood autism. Am J Psychiatry 136:1055–1057, 1979

Young JG, Newcorn JH, Leven LI: Pervasive developmental disorders, in Comprehensive Textbook of Psychiatry, Vol 2, 5th Edition. Edited by Kaplan HI, Sadock BJ. Baltimore, MD, Williams & Wilkins, 1989, pp 1772–1787

Zappella M: Young autistic children treated with etiologically oriented family therapy. Family Systems Medicine 8:14–27, 1990

Zentall SS: Effects of color stimulation on performance and activity of hyperactive and nonhyperactive children. Journal of Educational Psychology 78: 159–165, 1986

Zilbovicius M, Garreau B, Tzourio N, et al: Regional cerebral blood flow in childhood autism: a SPECT study. Am J Psychiatry 149:924–930, 1992

6

NEUROPSYCHOLOGICAL FUNCTIONS IN PERSONALITY DISORDER

Gregg E. Gorton, M.D., Thomas Swirsky-Sacchetti, Ph.D.,
Richard Sobel, M.D., Steven Samuel, Ph.D., and
Amy Gordon, M.A.

ALTHOUGH BRAIN DYSFUNCTION in personality disorder (PD) has long been suspected, only over the past 15 years have research findings begun to clearly delineate cognitive patterns that may reflect neuropsychological dysfunction in at least a subset of patients from among those meeting DSM criteria for PD. Some of these patients are among those often identified as *difficult to treat* (Colson and Allen 1986), and if frank brain dysfunction is identified, this apparent treatment resistance can be understood not simply as psychodynamically or interpersonally based pathology but as something in the realm of fixed deficit. The patient who "won't" then becomes, in a different treatment perspective, the patient who "can't." Such patients, viewed initially as uncooperative, resistant, manipulative, untreatable, and so forth, can now be more usefully seen as struggling and incapable, in need of empathic support and alternative therapeutic strategies rather than persistent psychodynamic interpretation, stern confrontation, or even dismissal from treatment (Anscombe 1986).

Although such a shift in the clinician's perspective on the patient with PD begs questions such as the degree to which there is plasticity in brain structure (see Spreen et al. 1995 for a review) and how much capacity such patients have for compensatory or even restorative learning (Jaeger et al. 1992; Keefe 1995), it may at the same time suggest modification of traditional treatment approaches in order to take into account neuropsychological weaknesses and strengths.

But how many patients with PD appear to have neuropsychological disturbances, and what is the patterning of such disturbances? We examine in depth only those PDs for which a body of neuropsychological research data exists. Neuropsychological assessment of cognitive strengths and weaknesses—what has been called the *cognitive profile*—can be useful for making an accurate diagnosis, determining the patient's prognosis, planning treatment, recommending appropriate psychoeducation, and formulating a particular psychotherapeutic approach.

Care must be taken neither to assume nor to conclude that differences in cognitive profiles among patients in a given study, between patients and control subjects, or among patients in different studies necessarily signify some sort of brain dysfunction. Such differences are not necessarily the result of something that is unchangeable, such as a localizable, anatomic-structural, "hardware" lesion. Consider, for example, patients who have both a PD and a long-term, comorbid Axis I disorder such as obsessive-compulsive disorder or substance dependence (see O'Donnell and Calev, Chapter 4, and Bates and Convit, Chapter 9, in this volume). In such cases, the apparent PD may seem to remit after successful treatment of the Axis I condition (Gorton and Akhtar 1994). Naturally, this response raises the question of whether the PD was validly diagnosed in the first place, but an alternative conceptualization of a PD casts its manifestations as deriving from a long-term *functional* central nervous system (CNS) process or a *software deficit* that is somewhat plastic. This view should be familiar to devotees of psychodynamic theories of PD etiology and treatment. In the discussion that follows, we hope to contribute to a dialectical, structural-functional approach to PD (and personality, broadly speaking) that acknowledges the stark uncertainties in the details of how variations either within an individual's brain-functional domains or between two or more individuals' patterns of neuropsychological function contribute to what we understand to be their disparate personalities.

It is hoped that future research will delineate not only neuropsychological differences between patients who have PD and control subjects but also reproducible, localizable deficits in brain function in at least some of the same patients, as measured by structural and functional brain imaging. Only then will we be able to argue with greater certainty that distinct cognitive profiles in patients with PD or any other disorder are validly related to brain dysfunction rather than to confounding states such as anxiety, poor motivation, fatigue, or acute stress.

Before we review the research literature for each of the PDs that have undergone substantive neuropsychological investigation, we must note some relevant methodological issues that these studies have not always addressed rigorously. First, until the advent of DSM-III (American Psychiatric Association 1980), the field lacked a broad consensus regarding diagnostic criteria for PDs. Therefore, it is difficult to make meaningful comparisons between studies of PDs conducted before 1980 and more up-to-date studies. We focus this chapter largely on those studies that used criteria from DSM-III, DSM-III-R, or DSM-IV (American Psychiatric Association 1987, 1994).

Second, valid and reliable diagnosis of PDs depends on rigorous application of both the general criteria required for diagnosis of any PD and the particular set of criteria for a specific PD. Rigorous application of the criteria involves excluding cases from PD diagnosis if an identifiable medical factor exists—such as complex partial seizures—that can be correlated temporally with the apparent PD symptoms. In such cases, the proper diagnosis would be either "organic personality syndrome" (DSM-III/DSM-III-R) or "personality change due to [specify identified general medical condition]" (DSM-IV).

A general exclusionary criterion regarding substance abuse that was added to DSM-IV affects the PD criteria. This criterion should be applied whenever a substance-related disorder is present and its onset is believed to correlate with apparent PD symptoms. This landmark alteration, as applied to the PD criteria, can minimize false-positive inclusion in a PD category (e.g., antisocial or borderline) of individuals whose PD symptoms correlate temporally with intoxicant use. Some pre-DSM-IV studies included patients who had what should more properly have been labeled "personality change due to a [name of substance]-related disorder" or "[name of substance]-related [name of disorder]." (For a review of the relationship between addiction and PD, see Gorton and Akhtar 1994.)

Third, as other chapters in this book demonstrate, many other Axis I conditions may confound etiological attribution of the neuropsychological differences found in patients with PD. Ideally, clinically significant anxiety and mood disorders, substance-related disorders, psychosis, and attention-deficit disorder, at the very least, should be excluded (see Calev, Chapter 2; Calev et al., Chapter 3; O'Donnell and Calev, Chapter 4; and DeCaria et al., Chapter 5, in this book). In addition, because some medications may either impair or improve an individual's cognitive function, patients should ideally be medication free.

Fourth, a subject's particular PD symptoms often do not fit neatly into one PD category, so that multiple PD diagnoses may be present simultaneously, or only a mixture of several PDs may be apparent without a single PD's being fully present (i.e., PD not otherwise specified). Indeed, the specific PDs we examine in this chapter often overlap one another. Thus, when performing research on a specific PD, it is not enough to validate that diagnosis. One must also exclude all other PDs. However, the more homogeneous the research sample, the less potentially generalizable any significant findings will be as far as elucidating what is happening in typical, more heterogeneous clinical populations, because such research subjects will represent a relatively uncommon patient type.

Fifth, some studies use control groups, whereas others rely on historical neuropsychological test norms to assess the significance of study findings. The use of historical norms in this research is problematic if one is attempting to identify subtle variability within a study population (Swirsky-Sacchetti et al. 1993). Yet in this area of psychopathology, the clinical usefulness and degree of generalizability of research findings involving control groups is problematic because in the clinical setting the use of comparative control subjects is impractical and costly. It may be nearly impossible in the clinical setting to disentangle the multiple possible causes of cognitive dysfunction (e.g., Colson and Allen 1986; Hamilton and Allsbrook 1986).

With regard to possible cognitive dysfunction in PDs, significant bodies of research data exist only for antisocial PD (ASPD), borderline PD (BPD), and schizotypal PD (SPD). We address each of these PDs separately, beginning each section with a case vignette, followed by reviews of neurological, neurophysiological, neuroimaging, and neuropsychological studies. After comparing the findings in ASPD, BPD, and SPD, we conclude with a discussion of the clinical implications of the data we have reviewed.

◈ ANTISOCIAL PERSONALITY DISORDER

The following case vignette illustrates ASPD associated with a variety of neuropsychological deficits representative of those identified in research on cognitive function in this PD. The vignette also suggests how a stagnant treatment approach can be enlivened by considering the cognitive test profile.

Mr. A, a 22-year-old man, was referred for neuropsychological testing by his father, who felt "at the end of my rope" in trying to help his son to establish stable, independent adult functioning. The father's call was prompted by his having seen a television program that mentioned a possible "organic cause" of "impulsive, reckless children who are unable to establish normal emotional bonding with their parents."

Mr. A had been adopted as an infant. At an early age, he was unable to meet normal expectations for socialized behavior. He was frequently involved in fighting, stealing, lying, and reckless behavior, and he was given to intermittent drunkenness. Despite normal intelligence, he received special education in the public schools but dropped out in eleventh grade. The father said that Mr. A never seemed to feel "true remorse" for any of his hurtful actions.

Mr. A's adoptive mother had died when he was 14 years old. Several years later, the father married a woman who tried to become a second mother to Mr. A. Two years before the referral, Mr. A had stolen his new mother's camera equipment, prompting her finally to declare the home "off limits" to Mr. A. Traditional therapeutic approaches that explored Mr. A's issues of anger and loss at his adoptive status, the death of his adoptive mother, and his father's remarriage were unsuccessful. Two weeks before the referral, Mr. A was fired from his fifth job since leaving school and lost his driver's license as a result of numerous legal infractions. Clinical evaluation revealed that he met criteria for ASPD and had no concurrent Axis I diagnosis except possible alcohol abuse.

Neuropsychological testing indicated that Mr. A had a normal level of intelligence, with slightly higher nonverbal, visuospatial problem-solving abilities relative to his verbal intelligence. Among the verbal IQ subtests, Mr. A's fund of information, expressive word knowledge, and verbal abstraction skills were below average. He was mildly impaired on vigilance tasks in which target stimuli had to be identified through careful visual scanning. His verbal memory skills were mildly impaired, especially for tasks that required rapid planning and organization. His memory for short stories and designs was at the borderline level of mild impairment. Mr. A's basic skill levels in reading, spelling, and written arithmetic were generally commensurate with his IQ. No specific learning disability was identified.

Motor and sensory-perceptual skills were within normal limits, with the exception of complex motor regulatory skills. Mr. A was impaired on rapid alternating hand sequences and verbal regulation of motor responses. On measures of complex problem solving, the results were mixed. Mr. A performed within normal limits on a fairly structured task requiring speed, concentration, sequencing, and set-shifting, but his performance was mildly impaired on a task requiring mental flexibility, hypothesis generation, and abstract reasoning. Overall, the results were consistent with mildly deficient performance on tasks likely to involve the left frontotemporal region.

A family feedback session was held, with the goal of reframing Mr. A's behavior. Rather than viewing Mr. A simply as a defiant, belligerent youth who was acting out long-standing feelings of anger and loss, the parents were encouraged to accept a more comprehensive view of his behavior that included deficiencies in certain aspects of cognitive performance. Mr. A agreed to participate in a structured, cognitive-behavioral type of therapy with the specific goal of helping him to identify situations in which he was at risk for impulsive or reckless behavior. Mr. A's use of *self-talk* was encouraged, the goal being to help him to think before acting. Time-limited and structured activities with both parents were encouraged, and individual treatment was supplemented with occasional family sessions. The parents were included in a behavioral plan to shape Mr. A's behavior with concrete rewards. With this approach, he began to show increased self-esteem and gradual behavioral improvement.

Literature Review

The literature pertaining to neuropsychological function in ASPD encompasses findings from a potpourri of related disorders, including psychopathy, psychopathic disorder, criminality, juvenile delinquency, impulse-control disorder, conduct disorder, substance abuse, attention-deficit/hyperactivity disorder, and traumatic brain injury. Although in this section we emphasize studies using DSM-III criteria, we also include some studies from the large non-DSM-III literature on brain-related mechanisms involved in antisocial behavior. Our goal is to understand the nature and extent of neuropsychological impairment in patients with a behavioral disorder characterized by impulsive, aggressive, and antisocial behavior.

Despite many methodological problems, several trends emerge from the literature on neuropsychological function in ASPD:

◆ Apparent dysfunction lateralizable to the dominant or left hemisphere

♦ Apparent dysfunction localizable to the frontal lobes
♦ Deficient performance suggestive of possible brain dysfunction but that is not even tentatively localizable
♦ No consistently demonstrated neuropsychological impairment

We review studies supporting each trend in the next four sections. These results are summarized in Table 6–1.

Left-hemisphere dysfunction. Before the question of brain dysfunction in ASPD was considered seriously, the prevailing conceptualization was that psychopathic individuals had a defect in moral character rather than an intellectual or cognitive deficit. Flor-Henry (1976) was among the first modern brain scientists to postulate an organic basis of psychopathic behavior. Yeudall (1977) noted that failure to censor behavior under consideration could be related to specific functions normally attributed to the left or dominant hemisphere, such as the use of internalized language or emotionally laden memories in anticipation of response to one's behavior.

Hare and McPherson (1984) studied differences in brain function between two groups of prison inmates, one meeting the DSM-III criteria for ASPD and high psychopathy and one having neither disorder. The ASPD/high- psychopathy group showed significantly less right ear advantage on a dichotic listening task, a finding often associated with damage to the left hemisphere. Nachshon (1988) also observed left-hemisphere dysfunction in violent offenders, based on a dichotic listening task.

Jutai and Hare (1983) found a similar pattern of abnormal asymmetry in processing of verbal information presented to both visual fields simultaneously. This finding indicates a more generalized left-hemisphere abnormality. A poorly organized left hemisphere might lead to psychopathic behavior to the extent that rational, logical, and verbal thought processes are underutilized in the modulation of behavioral expression.

Research into the nature of psychopathic behavior has also focused on affective information processing. Hare et al. (1988) found that nonpsychopathic subjects respond more rapidly to affective words in a lexical decision task than to neutral words and that this affective facilitation is not present in psychopathic individuals. Gillstrom and Hare (1988) studied hand gestures in psychopathic individuals during speech and found that these individuals have more movements during speech that bear no relation to speech content than do nonpsychopathic subjects, suggesting they have difficulty with integration of language and affect.

Table 6–1. Methodology and characteristics of antisocial personality disorder (ASPD) neuropsychological studies

Study	Participants	Setting/mean age/ comorbid diagnosis	Tests administered	Significantly different tests and/or significant findings
Yeudall et al. (1982)	Delinquency (64 M/ 35 M), control subjects (29 M/18 W)	Residential/14.6 years/80% had drug or alcohol abuse	HRNB, Ravens, WISC-R or WAIS, COWAT	84% = abnormal profile WAIS
Fedora & Fedora (1983)	Psychopathy (28 M), control subjects (31 M)	Prison/25 years	HRNB, WAIS, COWAT, WCST, Category, Stroop, Ravens	Trails B; left-hemisphere markers
Jutai & Hare (1983)	DSM-III-R ASPD, high vs low psychopathy checklist	Prison/28.6 years	Atari video games, skin conductance, heart rate, eye movements, EEG	"High" group poorer in allocating attentional resources
Hare & McPherson (1984)	DSM-III ASPD (45 M), mixed diagnosis group (58 M), control subjects (43 M)	Prison/29 years	Dichotic listening task	Language is weakly lateralized and poorly organized
Sutker & Allain (1987)	DSM-III-R ASPD (19 M), control subjects (15 M)	Outpatients/ 33 years/drug or alcohol abuse	MMPI, WAIS-R, WCST, Porteus mazes	NS
Moffitt (1988)	Delinquency (76 M/61 W)	Cohort study in New Zealand/13 years	WISC-R, AVLT, Rey Figure, Trails, Grooved Pegboard, COWAT	Boys: COWAT, AVLT, Trails, VIQ, PIQ; Girls: Rey Figure, Grooved Pegboard

Study	Subjects	Setting/Age	Tests	Results
Nachshon (1988)	Murderers (17 M), violent offenders (22 M), nonviolent offenders (54 M)	Prison/25.04 years	Lateral preference, dichotomous listening task	Violent offenders: left-hemisphere dysfunction
Hart et al. (1990)	Psychopathy checklist: high (52 M), medium (136 M), low (67 M)	Prison/30 years	Trails, AVLT, COWAT, BD, WRAT-reading	NS
Malloy et al. (1990)	DSM-III-R ASPD (29 M/1 W), control subjects (29 M/1 W)	Outpatients/32 years/ alcohol dependence	Category, TPT, Trails, BD, DSy, WMS-Russel Rev, BAQ	BAQ, BD, Trails B, WMS Verbal/Nonverbal, drinking history
Burgess (1991)	DSM-III-R PD: BPD (37 T), ASPD (7 T), HPD (4 T), NPD (2 T), DP (2 T), OCPD (2T), schizoid (1 T); DSM-III-R major depression (17 T); DSM-III-R schizophrenia (20 T)	Psychiatric patients /36 years	Neuropsychiatric screening exam	NS; PD patients reported more depression than the other two groups; depression correlated with motor planning and sequencing impairment

(continued)

Table 6–1. Methodology and characteristics of antisocial personality disorder neuropsychological studies *(continued)*

Study	Participants	Setting/mean age/comorbid diagnosis	Tests administered	Significantly different tests and/or significant findings
Burgess (1992)	DSM-III-R PD: HPD (5 T), NPD/BPD (1 T), ASPD (1 T), HPD/BPD (4 T), NPD/BPD (6 T), BPD/ASPD (5 T); control subjects (20 M/20 W)	Psychiatric patients/ 34.3 years	Neuropsychiatric screening examination	Patients with Cluster B PDs had overall impairment in Delayed Memory, Naming Similarities and Differences, Serial 7s, Luria Motor, Perseveration, Omissions
Gillen & Hesselbrock (1992)	DSM-III-R ASPD (34 M)	Volunteers with family history of alcoholism/ 23 years	Luria Motor, Trails, CVLT, WMS-Russel Rev, COWAT, JLO, WCST, WAIS-R, Porteus mazes	WCST: perseverative errors, complex motor, similarities; WAIS-R: response inhibition
Glenn et al. (1993)	DSM-III-R alcohol dependence (83 M/ 48 W), control subjects (47 M/36 W); ASPD symptoms based on antisocial personality section of SADS	Outpatients in alcoholism treatment/ 35 years	Shipley Vocabulary, BDI, SADS, SAI, CPI, BD, Figure Memory, COWAT, Semantic Memory, Grooved Pegboard, Trails, Category, Analogies	Alcoholic patients reported more antisocial behaviors (ASB), affective, and childhood behavioral symptoms (CBD); CBD predicted poorer neuropsychological performance, ASB predicted flexibility in males

Study	Sample	Subjects	Tests	Findings
Stein et al. (1993)	DSM-III-R (10 M/8 W): BPD (10 T), ASPD and BPD (8 T)	Inpatients and outpatients/ 31.2 years	Vocabulary, Trails, WCST, Rey Figure, Familiar Figures	Left soft signs (ss) correlated with Trails, Familiar Figures; right ss correlated with WCST errors and aggression
Fals-Stewart & Lucente (1994)	DSM-III-R substance abuse (180 M/66 W), subset with elevated score in MCMI-II antisocial category	Inpatient substance abuse treatment/ 27.4 years	MCMI-II, Category, TPT, Trails, BD, DSy, Vocabulary	ASPD symptoms and lower cognitive status negatively correlated with length of stay

Note. AVLT = Auditory-Verbal Learning Test, BAQ = Brain Age Quotient, BD = Block Design, BDI = Beck Depression Inventory, BPD = borderline personality disorder, Category = Category Test, COWAT = Controlled Oral Word Association Test, CPI = California Psychological Inventory, CVLT = California Verbal Learning Test, DP = dependent personality disorder, DSy = Digit Symbol, EEG = electroencephalography, HPD = histrionic personality disorder, HRNB = Halstead-Reitan Neuropsychological Battery, JLO = Judgment of Line Orientation, M = men, MCMI = Million Clinical Multiaxial Inventory, MMPI = Minnesota Multiphasic Personality Inventory, NPD = narcissistic personality disorder, NS = no significantly different tests or findings, OCPD = obsessive-compulsive personality disorder, PD = personality disorder, PIQ = Performance IQ, Ravens = Raven's Progressive Matrices, Rey Figure = Rey-Osterrieth Complex Figure, SADS = Schedule of Affective Disorders and Schizophrenia, SAI = Spielberger State Anxiety Inventory, Stroop = Stroop Color and Word Test, T = total, TPT = Tactual Performance Test, Trails = Trail Making Test, VIQ = Verbal IQ, W = women, WAIS-R = Wechsler Adult Intelligence Scale—Revised, WCST = Wisconsin Card Sorting Test, WISC-R = Wechsler Intelligence Scale for Children—Revised, WMS = Wechsler Memory Scale, WRAT = Wide Range Achievement Test.

Few studies of ASPD have used neuroradiological or brain metabolic measures. Volkow and Tancredi (1987) used brain computed tomography (CT), positron-emission tomography (PET), and electroencephalography (EEG) to study four patients who had a history of repetitive, violent, purposeless behavior. The results were generally suggestive of left-hemisphere dysfunction, especially of the frontal and temporal lobes.

Frontal-lobe dysfunction. Jutai and Hare (1983) used auditory evoked potentials and simultaneous video games to investigate attentional processes in two groups of prison inmates rated high and low on a psychopathy scale. The results indicated that psychopathic individuals are able to "allocate a relatively large proportion of their attentional resources to things of immediate interest, effectively ignoring or screening out other stimuli" (p. 150).

In a similar vein, when Fedora and Fedora (1983) predicted that psychopathic individuals would perform better than control subjects on the Stroop Color and Word Test, which requires the subject to screen out an overlearned response in favor of a less automatic one, the results showed a trend in the predicted direction, suggesting frontal hyperfunction.

Yeudall et al. (1982) found a pattern of apparent frontal-lobe dysfunction when they tested a large sample of inpatient juvenile delinquents. Compared with the nondelinquent group, a much greater percentage of the delinquent group had abnormal neuropsychological profiles, especially nondominant-hemisphere impairment. This lateralized finding may reflect the low incidence of violent criminals in the sample, in contrast to other studies of violent criminals that reported a greater left-anterior dysfunction (Krynicki 1978).

Gorenstein (1990) theorized that in delinquents, dysfunction is localized to the prefrontal cortex and its limbic connections, which affects the individuals' capacity for avoiding incidental punishment, anticipating aversive events, mediating temporal intervals, and seeking stimulation. Gorenstein relied on Luria's (1973) work to explain the behavior problems of unsocialized delinquents. In the Lurian model, prefrontal damage disrupts one's internal plan or intentional set, which is normally used to inhibit a potential response based on biological drive, stimulus cuing, or prior exposure. Individuals with prefrontal damage thus have *disinhibitory* deficits. Gorenstein noted that Luria's prefrontal deficit theory explains not only the decreased responsiveness to punishment but also the enhanced responsiveness to reward that characterizes antisocial behavior. First, a delinquent's ability to generate an internalized representation of a hypothetical punishing event is lacking. Second, an individual with a prefrontal deficit cannot initiate and maintain higher-order activity that facilitates moving away from an immediately rewarding activity.

In an earlier controlled study, Gorenstein (1982) reported significant deficits on measures of frontal-lobe function in a group of psychopathic patients who met DSM-III criteria for ASPD. The ASPD group had more perseverative errors on the Wisconsin Card Sorting Test (WCST) and more errors on the Sequential Matching Figures Test. One additional test measure, spontaneous reversals of the Necker Cube, was also significantly higher in the ASPD group than in a psychiatric control group and a group of normal college students. Previous research had shown patients with bilateral frontal lesions to have significantly more reversals than patients with unilateral frontal lesions or control subjects (Teuber 1964).

Raine et al. (1992a) used PET to evaluate regional patterns of glucose metabolism in convicted murderers. In comparison with control subjects, the murderers had a decrease in glucose metabolic rate localized to the orbital frontal and prefrontal cortex. Goyer et al. (1994) used PET to study 17 patients who met DSM-III-R criteria for PD. They noted a significant inverse correlation between a life history of aggressive impulse-control difficulties and regional glucose metabolism in the frontal cortex, but significant differences were not found when the six ASPD patients were compared with control subjects.

Nonlocalizable neuropsychological dysfunction. With regard to the danger in ascribing poor performance on any particular neuropsychological test to a structural defect in a particular brain region (Keefe 1995), Luria (1980) maintained that the score on a particular task was not as important in determining underlying localization as was the qualitative nature of the mistake.

Although few would argue with the lateralization of the linguistic aspects of language function to the left hemisphere, the assignment of particular tasks to the frontal lobes is subject to more controversy and may be responsible for inconsistent results. For this reason, the studies described in this section, which are largely suggestive of some type of brain dysfunction in ASPD that is not clearly localizable, are presented separately.

Malloy et al. (1990) compared alcoholic inpatients who met DSM-III criteria for ASPD with those who did not. The ASPD patients performed significantly worse on measures of visuoanalytical problem-solving and on a task requiring speed, concentration, set-shifting, and visuomotor integration. There was an insignificant trend for the ASPD group to perform more poorly on additional tests of complex problem-solving and memory.

Gillen and Hesselbrock (1992) found that patients with ASPD had significantly more errors on a complex motor task and greater deficits in verbal abstraction and concept formation than did patients who did not have ASPD, findings believed to be consistent with left frontal-lobe deficits.

In a study of juvenile delinquents, Moffitt (1988) reported that the boys were significantly worse than control subjects on several language and memory measures, whereas the girls were significantly worse on visuospatial skills and those skills requiring visuomotor integration and executive functions. Gender appears to be an important variable all too often overlooked in ASPD research.

No significant neuropsychological dysfunction.   Glenn et al. (1993) administered a comprehensive battery of neuropsychological tests to alcoholic patients with and without ASPD and found that ASPD was not a significant predictor of overall neuropsychological performance.

Hart et al. (1990) studied inmates who were divided into three groups reflecting severity of psychopathy but found no differences among the groups on two 60-minute test batteries.

Sutker and Allain (1987) compared psychopathic inpatients who met DSM-III criteria for ASPD with nonpsychopathic inpatient control subjects but found no significant differences in abstraction, flexibility, control, and planning.

Summary of ASPD Research

Research to date indicates numerous methodological problems that severely limit conclusions regarding brain dysfunction unique to ASPD (Kandel and Freed 1989). Even so, the overwhelming majority of data suggests the presence of at least mild brain dysfunction tentatively localized to the left hemisphere or to the frontal lobes, as our introductory case vignette illustrates. As a general rule, findings that are relatively consistent across multiple studies are more likely to be unrelated to transient states of distress, anxiety, and so on, yet these findings cannot be ruled out entirely as contributing factors in the currently available data.

Deficient language organization in the left hemisphere might facilitate impulsive-aggressive behavior in ASPD by reducing the individual's capacity to use logical, rational thought processes to modulate emotionally charged behavior. Deficient dominant temporal-lobe functioning might also disrupt appropriate learning or access to remote memories, thereby making it more difficult for an ASPD individual to learn from past mistakes.

The dysfunctional behavior of ASPD also appears consistent with a frontal-lobe dysfunction hypothesis, but the research we have reviewed does not consistently support this possibility. Subtypes of ASPD may be represented by the left-hemisphere or frontal-lobe dysfunction hypotheses, but other subtypes of ASPD that do not necessarily involve frank neuropsychological dysfunction are also highly likely. We cannot exclude the possibility that the learned acquisition of an antisocial response pattern might result in a distinguishable cognitive profile that does not presuppose identifiable brain dysfunction.

Delineation of ASPD subtypes requires further research with large samples of patients who meet the DSM-IV criteria for ASPD. Such research would permit statistical analysis to identify within-group clusters and to compare subgroups defined by age, gender, education, and IQ. Prospective neuropsychological study of young adult populations at risk for ASPD who have not yet had significant exposure to drugs and alcohol would also be useful.

◈ BORDERLINE PERSONALITY DISORDER

The following case vignette illustrates BPD in an individual who has some of the cognitive performance problems found in neuropsychological studies of BPD subjects.

Ms. B, a 32-year-old former secretary with a diagnosis of BPD, was being treated with intensive individual and group psychotherapy in a partial hospitalization program. The fifth child of a schizophrenic mother and alcoholic father, she had been raped by an uncle as a child. First hospitalized at age 19 after a nearly fatal suicide attempt by drug overdose, she had been hospitalized 12 times during the intervening 13 years and had had seven different outpatient therapists. Medication trials had included antidepressants, antipsychotics, lithium, and lorazepam.

Ms. B's treatment team at the partial hospitalization program reported that she was one of their most difficult patients. Her therapist, who noted Ms. B's great difficulty sustaining a sense of connectedness, said "she often calls between sessions just to hear my voice." Ms. B had trouble recalling themes in the therapy from session to session and showed extremes of all-or-nothing thinking. Overall, her progress was extremely slow, and she was considered quite uninsightful.

During a stagnant period in her treatment, Ms. B coincidentally agreed to participate in a research study of neuropsychological performance in BPD patients. She had no Axis I diagnosis at the time of testing. Neuropsychological testing revealed a Full-Scale IQ of 85, with a Verbal IQ of 96 and a Performance Scale IQ of 74. She did especially poorly on the Picture Arrangement, Object Assembly, and Digit Symbol tests of the Wechsler Adult Intelligence Scale—Revised (WAIS-R); on the Trail Making Test Part A and B; on the Wechsler Memory Scale—Revised (WMS-R) Figural Memory test; and on the Rey-Osterrieth Complex Figure (copy and recall).

When results of the neuropsychological testing were made available to the treatment team, they felt some disappointment and hopelessness because Ms. B, with whom they had worked so hard for many months, showed significant cognitive limitations. With input from the research team, however, they were able to link the cognitive difficulties to Ms. B's object constancy issues and her slowness to learn.

After Ms. B was educated by the neuropsychologist about her cognitive trends—both strengths and weaknesses—she underwent a brain CT and EEG. Both tests were within normal limits. She had been upset initially by the cognitive test findings, but her mood gradually brightened as she realized that her self-hatred and poor self-esteem were reflective of adaptive deficiencies linked to her *preferred cognitive modes.* She was advised that although she should not assume that the test findings would necessarily remain constant over time, she should continue to learn to cope and compensate through further treatment, including cognitive remediative strategies such as memory cuing.

Several months later, Ms. B required hospitalization for worsening depression and suicidality. She was now viewed by her care providers as having significant difficulties in her ability to cope and function in her environment because of impairment in her abilities to plan and to sequence, recall, and process complex information. No longer was Ms. B viewed simply as an "impossible" patient who had evoked a great deal of frustration and hopelessness. Her treatment was structured more carefully to take into account her struggles to maintain internal and external consistency, and her inpatient stay was much shorter than before. Afterward, she made slow but much steadier progress in the outpatient setting.

Literature Review

Patients with BPD often present extreme challenges to treatment providers. In addition to manifesting the well-known DSM-III, DSM-III-R, or DSM-IV behavioral criteria for this disorder [Gorton (1996) has proposed a mnemonic device[1] for the DSM-IV BPD criteria set: BP: AAIILRS], these patients frequently appear to have cognitive and perceptual disturbances including memory impairment (Adler and Buie 1979; Kroll 1988), poor object constancy (Adler and Buie 1979), dichotomous thinking, unpredictable alternation between a global viewpoint and a particularistic focus (O'Leary and Cowdry 1994), difficulty drawing logical correlations, perceptual integrative difficulty, odd reasoning (Judd and Ruff 1993; Sternbach et al. 1992), confusion (Burgess 1991; Kroll 1988), attentional difficulty, learning problems (Andrulonis et al. 1980), failure to anticipate the consequences of their actions (O'Leary and Cowdry 1994), episodic misperception (Vela 1991), and "capricious" cognition (Millon 1996).

The psychodynamic model traditionally has been used to account for such disturbances, which are viewed as defensive and desperately adaptive. As speculation about the neurological underpinnings of psychodynamic processes began to emerge more than a decade ago (for review, see Erdelyi 1985), some researchers advanced theories that had specific application to BPD. For example, Muller (1992) proposed a defect in interhemispheric communication as the neurophysiological basis of the splitting defense that figures so prominently in BPD. However, many clinicians and theorists (e.g., see Frayn 1996; Viederman 1996) still do not appreciate that the cognitive profiles of patients with BPD may have both explanatory and therapeutic value in the clinical setting.

Simultaneous with the emerging interest in brain mechanisms underlying psychodynamics, a number of research studies and reports were published that involved groups of children with BPD (Aarkrog 1981;

---

[1]Gorton (1996) has proposed a mnemonic device for the DSM-IV BPD criteria set, which emphasizes that patients with BPD are truly "ailing." Thus, "BP: AAIILRS"—**B:** boredom/emptiness, **P:** paranoid or dissociative periods, **A:** anger, **A:** abandonment anxiety, **I:** identity disturbance, **I:** impulsivity, **L:** labile mood, **R:** relationship ruptures, **S:** suicidality and self-mutilation.

Bemporad et al. 1982; Murray 1979; Palombo and Feigon 1984; Wergeland 1979) and adults with BPD (Andrulonis and Vogel 1984; Andrulonis et al. 1980, 1982; Quitkin et al. 1976). The range of indicators of brain dysfunction in these studies included neurological soft signs; abnormal EEG findings; visuomotor problems; hyperactivity; attentional problems; speech and language problems; reading disability; tics; motor incoordination; and histories of developmental delay, head injury, or encephalitis (see Vela 1991 for a summary).

Soloff and Millward (1983) were unable to confirm a higher prevalence of neurodevelopmental disturbance in BPD inpatients but called for further neurological and neuropsychological BPD research. Zanarini et al. (1994) found no greater prevalence of CNS disturbance in patients with BPD than in control patients with other PDs. In contrast, van Reekum et al. (1993) detected a significantly greater prevalence of developmental CNS problems, acquired CNS disturbance, and total brain injuries among BPD patients than among control subjects.

Andrulonis and Vogel (1984) postulated two subcategories of BPD involving frank evidence of brain dysfunction: an attentional deficit–learning disabled subcategory and an organic subcategory. These subcategories appear to comprise only a minority of all BPD patients and perhaps include an overabundance of men with BPD. Although it has begun to shed light on the heterogeneity within groups of BPD patients, this work does not appear to address the role of neurocognitive disturbance in most of these patients, who show no overt "organicity." Could such disturbance be subclinical yet play a significant role in the etiology of BPD?

The consensus is that a multidimensional model involving interactions among a combination of genetic, biological, developmental, and environmental factors best accounts for the disturbed cognition, affect dysregulation, and impulse dyscontrol that together are both cause and effect of borderline ego development and behavior (Marziali 1992). Judd and Ruff (1993) delineated two possible etiological developmental models that can be used to explain the origin of BPD: 1) interaction between a cognitively vulnerable child and abuse and/or biparental failure, and 2) early and prolonged childhood trauma that interferes with neurocognitive development. In either model, resultant deficits would be expected to interfere with cognitive-affective development and integration.

van Reekum (1993) postulated four complex models in which brain dysfunction interacts with psychodynamic etiological variables to produce BPD:

1. Brain injury may initiate a disorder of impulse control, affective dysregulation, cognitive disability, and predisposition to psychotic decompensation, with resultant interpersonal dysfunction.
2. Developmental disturbance may be initiated and exacerbated by developmentally disturbed parents and other family members, with the effects of direct and indirect trauma being additive.
3. An inherited tendency to impulse dyscontrol may lead to higher risk of traumatic brain injury and substance abuse, with resultant cognitive impairment and social dysfunction.
4. Any combination of insults to ego and/or cognitive functioning that surpasses some cumulative threshold may lead into a common pathway of borderline personality development.

These models do not always clearly distinguish between BPD patients with frank, identifiable brain injury and those lacking such a history but who nevertheless show significant differences in neurocognitive function. The causal directionality of cognitive dysfunction is part of what is at issue in these models, yet none of van Reekum's models address the possibility of subtle, congenital cognitive disturbance or congenital vulnerability to environmentally induced disturbance of normal neurodevelopment, models that Judd and Ruff (1993) allow and that would encompass Muller's hypothesis (1992), mentioned earlier in this chapter.

The identification of cognitive dysfunction and long-lasting brain changes in patients with posttraumatic stress disorder is relevant here (Gil et al. 1990). However, though the behavioral phenomenology of BPD overlaps with that seen after brain injury, a recent retrospective study by Zanarini et al. (1994) failed to support an association between childhood trauma (with or without frank head trauma) and brain dysfunction in BPD. This possibility bears further investigation.

Until the late 1980s, disturbance in cognition was not investigated specifically in BPD patients, largely because of the tenacity of a long-held belief in the "intact WAIS, disturbed Rorschach" pattern of test results in BPD (see O'Leary and Cowdry 1994 for a review). However, this belief has been shown to be misguided (Widiger 1982).

The first studies using neuropsychological tests in BPD patients typically used the WAIS. For example, Berg (1983) noted the presence of significant scatter between WAIS subtests among BPD subjects and suggested "a temporary decline in cognitive efficiency or a developmental lapse of unknown origin" (p. 122). However, because he based these observations on a review of many studies conducted before DSM-III, results from these study populations cannot validly be compared with subsequent studies.

In this section, we review studies examining various neurological parameters in BPD. As a group, four studies using EEG in BPD patients found no pattern of localization, no consistent type of EEG abnormality, and no clear relation between EEG abnormalities and BPD symptoms (Cornelius et al. 1986; Cowdry et al. 1985–1986; Snyder and Pitts 1984; van Reekum et al. 1993).

Gardner et al. (1987) found neurological soft-sign abnormalities to have greater-than-expected prevalence in BPD patients, suggesting that subtle, nonfocal neurological dysfunction may be associated with a predisposition to developing BPD. Stein et al. (1993) found no significant difference between patients with BPD only and patients with BPD and ASPD on soft-sign scores, suggesting that soft-sign abnormalities may be a nonspecific finding in some PDs.

Six studies to date have used CT or magnetic resonance imaging (MRI) of the brain to examine BPD patients, but they identified no significant differences between patients with BPD and control subjects (Lucas et al. 1989; Parnas and Teasdale 1987; Schulz et al. 1983; Snyder et al. 1983; van Reekum et al. 1993; Zanarini et al. 1994).

Using auditory evoked potentials, Kutcher et al. (1987) found that patients with BPD differ from patients without BPD but not from patients with schizophrenia, suggesting that patients with BPD and patients with schizophrenia may share a dysfunction in auditory neurointegration. Kutcher et al. (1989) extended this finding to include similarity in auditory evoked potential responses between patients with BPD and patients with SPD but not between patients with BPD and patients with other PDs nor between patients with BPD and control subjects without PDs. The neurological measure used in this study indicated that although BPD may represent a schizophrenia spectrum disorder, at the very least some degree of subtle difference in brain function may be present in BPD. Drake et al. (1991) reported a similar finding.

In a study involving a visual backward masking task, Schubert et al. (1985) reported no difference between inpatients with BPD and normal control subjects, suggesting that information-processing speed is unimpaired in BPD.

Two studies have used PET to assess brain function in BPD. Goyer et al. (1994) used PET assessment of cerebral metabolic rates of glucose to study BPD patients. They found significant differences in some areas of the frontal lobes, but the findings are extremely preliminary. De la Fuente et al. (1994) used PET to compare BPD patients with nonimpaired control subjects. They found no evidence of seizurelike asymmetry in brain function, but they did detect a trend toward higher right- than left-posterior temporal metabolic activity in the BPD group, suggesting possible dysfunction in that cortical area.

Taken together, these studies diverge with regard to whether BPD subjects differ from either normal control subjects or other psychiatric populations. Recall that BPD is almost certainly a heterogeneous diagnostic category and that DSM allows for many different symptomatic presentations that can be validly diagnosed as BPD by using the polythetic BPD criteria. Thus when small sample sizes are used, researchers run the risk of including or excluding one or another subgroup from within the larger universe of BPD, possibly producing great divergence in test results. Larger study samples are needed both to define subgroups within BPD and to identify phenomenological and diagnostic overlap between BPD and other PDs.

Neuropsychological Studies

We have identified eight neuropsychological studies of BPD patients, all of them published or presented at national meetings since 1988. Tables 6–2 and 6–3 summarize six of these studies.

Cornelius et al. (1989) performed the Pittsburgh Initial Neuropsychological Testing System (PINTS) on 24 consecutive inpatients with acute BPD who had been medication free for at least 1 week. The PINTS consists of a series of widely used tests of memory, language, and motor and spatial-constructional functions, although in general these tests are relatively insensitive to frontal system function. Because the PINTS scores all fell between the 33rd and 72nd percentiles for the 24 tests performed, no consistent pattern of abnormalities was demonstrated. This study cannot be taken as definitive because Cornelius et al. did not use DSM to diagnose BPD in their subjects, they did not control for acute depression or anxiety states, and they did not use a matched control group to assess their subjects' neuropsychological test results (using instead historical norms).

Burgess (1990) compared neurocognitive information processing in 18 patients who had BPD with 14 matched control subjects. He used an

Table 6–2. Methodology and characteristics of BPD neuropsychological studies

Characteristics	Cornelius et al. (1989)	Burgess (1990)	O'Leary et al. (1991)	Swirsky-Sacchetti et al. (1993)	Carpenter et al. (1993)	Judd and Ruff (1993)
Diagnosis		DSM-III-R	DSM-III-R	DSM-III-R	DSM-III-R	DSM-III
Diagnostic method	DIB	Interview	Interview, DIB	Interview, DIB + MCMI	Interview	Interview
Current Axis I included	Some	No	Yes	No	Yes	No
Number of patients	24	18	16	10	17	25
Gender (% male/ % female)	34/66	67/33	19/81	0/100	0/100	20/80
Setting	Inpatient acute	Outpatient acute	Inpatient research	Outpatient nonacute	Inpatient long-term	Outpatient nonacute
Medication status (medication free)	>1 week	Unknown	>2 weeks	No	No	>2 weeks
Substance abuse	No current, some prior	No current, some prior	No current, some prior	No current, some prior	No current, some prior	No current, some prior
IQ assessed	Yes	No	Yes	Yes	Yes	Yes
Attention assessed	Yes	No	Yes	Yes	Yes	Yes
Psychomotor skill assessed	Yes	No	Yes	Yes	Yes	Yes

Note. BPD = borderline personality disorder, DIB = Diagnostic Interview for Borderlines, MCMI = Millon Clinical Multiaxial Inventory.
Source. Adapted from O'Leary and Cowdry 1994.

11-item, 10-minute screening examination to assess memory, language, abstract operations, and behavior sequencing. Significant differences were found on the Delayed Memory, Serial 7s, Rhythm Reproduction, and Perseveration subtests. This particular pattern of cognitive deficiencies was viewed as fitting the Das et al. (1979) model of deficient sequential (as opposed to simultaneous) information processing and was thought to implicate mild frontotemporal brain deficits of the kind typically seen following frontal brain injury. However, as we have pointed out elsewhere (Gorton et al. 1991), this study has significant methodological flaws, so the findings must be interpreted with great caution.

In a related study (not shown in Tables 6–3 and 6–4 because it used neither normal control subjects nor historical norms), Burgess (1991) used a test battery of his own design to compare neurocognitive performance by patients who had BPD with that of subjects with schizophrenia and major depression. Patients with BPD made significantly more errors on the Delayed Memory and Omission Errors subtests than did those with major depression, but they made fewer errors on the Similarities and 3-Step Command subtests than did the patients with schizophrenia. These findings suggest that neurocognitive impairment in BPD, albeit limited to certain domains of function, is not simply the result of concomitant depression, yet it is not as severe as that seen in schizophrenia (see Calev, Chapter 2, in this volume). Burgess's additional finding from this study was that the degree of self-injurious behavior in BPD correlates with the degree of neurocognitive impairment but not with the degree of depression, a groundbreaking finding that requires confirmation.

O'Leary et al. (1991) studied 16 research outpatients who had BPD and 16 "healthy volunteers." The two groups showed no difference in Full-Scale IQ, but the patients with BPD had significantly worse performance than the volunteers on the following tests: WAIS-R Digit Symbol, WMS-R Logical Memory and Delayed Logical Memory, Rey-Osterrieth Recall and Delayed Recall, Corsi Blocks, Embedded Figures, and the timed Road-Map Test. These results reveal difficulty with uncued retrieval from memory and the process of visual discrimination and filtering, both of which involve temporal-lobe function.

Swirsky-Sacchetti et al. (1993) administered a neuropsychological test battery to a small group of outpatients with rigorously diagnosed BPD who were free of significant substance abuse but not free of medication. The BPD group's results, compared with those of a non-BPD volunteer control group, showed significantly lower performance on WAIS-R Picture Arrangement, Luria Motor Skills, WMS-R Figural Memory,

Table 6–3. Significant neuropsychological test findings in BPD (versus control subjects[a])

Characteristics	Cornelius et al. (1989)	Burgess (1990)	O'Leary et al. (1991)	Swirsky-Sacchetti et al. (1993)	Carpenter et al. (1993)	Judd and Ruff (1993)
WAIS-R subtests	Digit Span Block Design	NA	Digit Symbol* Block Design Vocabulary Information Digit Span Arithmetic Comprehension Similarities Picture Completion Picture Arrangement Object Assembly	Digit Symbol Block Design Vocabulary Information Digit Span Comprehension Similarities Picture Completion Picture Arrangement* Object Assembly	Digit Symbol* Block Design* Vocabulary	Digit Symbol* Block Design Vocabulary Information Digit Span Comprehension Similarities Picture Completion
Visuospatial skills						
Copy a design	NA	NA	Rey-Osterrieth	Rey-Osterrieth*	Rey-Osterrieth* (Block Design*)	Rey-Osterrieth*
Attention, perception, disembedding	NA	NA	Embedded Figures Test* Road-Map* Corsi Blocks* Visual Search	Symbol Digit (Digit Symbol) Trails A and B	Trails A and B* (Block Design*) (Digit Symbol*) Continuous Performance Task	Ruff Figural Fluency Test* Corsi Blocks* (Digit Symbol*)
Memory						
Simple visual	WMS Visual Memory	NA	WMS-R Visual Reproduction	WMS Visual Memory*	WMS-R Visual Reproduction*	NA

Complex visual	Crosses Star Drawing	NA	Rey-Osterrieth* (Embedded Figures*) (Corsi Blocks*)	Rey-Osterrieth*	Rey-Osterrieth*	Rey-Osterrieth* (Corsi Blocks*)
Simple verbal	WMS Associate Learning	NA	WMS Associate Learning	NA	NA	Selective Reminding
Complex verbal	WMS Logical Memory	NA	WMS-R Logical Memory*	WMS-R Logical Memory	WMS-R Logical Memory	WMS-R Logical Memory*
Motor functions	Grooved Pegboard Finger Tapping Test	Luria Motor Rhythm Reproduction	NA	Luria Motor Skills*	NA	Finger Tapping Test Grooved Pegboard
Abstraction	NA	Proverbs	WCST (Similarities)	Stroop* WCST (Similarities)	WCST	Stroop (Similarities)

Note. BPD = borderline personality disorder, NA = not administered, Stroop = Stroop Color and Word Test, WAIS-R = Wechsler Adult Intelligence Scale—Revised, WCST = Wisconsin Card Sorting Test, WMS-R = Wechsler Memory Scale—Revised. Parentheses indicate that the test also has been listed for that study in a prior category.

[a]Cornelius et al. (1989) used historical percentile norms rather than control subjects. They found no abnormalities.

*The performance of the patients with BPD was worse than that of the control subjects in all cases at a significance level of $P < .05$.

Source. Adapted from O'Leary KM, Cowdry RW: "Neuropsychological Testing Results in Borderline Personality Disorder," in *Biological and Neurobehavioral Studies of Borderline Personality Disorder.* Edited by Silk KR. Washington, DC, American Psychiatric Press, 1994, pp. 127–157. Copyright 1994, American Psychiatric Press. Used with permission.

Rey-Osterrieth Recall and Delayed Recall, and the Stroop Color and Word Test. These findings are consistent with dysfunction in temporal, frontal or prefrontal, and nondominant parietal areas. They are even more pronounced in a subgroup analysis revealing that five patients accounted for all of the significant variance. This study's findings support those of O'Leary et al. (1991) in confirming deficits in memory and in certain types of visual skills that require the patient to distinguish relevant visual detail from complex stimuli. The study's small sample size and the non-medication-free status of its subjects are limiting factors.

Carpenter et al. (1993) compared 17 female inpatients who had BPD with 17 nonpsychiatric control subjects. The BPD patients had significantly lower performance than the control subjects on a number of tests, including the WAIS-R Digit Symbol and Block Design tests, the Trail Making Test Part A and B, the WMS-R, the Visual Reproduction I and II tests, and the Rey-Osterrieth Figure (Recall) subtest. The Figure Recall and Digit Symbol subtest results echoed those in the O'Leary et al. (1991) study. Overall, the results suggested deficits in visuospatial processing, visual memory, and graphomotor speed, again implicating frontotemporal and possibly nondominant parietal areas.

Judd and Ruff (1993) studied 25 medication-free outpatients who had BPD. Study subjects were given the San Diego Neuropsychological Battery and were compared with 25 matched archival control subjects. Significant differences were observed on the WAIS-R Digit Symbol test, the Rey-Osterrieth Figure (Recall) subtest, the Ruff Figural Fluency Test, and the WMS-R Logical Memory and Delayed Recall tests. These findings suggested difficulty in encoding or learning new complex information, especially visuospatial information, and in visuospatial discrimination, processing speed, fluency, and verbal recall. Again, frontotemporal and nondominant parietal deficits were implicated in these findings.

Finally, van Reekum et al. (1993) performed an uncontrolled, non-blinded, limited neuropsychological test battery on nine BPD patients who were part of a larger neurobehavioral study of BPD. Unfortunately, they did not report the results in detail (therefore, this study is not included in Tables 6–3 and 6–4), except to state that seven of the nine patients "showed evidence of frontal system dysfunction" and that the deficits most often observed were "impulsive cognitions, cognitive inflexibility, poor self-monitoring, poor set-maintenance and perseveration" (p. 125). Apparently, these problems were noted most often on the WCST, Trail Making Test Part B, and Rey-Osterrieth Complex Figure test.

Summary of BPD Research

Despite the methodological challenges in BPD research and the small sample sizes, these studies have notably consistent findings. Patients who have BPD tend to be impaired on tasks requiring visuospatial skills, memory, and certain types of motor output. The consistency and selectivity of these deficits argues against their being the result of medication side effects, comorbid Axis I disorders, patient status, substance abuse, or learning disabilities, despite differences in these variables across the studies.

Several studies report significantly worse performance by BPD patients on the Rey-Osterrieth Complex Figure test. Successful completion of this task requires simultaneous attention to the gestalt of the complex figure and to its internal detail. One must continually shift perceptual set to process both aspects of this information. BPD patients seem to have particular difficulty with this type of ongoing mental flexibility, in which perceptual set must be shifted in order, for example, to integrate good and bad, or to maintain object constancy. This may contribute to the predominant use of splitting as a cognitive strategy, with resultant disturbance in affective stability and identity consolidation.

Several studies also report impaired WAIS-R Digit Symbol test performance. This subtest requires sustained attention, motor persistence, and efficient visuomotor coordination and is consistently sensitive to even minimal brain damage (see Lezak 1983).

Most of these studies report memory impairment, although inconsistencies occur in whether immediate or delayed recall is significantly impaired or whether the memory impairment includes both verbal and figural material. BPD patients may have a mild memory-encoding problem that becomes especially problematic when large amounts of information must be encoded. This problem may contribute to disturbance in the temporal sense of continuity of the self, which is an aspect of identity consolidation.

Several studies report significant differences that remain unconfirmed. O'Leary et al. (1991) found deficits on the Corsi Blocks test, a different type of nonverbal memory task that taxes spatial functioning. Swirsky-Sacchetti et al. (1993) found significant differences on the WAIS-R Picture Arrangement test, which requires the visual filtering of essential from nonessential detail that O'Leary and Cowdry (1994) postulated may be responsible for the pattern of visuospatial deficits found in BPD patients.

The role of emotional stimulation in the *kindling* of mild problems in neuropsychological function requires further investigation. Cognitive dysfunction may be most readily observable under conditions of differential state stimulation, retreating at other times to an underlying trait that may or may not be detected on comprehensive neuropsychological testing. Swirsky-Sacchetti et al. (1993) attempted to assess the role of emotional interference on list learning. The results were in the predicted direction but did not reach significance, perhaps because of the varying emotive value of the stimuli used. This is a promising area for future research.

Another way to summarize these studies is to look at the areas of brain function that are most often implicated as having relative deficiencies in BPD, such as frontal or prefrontal, temporal, and nondominant parietal areas. But as we have emphasized, conclusions about localization must be stated cautiously (Keefe 1995). Ongoing studies involving the correlation of cognitive tasks with PET imaging of brain function will help sort out structural-functional correlations. Meanwhile, clinicians would be wise to interpret cognitive test findings as being most usefully reflective of a patient's specific functional strengths and weaknesses in order best to assess the clinical picture and adjust the treatment approach.

◈ SCHIZOTYPAL PERSONALITY DISORDER

The following case vignette depicts a patient with SPD who has a cognitive profile of a type identified in neuropsychological research on this PD.

Mr. C is a 24-year-old man who lives with his parents. He has always been very shy and introverted, and he has no close friends and few acquaintances. He maintained average to low-average grades in school and did not go to college after finishing high school. He has had difficulty maintaining steady employment and often feels undermined by co-workers. When one of Mr. C's jobs required increased interaction with the public, he became very anxious, suspicious, and preoccupied with magical rituals through which he hoped to avoid harm to himself. Although Mr. C did somewhat better at jobs allowing isolation from people, he tended to have difficulty with changes in his routine. His father was very upset about his son's lack of achievement and wanted treatment for what he perceived to be his son's "laziness and lack of motivation."

After a psychiatric evaluation identified SPD, Mr. C was referred for neuropsychological testing as part of a vocational assessment. His overall IQ was average, without significant skew between verbal and performance scores. Verbal fluency was the only impaired language measure. Most memory measures were within normal limits, although when Mr. C was presented with a list of words to learn through repeated exposures, his lack of an adequate strategy resulted in a mildly impaired performance. He was impaired on the Trail Making Test Part B and moderately impaired on the WCST.

In general, Mr. C's pattern of cognitive processing suggested that he was average to above average on fairly structured tasks that depended on speed, learning, and basic perceptual processes. In less structured tasks requiring greater levels of abstraction, mental flexibility, planning and organization skills, and use of feedback to alter his pattern of responding, Mr. C was mildly to moderately impaired. This information led his therapist to simplify and more concretely structure the treatment approach. In addition, once this information was provided to Mr. C's parents in the context of psychoeducational meetings, they were better able to develop more appropriate expectations for their son's treatment, his future, and his vocational options.

Literature Review

SPD patients have long been identified as manifesting perceptual and cognitive distortions. Millon (1996) noted that they have particular difficulty in organizing their thoughts "in the realm of interpersonal understanding and empathy," with an inability to "differentiate what is salient from what is tangential." He noted that their "distortions and deficiencies appear limited to the interpersonal facets of the cognitive domain" (p. 625). He described their superstitions, referential ideas, and illusions as an effort at coping with feelings of underlying emptiness and alienation. Might neuropsychological dysfunction underlie these apparently psychodynamic phenomena?

Neurological, neurophysiological, and neuroimaging studies. Patients with SPD have increased ventricular size and increased lateral and frontal ventricular-to-brain ratios (Siever et al. 1993). In contrast, Cannon et al. (1994a) suggested that similar cortical sulcal enlargement would be found in individuals who had schizophrenia or SPD and were the offspring of schizophrenic mothers, but ventricular enlargement was present only in schizophrenic offspring. Patients who met DSM-III-R criteria for SPD were found to have smaller prefrontal areas on MRI, compared with a nonmedicated, noninstitutionalized normal control group (Raine et al. 1992b).

Functional imaging studies have shown increased activation of prefrontal cortex, in particular on the right side, in SPD patients compared with control subjects without SPD, suggesting that this increase may compensate for left-sided dysfunction and inefficient processing (Siever 1994). Higher left than right activation correlated with positive symptoms, and higher right than left activation correlated with negative symptoms in schizophrenic patients and SPD patients (Gruzelier and Raine 1994).

SPD patients share with schizophrenic patients impairments in smooth pursuit eye movement, a defect that seems to be associated selectively with negative symptoms (Siever et al. 1993).

Kelley and Coursey (1992) compared male undergraduates who had high scores on schizotypy questionnaires with those who scored on the low end on the same questionnaires. Among those with high scores, they found increased lateral preference for left foot and hand dominance in the absence of lateral preference for cognitive function but without differences in motor speed or smooth eye pursuit.

Finally, EEG assessment of SPD patients using evoked potentials revealed abnormalities in P300 and N220 amplitude that were intermediate between those of control subjects and schizophrenic patients (Siever et al. 1993).

Neuropsychological testing. Interest in studying neuropsychological deficits in SPD patients emerged out of research on cognitive deficits in schizophrenic patients (see Chapter 2 in this book). Many of the studies on SPD compare these two groups with control subjects and with family members of schizophrenic patients (Battaglia et al. 1994; Cannon et al. 1994a; Condray and Steinhauer 1992; Keefe et al. 1994). As shown in Tables 6–4 and 6–5, the neuropsychological findings vary somewhat among the studies.

Keefe et al. (1994) studied first-degree relatives of schizophrenic probands and control subjects matched for age and education. Eight relatives who met DSM-III-R criteria for SPD were more impaired than the other 46 relatives on letter fluency but otherwise performed similarly to the relatives who did not meet DSM-III-R criteria for SPD. Of greater note, all the relatives performed worse than did control subjects on Trail Making Test Part B and in verbal fluency, but these two tests did not distinguish between the relatives with or without SPD.

Table 6–4. Methodology and characteristics of SPD neuropsychological studies

Study	Diagnostic criteria	Population	Number of subjects (men/women)	Control group characteristics	Setting	Exclusion criteria
Battaglia et al. (1994)	DSM-III-R, SIDP-R	Consecutive psychiatric outpatients	15 (6/9)	25 normal control subjects, 35 patients with schizophrenia	Consecutive outpatients	DSM-III-R schizophreniform, schizoaffective, or delusional disorder; dementia; organic mental disorder; mental retardation
Cannon et al. (1994a)	SADS, Present State Examination, Personality Disorders Examination	High- and low-risk individuals with SPD or schizophrenia	207	Same population, no psychiatric disorders and nonschizophrenia-spectrum disorders	Prospective longitudinal study of 207 high-risk children (with severely schizophrenic mothers) and 104 matched control subjects	None noted

(continued)

Table 6–4. Methodology and characteristics of SPD neuropsychological studies (*continued*)

Study	Diagnostic criteria	Population	Number of subjects (men/women)	Control group characteristics	Setting	Exclusion criteria
Condray and Steinhauer (1992)	DSM-III, SADS-L, SIDP	Individuals who had SPD with and without schizophrenic relatives	25 (25/0)	24 normal control subjects	General population	Major medical disease, neurological injury or disorder, neuroleptic medication
Keefe et al. (1994)	SADS, CASH, DSM-III-R	54 relatives of schizophrenic patients, 8 with SPD	54 (22/32)	18 control subjects from the community (15/3)	Community	Non–English speaking, psychosis
Kelley and Coursey (1992)	MMPI, schizotypy questionnaires	266 white undergraduate students	33 (33/0)	40 on low end of screening	College	Nonwhite
LaPorte et al. (1994)	Chapman Scale for psychosis proneness	College students	409	None	College outpatient	None noted
Lyons et al. (1991)	Kendler Structured Interview, MMPI	Recruited undergraduate students having "ESP"	5 (3/2)	13 student volunteers (4/9)	College undergraduates	Not described

Park et al. (1995)	PAS	Normal students	28 (14/14)	23 students with low PAS scores (11/12)	College	>3 on Infrequency Scale of Jackson Personality Research Scale
Raine et al. (1992b)	DSM-III-R	Outpatient	17 (8/9)	Normal	Hospital employees	Mental retardation, drug or alcohol abuse, neurological illness
Siever et al. (1993)	DSM-III-R	Outpatient	13	Normal, other PD	Research laboratory	None noted

Note. SPD = schizotypal personality disorder, CASH = Comprehensive Assessment of Symptoms and History, MMPI = Minnesota Multiphasic Personality Inventory, PAS = Perceptual Aberration Scale, SADS = Schedule for Affective Disorders and Schizophrenia, SIDP-R = Structured Interview for DSM-III Personality Disorders, Revised, PD = personality disorder.

Table 6–5. Neuropsychological test findings in SPD

Study	WCST	Trails B	Verbal Fluency	WAIS-R	Continuous Performance Test	Vigilance Performance	Logical Memory	Wechsler Memory Scale
Battaglia et al. (1994)[a]	**	NA	NA	NA	NA	NA	NA	NA
Cannon et al. (1994a)[b]	*	*	*	[c]	*	*	*	*
Condray and Steinhauer (1992)	**	**	NA	**[d]	**	*	NA	NA
Keefe et al. (1994)	NA	*[e]	*	NA	NA	NA	NA	NA
Kelley and Coursey (1992)	NA	NA	NA	**[f]	NA	NA	NA	NA
LaPorte et al. (1994)	NA	NA	NA	NA	NA	NA	**	**
Lyons et al. (1991)	*	NA	NA	NA	NA	NA	NA	NA
Park et al. (1995)	*[g]	NA	NA	NA	NA	NA	NA	NA
Raine et al. (1992b)	**[h]	NA	NA	NA	NA	NA	NA	NA
Siever et al. (1993)	*	*	NA	NA	*	NA	NA	NA

Note. SPD = schizotypal personality disorder, WCST = Wisconsin Card Sorting Test, Trails B = Trail Making Test Part B, WAIS-R = Wechsler Adult Intelligence Scale—Revised. * = significant impairment compared with control group (P > .05); ** = no significant impairment compared with control group (P > .05); NA = not assessed.

[a] Schizophrenic relatives impaired, SPD relatives not.

[b] This study used multiple tests in each of seven functional domains and reported results only for these domains.

[c] Subtest: Digit Span and Digit Symbol.

[d] Subset: Block Design.

[e] Versus normal control subjects. No significant difference in SPD relatives of schizophrenic patients versus non-SPD relatives of schizophrenic patients. Trails A showed no difference among any groups.

[f] Subsets: Block Design, Similarities, Object Assembly, Vocabulary.

[g] Deficit found in set maintenance.

[h] Deficit found in perseveration, proportional to reduced prefrontal area.

In contrast, most other neuropsychological studies found differences in prefrontal performance in patients who had SPD compared with control subjects, specifically on the WCST (Battaglia et al. 1994; Condray and Steinhauer 1992; Lyons et al. 1991; Raine et al. 1992b; Siever et al. 1993), the Trail Making Test Part B (Condray and Steinhauer 1992; Siever et al. 1993), the Continuous Performance Test (Condray and Steinhauer 1992), the Verbal Fluency Test (Siever et al. 1993), and the Stroop Color and Word Test (Siever et al. 1993). In general, these problems could not be accounted for by general poor intelligence or global deficits, as SPD patients could not be distinguished from control subjects on tests such as the WAIS-R Vocabulary and Block Design subtests. Condray found that neurocognitive vulnerability seemed to increase as a function of the degree of family penetrance of schizophrenia (Condray and Steinhauer 1992).

Park et al. (1995) found that college students who scored high on a measure of psychosis proneness had a reduced ability to hold material in spatial working memory. LaPorte et al. (1994) studied verbal memory and verbal intelligence function in psychosis-prone college students but found no relationship between schizotypal features and recall/retention measures. Cannon et al. (1994b) tested nonschizophrenic siblings against their schizophrenic siblings and normal control subjects using measures of verbal and spatial memory, abstraction, attention, and language and sensory-motor function. Nonschizophrenic siblings with probable and certain diagnoses of SPD were more impaired, although not as impaired as were the schizophrenic siblings.

Summary of SPD Research

Although SPD has not been studied extensively from a neuropsychological perspective, the neurocognitive profile of patients with SPD can, at least tentatively, be understood on several levels. The most consistent findings are of deficits in executive functions believed to be mediated by frontal and prefrontal cortex, with some evidence of a greater level of dysfunction on the left side. How these deficits may contribute to the oddities in thinking observed in patients with SPD is unclear. Green (1996) argued that deficits in vigilance and verbal memory may act as "neurocognitive rate-limiting factors" in schizophrenic patients. Perhaps these findings can be extended to SPD patients, giving direction to further research.

◈ COMPARATIVE NEUROPSYCHOLOGICAL PROFILES IN ASPD, BPD, AND SPD

We are not aware of any studies that meaningfully compare neuropsychological function in pure populations of patients with ASPD, BPD, or SPD. Therefore, for comparative discussion, we must rely on the findings from the relevant literature we have already reviewed.

The SPD literature is most consistent in suggesting possible frontal or prefrontal disturbance on neuropsychological measures. This possibility is supported by PET abnormalities and MRI findings localizing to frontal regions.

The ASPD literature suggests both diffuse left-hemisphere and frontal or prefrontal deficits. These findings may reflect at least two subtypes of ASPD. Alternatively, the left-hemisphere findings suggested earlier may have been unduly biased by the high prevalence of learning disabilities or attention-deficit/hyperactivity disorder in the population studied.

The BPD studies consistently point to deficient visuospatial skills that normally allow fluid shifting of perspective from detail to overall gestalt. In addition, findings of dysfunction in verbal and nonverbal memory, simultaneous processing, and susceptibility to interference all suggest diffuse, nonlocalizable deficits.

We are left with tantalizing but highly tentative patterns of apparent dysfunction, yet clear and consistent evidence indicating some subtle neurocognitive differences in at least subgroups of all three PDs (see Table 6–6 for a summary). It is unclear whether findings suggestive of frontal dysfunction, for example, will turn out to be specific to the PDs we have reviewed or whether they reflect something about PD generally, perhaps as part of a final common pathway to a disturbed personality or even to broader psychiatric disturbance.

◈ CLINICAL IMPLICATIONS OF NEUROPSYCHOLOGICAL DIFFERENCES

We believe, as do other researchers in this area (Burgess 1992; Carpenter et al. 1993; Docherty 1992; Gabbard 1994; Palombo and Feigon 1984; Ratey 1995; Silk 1994), that strong consideration should be given to neuropsychological screening of all patients who have severe PD. This is especially true of PDs in the *odd* DSM-IV cluster (SPD, paranoid PD, and schizoid PD) and the *dramatic* DSM-IV cluster (ASPD, BPD, histri-

Table 6–6. Tentative comparative neuropsychological dysfunctions in ASPD, BPD, and SPD

Disorder	Tests most commonly impaired	Impaired functions	Hypothetical localization[a]
ASPD	Trail Making Verbal learning COWAT WMS-R (Logical and Figural Memory) Complex Motor WCST	Simultaneous processing Verbal fluency Verbal and figural memory Abstract verbal reasoning Motor output	Left hemisphere Frontal/prefrontal
BPD	Complex Figure Symbol Digit Modalities WMS-R (Logical and Figural Memory) Trail Making Test Part A & B Stroop Embedded Figures	Complex visuospatial skills Speed/motor perseveration Visuomotor integration Verbal and nonverbal learning Susceptibility to interference	Diffuse (nonlocalized) Right and left hemisphere
SPD	WCST Trail Making Test Part B Stroop COWAT	Mental flexibility Abstract problem solving Simultaneous processing Verbal fluency Susceptibility to interference	Frontal

Note. ASPD = antisocial personality disorder, BPD = borderline personality disorder, SPD = schizotypal personality disorder, WCST = Wisconsin Card Sorting Test, COWAT = Controlled Oral Word Association Test, WMS-R = Wechsler Memory Scale—Revised, Stroop = Stroop Color and Word Test.

[a]We emphasize the danger in premature conclusions about structural-functional correlation, so this column is provided only to stimulate hypotheses for further functional-anatomical research (e.g., via positron-emission tomography).

onic PD, and narcissistic PD), and in patients with PD who appear self-defeating, noncompliant, or treatment resistant, or whose treatment is stagnating despite consultation and review.

The cost-effectiveness of treatment with or without neuropsychological screening should be considered carefully given that severely disturbed patients with PD often use a larger-than-average share of treatment resources and are also at high risk for catastrophic outcomes such as suicide (Plakun 1996). We have reviewed research related to what are almost certainly the two most common severe PDs in the general population: ASPD and BPD. Even though neuropsychological research assessment of PDs has been limited largely to three disorders, the findings we have summarized have tremendous potential relevance to many so-called difficult patients.

◈ RECOMMENDATIONS FOR A NEUROPSYCHOLOGICAL SCREENING BATTERY

Table 6–7 is offered with the hope that more patients with PD will receive a multifaceted diagnostic evaluation, even if a comprehensive neuropsychological battery is not feasible for all such patients. This battery was designed to assess all major areas of cognitive function, including attention, memory, motor skills, language, visuospatial skills, and complex problem-solving skills. It takes approximately 70–90 minutes to adminis-

---

Table 6–7. Recommendations for a brief neuropsychological screening battery for personality disorders

---

Wechsler Adult Intelligence Scale—Revised

  Vocabulary and Digit Symbol tests

Continuous Performance Test

Luria's Complex Motor Skills

Controlled Oral Word Association Test

Wechsler Memory Scale (Russell Revision)

  Logical and Figural Memory tests

Rey-Osterrieth Complex Figure (with Recall)

Stroop Color and Word Test

Short Category Test

Note. See Lezak (1983, 1995) for sources, administration instructions, and normative data.

ter. Sources for test materials, detailed administration instructions, and norms can be found in Lezak (1983, 1995), unless otherwise noted. The specific tests were selected as those most likely to reveal significant differences, based on our review of this literature.

◈ CLINICAL APPLICATION OF NEUROPSYCHOLOGICAL FINDINGS IN PERSONALITY DISORDER

The first task following neuropsychological assessment is the presentation of the findings to the primary treatment team so that those performing the assessment and those performing the treatment can enrich one another's interpretations not only of test results but also of how and when it would be best to present them to the patient and family. The therapist and other providers would do well to take note of any strong reactions of their own to test findings, as conscious and unconscious interaction with preexisting attitudes and countertransference is to be expected.

Extremes of hopelessness and therapeutic nihilism may be seen in treatment providers working with especially difficult patients who have BPD or ASPD or patients with other PDs whose test batteries show significant deficiencies. In contrast, therapists may be relieved to find that their often heroic but frustrating struggles with so-called impossible patients were in part the result of previously unidentified cognitive problems and not necessarily the result of therapists' lack of skill or patients' refusing, resisting, or sabotaging treatment efforts.

Setting aside time for the treatment team to explore the meanings of the test results along with their implications for the patient, family, and other clinicians is a crucial first step in the process of integrating the neuropsychological data into the clinical work, reformulating the case, and amending the treatment plan.

The second step involves thoughtful and sensitive presentation of neuropsychological findings to the patient and family. Given these patients' propensity for regression and other extreme reactions, clinicians must proceed deliberately but cautiously. Allen et al. (1986) provide useful general guidelines for the neuropsychoeducational process, which should never be conceived of as a single event but rather as an ongoing integration of information and reaction within the therapeutic framework. Although an ideal outcome of this therapeutic- educational process involves acceptance by the patient and concerned parties of the concept of some degree of functional disadvantage (albeit not necessarily a fixed deficit), the presence of functional strengths and compensatory adaptations should also be stressed.

When presented empathically, the neuropsychological findings may serve as a new schema for self-understanding that often has the apparently paradoxical effect of relieving shame, guilt, self-blame, and poor self-esteem rather than adding to the patient's self-perceived burden of fault, incapacity, ineffectiveness, failure, and so forth. Patients who have struggled unsuccessfully for years to adapt sometimes have an "Ah-ha!" response to learning that at least some of their difficulties can be defined, named, and understood—even if not necessarily compensated for—in a way that can be empowering rather than further traumatizing.

The third step involves delineation of cognitive weaknesses and strengths as additional dimensions of psychopathology (Silk 1994) and dimensions of psychological health, respectively, which should lead to reconsideration of the treatment approach and structure. In general, more supportive, structured, rehabilitative treatment appears most helpful in the presence of significant impairment that is often the virtual equivalent of a learning disability (Links 1993). Even when a question of subtle impairment exists, a shift away from a purely insight-oriented, reconstructive, expressive psychotherapeutic approach toward a more educational, instructive, cognitive-behavioral, or psychopharmacological approach (albeit still insight-oriented) may be helpful (Andrulonis and Vogel 1984; Burgess 1992; Murray 1979; Ratey 1995).

In addition, aspects of cognitive remediation may be useful to patients with PD, although we are not aware of any research using such techniques in this patient population. In a review article, Green (1993) suggested that there may be some overlap between remediation of brain-injured patients and of patients with chronic psychiatric disorders, and many of the techniques found useful both with brain injury and with major mental disorders such as schizophrenia may have relevance to remedial treatment of neuropsychological problems in PD (Green 1996). In the absence of prospective outcome studies of attempted cognitive remediation in a PD population, we can only refer interested readers to relevant sections of this book and offer some of the information that we have found to be helpful with some patients who have PD.

In general, treatment should shift toward a more structured, problem-solving approach that has been found helpful in treating severe PDs

(Linehan 1993). For example, the teaching of rational self-talk such as is espoused in cognitive therapy may be especially helpful to patients who have PD, as illustrated in the ASPD case vignette. Training patients to delay impulsive action using self-talk techniques such as counting to 10 helped reduce maladaptive perseverative responding in psychopathic patients in one study (Newman et al. 1987). Focusing on the consequences of an action by fostering rational verbalizations may be generally helpful in patients with especially impulsive or inflexible PDs.

Memory disturbances, such as those observed in BPD, can be approached through use of concrete memory devices such as self-rating scales, written records, diaries, photographs, or other idiosyncratic cuing objects and through personalized mnemonic devices or other verbal cuing of complex material (O'Leary et al. 1991).

Finally, psychotropic medication that may impair cognitive function should be used with caution in patients with PDs who manifest neuropsychological difficulty. Use of medication in this population is often problematic in any case (Gorton and Akhtar 1990), but strongly anticholinergic agents and sedative-hypnotics seem particularly to disturb memory and efficient brain function in some patients and should be avoided if possible.

◈ CONCLUSION

We are only beginning to understand the role of cognitive differences in some of the PDs. They are etiologically and phenomenologically complex disorders that are highly unlikely to have neuropsychological impairment as their sole cause. Subtle, nondefinitively localizable brain dysfunction in the absence of gross structural change appears to be a consistent finding in at least some subgroups of these patients. Taken together, these subgroups may represent a segment of the PD population that is most challenged to change and learn in traditional treatment environments. Early identification of such patients can facilitate shifts in treatment approach that may be both helpful and cost-effective.

Further research is needed before we can be sure how neurocognitive differences correlate with PD criteria, whether these differences are truly rate limiting in terms of everyday function or response to treatment, and whether cognitive remediation will be useful for these patients. Although definitive recommendations regarding routine neuropsychological evaluation of all patients with PDs cannot be made at present, clinicians need not wait before integrating the neuropsychological perspective into their work with patients who have ASPD, BPD, or SPD or who have other PDs that respond poorly to treatment.

◈ REFERENCES

Aarkrog T: The borderline concept in childhood, adolescence and adulthood. Acta Psychiatr Scand 64 (monograph suppl 293), 1981

Adler G, Buie DH: Aloneness and borderline psychopathology: the possible relevance of child developmental issues. Int J Psychoanal 60:83–96, 1979

Allen JG, Lewis L, Blum S, et al: Informing neuropsychiatric patients and their families about neuropsychological assessment findings. Bull Menninger Clin 50:64–74, 1986

American Psychiatric Association: Diagnostic and Statistical Manual of Mental Disorders, 3rd Edition. Washington, DC, American Psychiatric Press, 1980

American Psychiatric Association: Diagnostic and Statistical Manual of Mental Disorders, 3rd Edition, Revised. Washington, DC, American Psychiatric Press, 1987

American Psychiatric Association: Diagnostic and Statistical Manual of Mental Disorders, 4th Edition. Washington, DC, American Psychiatric Press, 1994

Andrulonis PA, Vogel NG: Comparison of borderline patient subcategories to schizophrenic and affective disorders. Br J Psychiatry 144:358–363, 1984

Andrulonis PA, Glueck BC, Stroebel CF, et al: Organic brain dysfunction and the borderline syndrome. Psychiatr Clin North Am 4:47–66, 1980

Andrulonis PA, Glueck BC, Stroebel CF, et al: Borderline personality subcategories. J Nerv Ment Dis 170:670–679, 1982

Anscombe R: Treating the patient who "can't" versus treating the patient who "won't." Am J Psychother 40:26–35, 1986

Battaglia M, Abbruzzese M, Ferri S, et al: An assessment of the Wisconsin Card Sorting Test as an indicator of liability to schizophrenia. Schizophr Res 14:39–45, 1994

Bemporad JR, Smith HF, Hanson G, et al: Borderline syndromes in childhood: criteria for diagnosis. Am J Psychiatry 139:596–602, 1982

Berg M: Borderline psychopathology as displayed on psychological tests. J Pers Assess 47:120–133, 1983

Burgess JW: Cognitive information processing in borderline personality disorder: a neuropsychiatric hypothesis. Jefferson Journal of Psychiatry 8:34–48, 1990

Burgess JW: Relationship of depression and cognitive impairment to self-injury in borderline personality disorder, major depression, and schizophrenia. Psychiatry Res 38:77–87, 1991

Burgess JW: Neurocognitive impairment in dramatic personalities: histrionic, narcissistic, borderline, and antisocial disorders. Psychiatry Res 42:283–290, 1992

Cannon TD, Sarnoff SA, Mednick AS, et al: Developmental brain abnormalities in the offspring of schizophrenic mothers, II: structural brain characteristics of schizophrenia and schizotypal personality disorder. Arch Gen Psychiatry 51:955–962, 1994a

Cannon TD, Zorrilla LE, Shtasel D, et al: Neuropsychological functioning in siblings discordant for schizophrenia and healthy volunteers. Arch Gen Psychiatry 51:651–661, 1994b

Carpenter CJ, Gold JM, Fenton W: Neuropsychological test results in BPD inpatients. New Research Poster 316, presented at the 146th annual meeting of the American Psychiatric Association, Chicago, IL, May 1993

Colson DB, Allen JG: Organic brain dysfunction in difficult-to- treat psychiatric hospital patients. Bull Menninger Clin 50:88–98, 1986

Condray R, Steinhauer SR: Schizotypal personality disorder in individuals with and without schizophrenic relatives: similarities and contrasts in neurocognitive and clinical functioning. Schizophr Res 7:33–41, 1992

Cornelius JR, Brenner RP, Soloff PH, et al: EEG abnormalities in borderline personality disorder: specific or nonspecific. Biol Psychiatry 21:974–977, 1986

Cornelius JR, Soloff PH, George AWA, et al: An evaluation of the significance of selected neuropsychiatric abnormalities in the etiology of borderline personality disorder. J Personal Disord 3:19–25, 1989

Cowdry RW, Pickar D, Davies R: Symptoms and EEG findings in the borderline syndrome. Int J Psychiatry Med 15:201–211, 1985–1986

Das JP, Kirby JR, Jarman RF: Simultaneous and Successive Cognitive Processes. New York, Academic Press, 1979

De la Fuente JM, Lotstra F, Goldman S, et al: Temporal glucose metabolism in borderline personality disorder. Psychiatry Res: Neuroimaging 55:237–245, 1994

Docherty J: To know borderline personality disorder, in Borderline Personality Disorder: Clinical and Empirical Perspectives. Edited by Clarkin JF, Marziali E, Monroe-Blum H. New York, Guilford, 1992, pp 329–338

Drake ME, Phillips BB, Pakaluis A: Auditory evoked potentials in borderline personality disorder. Clinical Electroencephalography 22:188–192, 1991

Erdelyi MH: Psychoanalysis: Freud's Cognitive Psychology. New York, WH Freeman, 1985

Fals-Stewart W, Lucente S: Effect of neurocognitive states and personality functioning on length of stay in residential substance abuse treatment: an integrative study. Psychology of Addictive Behaviors 8:179–196, 1994

Fedora O, Fedora S: Some neuropsychological and psychophysiological aspects of psychopathic and non-psychopathic criminals, in Laterality and Psychopathology. Edited by Flor-Henry P, Gruzelier JH. North Holland, Elsevier, 1983, pp 41–48

Flor-Henry P: Lateralized temporal-limbic dysfunction and psychopathology. Ann NY Acad Sci 280:777–795, 1976

Frayn DH: Grief and object constancy (letter). Am J Psychiatry 153:297, 1996

Gabbard GO: Mind and brain in psychiatric treatment. Streckrer Monograph No 31. Philadelphia, PA, Institute of Pennsylvania Hospital, November 1994

Gardner D, Lucas PB, Cowdry RW: Soft sign neurological abnormalities in borderline personality disorder and normal control subjects. J Nerv Ment Dis 175:177–180, 1987

Gil T, Calev A, Greenberg D, et al: Cognitive functioning in post-traumatic stress disorder. J Trauma Stress 3:29–45, 1990

Gillen R, Hesselbrock V: Cognitive functioning, ASP, and family history of alcoholism in young men at risk for alcoholism. Alcohol Clin Exp Res 16:206–214, 1992

Gillstrom BJ, Hare RD: Language-related hand gestures in psychopaths. J Personal Disord 2:21–27, 1988

Glenn SW, Errico AL, Parsons OA, et al: The role of antisocial, affective, and childhood behavioral characteristics in alcoholics' neuropsychological performance. Alcohol Clin Exp Res 17:162–169, 1993

Gorenstein EE: Frontal lobe functions in psychopaths. J Abnorm Psychol 91:368–379, 1982

Gorenstein EE: Neuropsychology of juvenile delinquency. Forensic Reports 3:15–48, 1990

Gorton GE: A mnemonic device for efficient recall of DSM-IV borderline personality disorder criteria (letter). Am J Psychiatry 153:582, 1996

Gorton GE, Akhtar S: The literature on personality disorders, 1985–88: trends, issues and controversies. Hosp Community Psychiatry 41:39–51, 1990

Gorton GE, Akhtar S: The relationship between addiction and personality disorder: review and reflections. Integrative Psychiatry 10:185–198, 1994

Gorton GE, Samuel SE, Swirsky-Sacchetti T, et al: Reply to cognitive information processing in borderline personality disorder (letter). Jefferson Journal of Psychiatry 9:96–97, 1991

Goyer PF, Andreason PJ, Semple WE, et al: Positron-emission tomography and personality disorders. Neuropsychopharmacology 10:21–28, 1994

Green MF: Cognitive remediation in schizophrenia: is it time yet? Am J Psychiatry 150:178–187, 1993

Green MF: What are the functional consequences of neurocognitive deficits in schizophrenia? Am J Psychiatry 153:321–330, 1996

Gruzelier J, Raine A: Bilateral electrodermal activity and cerebral mechanisms in syndromes of schizophrenia and the schizotypal syndrome. Int J Psychophysiology 16:1–16, 1994

Hamilton NG, Allsbrook L: Thirty cases of "schizophrenia" reexamined. Bull Menninger Clin 50:323–340, 1986

Hare RD, McPherson LM: Psychopathy and perceptual asymmetry during verbal dichotic listening. J Abnorm Psychol 93:141–149, 1984

Hare RD, Williamson SE, Harpur RJ: Psychopathy and language, in Biological Contributions to Crime Causation. Edited by Moffitt TE, Mednick SA. Dordrecht, The Netherlands, Martinus Nijhoff, 1988, pp 68–92

Hart SD, Forth AE, Hare RD: Performance of criminal psychopaths on selected neuropsychological tests. J Abnorm Psychol 99:374–379, 1990

Jaeger J, Berns S, Tigner A, et al: Remediation of neuropsychological deficits in psychiatric populations: rationale and methodologic considerations. Psychopharmacol Bull 28:367–390, 1992

Judd PH, Ruff RM: Neuropsychological dysfunction in borderline personality disorder. J Personal Disord 7:275–284, 1993

Jutai JW, Hare RD: Psychopathy and selective attention during performance of a complex perceptual-motor task. Psychophysiology 20:146–151, 1983

Kandel E, Freed D: Frontal-lobe dysfunction and antisocial behavior: a review. J Clin Psychol 45:404–413, 1989

Keefe RSE: The contribution of neuropsychology to psychiatry. Am J Psychiatry 152:6–15, 1995

Keefe RSE, Silverman JM, Roitman SE, et al: Performance of nonpsychotic relatives of schizophrenic patients on cognitive tests. Psychiatric Res 55:1–12, 1994

Kelley MP, Coursey RD: Lateral preference and neuropsychological correlates of schizotypy. Psychiatric Res 41:115–135, 1992

Kroll J: The Challenge of the Borderline Patient. New York, WW Norton, 1988

Krynicki V: Cerebral dysfunction in repetitively assaultive adolescents. J Nerv Ment Dis 166:59–67, 1978

Kutcher SP, Blackwood DHR, St Clair D, et al: Auditory P-300 in borderline personality disorder and schizophrenia. Arch Gen Psychiatry 44:645–650, 1987

Kutcher SP, Blackwood DHR, Gaskell DF, et al: Auditory P 300 does not differentiate borderline personality disorder from schizotypal personality disorder. Biol Psychiatry 26:766–774, 1989

LaPorte DJ, Kirkpatrick B, Thaker GK, Psychosis-proneness and verbal memory in a college student population. Schizophr Res 12:237–245, 1994

Lezak MD: Neuropsychological Assessment, 2nd Edition. New York, Oxford University Press, 1983

Lezak MD: Neuropsychological Assessment, 3rd Edition, New York, Oxford University Press, 1995

Linehan MM: Cognitive-Behavioral Treatment of Borderline Personality Disorder. New York, Guilford, 1993

Links PS: Psychiatric rehabilitation model for borderline personality disorder. Can J Psychiatry 38 (suppl 1):S35–S38, 1993

Lucas PB, Gardner DL, Cowdry RW, et al: Cerebral structure in borderline personality disorder. Psychiatry Res 27:111–115, 1989

Luria AR: The Working Brain. New York, Basic Books, 1973

Luria AR: Higher Cortical Functions in Man. New York, Basic Books, 1980

Lyons MJ, Merla ME, Young L, et al: Impaired neuropsychological functioning in symptomatic volunteers with schizotypy: preliminary findings. Biol Psychiatry 30:424–426, 1991

Malloy P, Noel N, Longabaugh R, et al: Determinants of neuropsychological impairment in antisocial substance abusers. Addict Behav 15:431–438, 1990

Marziali E: The etiology of borderline personality disorder: developmental factors, in Borderline Personality Disorder: Clinical and Empirical Perspectives. Edited by Clarkin JF, Marziali E, Munroe-Blum H. New York, Guilford, 1992, pp 27–44

Millon T: Disorders of Personality: DSM-IV and Beyond, 2nd Edition. New York, Wiley, 1996

Moffitt TE: Neuropsychology and self-reported early delinquency in an unselected birth cohort: a preliminary report from New Zealand, in Biological Contributions to Crime Causation. Edited by Moffitt TE, Mednick SA. Dordrecht, The Netherlands, Martinus Nijhoff, 1988, pp 93–115

Muller RJ: Is there a neural basis for borderline splitting? Compr Psychiatry 33:92–104, 1992

Murray ME: Minimal brain dysfunction and borderline personality disorder adjustment. Am J Psychother 33:391–403, 1979

Nachshon I: Hemisphere function in violent offenders, in Biological Contributions to Crime Causation. Edited by Moffitt TE, Mednick SA. Dordrecht, The Netherlands, Martinus Nijhoff, 1988, pp 55–67

Newman JP, Patterson CM, Kesson DS: Response perseveration in psychopaths. J Abnorm Psychol 96:145–148, 1987

O'Leary KM, Cowdry RW: Neuropsychological testing results in borderline personality disorder, in Biological and Neurobehavioral Studies of Borderline Personality Disorder. Edited by Silk KR. Washington, DC, American Psychiatric Press, 1994, pp 127–157

O'Leary KM, Brouwers P, Gardner DL, et al: Neuropsychological testing of patients with borderline personality disorder. Am J Psychiatry 148:106–111, 1991

Palombo J, Feigon J: Borderline personality development in childhood and its relationship to neurocognitive deficits. Child and Adolescent Social Work Journal 1:18–33, 1984

Park S, Holzman PS, Lenzenweger MF: Individual differences in spatial working memory in relation to schizotypy. J Abnorm Psychol 104:355–363, 1995

Parnas J, Teasdale TW: A matched-paired comparison of treated versus untreated schizophrenia spectrum cases: a high-risk population study. Acta Psychiatr Scand 75:44–50, 1987

Plakun EM: Treatment of personality disorders in an era of limited resources. Psychiatr Serv 47:128–133, 1996

Quitkin F, Rifkin A, Klein DF: Neurologic soft signs in schizophrenia and character disorders. Arch Gen Psychiatry 33:845–853, 1976

Raine A, Buchsbaum MS, Stanley J, et al: Selective reductions in prefrontal glucose metabolism in murderers assessed with positron emission tomography. Psychophysiology 29:58, 1992a

Raine A, Sheard C, Reynolds GP, et al: Pre-frontal structural and functional deficits associated with individual differences in schizotypal personality. Schizophr Res 7:237–247, 1992b

Ratey JJ (ed): Neuropsychiatry of Personality Disorders. Cambridge, MA, Blackwell Scientific, 1995

Schubert DL, Saccuzzo DP, Braff DL: Information processing in borderline patients. J Nerv Ment Dis 173:26–31, 1985

Schulz SC, Koller MM, Kishore PR, et al: Ventricular enlargement in teenage patients with schizophrenia spectrum disorder. Am J Psychiatry 140:1592–1595, 1983

Siever L: Biological factors in schizotypal personality disorders. Acta Psychiatr Scand 90:45–50, 1994

Siever LJ, Kalus OF, Keefe RS: The boundaries of schizophrenia. Psychiatr Clin North Am 16:217–243, 1993

Silk KR (ed): Implications of biological research for clinical work with borderline patients, in Biological and Neurobehavioral Studies of Borderline Personality Disorder. Edited by Silk KR. Washington, DC, American Psychiatric Press, 1994, pp 227–240

Snyder S, Pitts WM: Electroencephalography of DSM-III borderline personality disorder. Acta Psychiatr Scand 69:129–134, 1984

Snyder S, Pitts WM, Gustin Q: CT scans of patients with borderline personality disorder (letter). Am J Psychiatry 140:272, 1983

Soloff PH, Millward JW: Developmental histories of borderline patients. Compr Psychiatry 24:574–588, 1983

Spreen O, Risser AH, Edgell D: Developmental Neuropsychology. New York, Oxford University Press, 1995

Stein DJ, Hollander E, Cohen L, et al: Neuropsychiatric impairment in impulsive personality disorders. Psychiatry Res 48:257–266, 1993

Sternbach SE, Judd PH, Sabo AN, et al: Cognitive and perceptual distortions in borderline personality disorder and schizotypal personality disorder in a vignette sample. Compr Psychiatry 33:186–189, 1992

Sutker PB, Allain AN: Cognitive abstraction, shifting, and control: clinical sample comparisons of psychopaths and nonpsychopaths. J Abnorm Psychol 96: 73–75, 1987

Swirsky-Sacchetti T, Gorton GE, Samuel S, et al: Neuropsychological function in borderline personality disorder. J Clin Psychol 49:385–396, 1993

Teuber HL: The riddle of frontal lobe function in man, in The Frontal Granular Cortex and Behavior. Edited by Warren JM, Akert K. New York, McGraw-Hill, 1964, pp 410–444

van Reekum R: Acquired and developmental brain dysfunction in borderline personality disorder. Can J Psychiatry 38 (suppl 1):S4–S10, 1993

van Reekum R, Conway CA, Gansler D, et al: Neurobehavioral study of borderline personality disorder. J Psychiatr Neurosci 18:121–129, 1993

Vela RM: Borderline disorder of childhood: clinical description and etiological considerations. Comprehensive Mental Health Care 1:109–118, 1991

Viederman M: Reply to Frayn (letter). Am J Psychiatry 153:297, 1996

Volkow ND, Tancredi L: Neural substrates of violent behavior. Br J Psychiatry 151:668–673, 1987

Wergeland H: A follow-up study of 29 borderline psychotic children 5 to 20 years after discharge. Acta Psychiatr Scand 60:465–476, 1979

Widiger TA: Psychological tests and the borderline diagnosis. J Pers Assess 46: 227–238, 1982

Yeudall LT: Neuropsychological assessment of forensic disorders. Canadian Mental Health 25:7–15, 1977

Yeudall LT, Fromm-Auch D, Davies P: Neuropsychological impairment of persistent delinquency. J Nerv Ment Dis 170:257–265, 1982

Zanarini MC, Kimble CR, Williams AA: Neurological dysfunction in borderline patients and Axis II control subjects, in Biological and Neurobehavioral Studies of Borderline Personality Disorder. Edited by Silk KR. Washington, DC, American Psychiatric Press, 1994, pp 159–175

7

NEUROPSYCHOLOGICAL FINDINGS IN CHRONIC MEDICAL ILLNESS

Elizabeth A. Gaudino, Ph.D., Dean A. Pollina, Ph.D., and
Lauren B. Krupp, M.D.

IN THIS CHAPTER, we summarize major neuropsychological findings in five
medical disorders that have psychiatric manifestations: multiple sclerosis
(MS), systemic lupus erythematosus (SLE), Lyme disease, chronic fatigue
syndrome (CFS), and epilepsy. These disorders were chosen because they
represent a broad range of diseases and illustrate the neuropsychological
and psychiatric problems found in primary neurological disease (MS and
epilepsy), rheumatological illness (SLE), multisystemic infection (Lyme
disease), and a medical disorder that overlaps with psychiatric illness
(CFS). We address the interrelation of neuropsychological abnormalities
with mood disorder, fatigue, and other disease symptoms, and we emphasize general issues regarding the recognition of cognitive dysfunction and
psychiatric disorders in chronic illness.

◈ MULTIPLE SCLEROSIS

Definition

MS is an organ-specific autoimmune disorder characterized by demyelination of the central nervous system (CNS). It is among the most common neurological diseases of young and middle-aged adults.

Pathogenesis

A combination of genetic predisposition and environmental factors are involved in the development of this immune disorder. The primary pathophysiological finding in MS is a T-cell-mediated inflammatory attack on the white matter of the CNS, which causes diverse neurological symptoms and signs.

Diagnosis

The diagnosis of MS requires clinical evidence of neurological dysfunction involving more than one area of the CNS. Attacks of neurological dysfunction must either occur over time or assume a progressive course over 6 months. When more than one area of CNS dysfunction is not apparent from clinical examination, magnetic resonance imaging (MRI) and electrophysiological tests such as visual evoked responses (VER), brain-stem auditory evoked responses (BAER), or sensory evoked responses (SER) may be used to document clinically silent lesions. Other etiologies for CNS dysfunction (such as B_{12} deficiency, vasculitis, CNS infection, or toxin exposure) must be excluded.

Clinical Manifestations

MS usually develops between ages 15 and 50 years. Rarely, younger or older patients may be afflicted. Early in the illness, exacerbations (so-called flare-ups) and remissions are common. A progressive course frequently follows. In approximately 15% of MS patients, the disease has a benign course with few exacerbations and little accumulating neurological deficit. In 10%–15% of patients, the disease has a progressive course from the onset.

Symptoms and signs of MS are varied and reflect both lesion site and lesion severity. The most common manifestations are weakness, gait disturbance, visual changes, urinary dysfunction, ataxia, paresthesias, and dysarthria or scanning speech (spasmodically paced speech). Mental disturbance, pain, vertigo, convulsions, hearing loss, tinnitus, and nonspecific symptoms such as fatigue or distractibility also occur. Symptoms may wax and wane.

Neuroradiological Findings

The most frequent neuroradiological findings in MS are discrete lesions scattered throughout the periventricular white matter and gray matter–white matter junction, widening of cortical sulci, and ventricular enlargement (Comi et al. 1993; Pozzilli et al. 1993). Callosal atrophy is sometimes found (Comi et al. 1993; Huber et al. 1992). Several MRI measures, including total lesion area (Pugnetti et al. 1993), ventricular dilation (Comi et al. 1993), and callosal atrophy (Comi et al. 1993; Huber et al. 1992), have been correlated with cognitive deficits.

Psychiatric Manifestations

Changes in the individual's ability to maintain emotional control have long been recognized as a characteristic of MS, and the association between MS, bipolar disorder, and major depression has been well documented (Schiffer et al. 1986; Whitlock and Siskind 1980). Psychiatric manifestations, including psychosis, can occur both early in the disease process and later. In rare instances it is the most obvious problem (Skegg 1993). Hence, psychiatrists should consider the diagnosis of MS when affective psychosis is accompanied by neurological signs (Pine et al. 1995).

Evidence indicates that brain lesions are responsible for some of the psychiatric symptoms in MS (Garland and Zis 1991; Goodstein and Ferrell 1977). Euphoria has been associated with cognitive impairment and MRI abnormalities (Möller et al. 1994).

Cognitive Manifestations

Although motor and sensory disturbances are the most commonly reported manifestations of MS, cognitive symptoms frequently have been documented (Peyser and Poser 1986; Rao 1986). Often cognitive deficits in MS are undetected by health care professionals who rely on insensitive measures of cognitive function such as bedside mental status examinations. These routine examinations are not sufficiently comprehensive to detect the moderate to severe deficits in attention, concept formation, and complex problem solving that are present in MS. (See Rao 1990a for more comprehensive coverage of the neurobehavioral aspects of MS.)

Neuropsychological studies have uncovered a greater incidence of cognitive impairment in MS than was suspected initially. Significant cognitive impairment may be the earliest manifestation of MS and represents one of the most functionally disabling symptoms (Franklin et al. 1989; O'Connor 1994). Approximately 40%–60% of MS patients have some type of deficit on neuropsychological tests. Strong evidence indicates that the pattern of cognitive decline in MS is heterogeneous (e.g., Beatty et al. 1996; Rao et al. 1991a, 1991b). Thus, group studies that report the mean performance of MS subjects on a variety of tests must be interpreted with caution. Research has shown that 22%–51% of MS patients show no evidence of cognitive impairment and 43%–56% show mild to moderate impairment. Severe, global cognitive impairment in MS may occur in 20%–32% of all MS subjects tested. Dementia secondary to MS is uncommon (3%–10%) (Fontaine et al. 1994). Although MS patients do not show one typical pattern of cognitive impairment, group analyses of neuropsychological test performance have helped to advance our understanding of the cognitive impairments that might be found in these patients.

General intelligence. Decreases in general intelligence in MS patients over time were first reported by Cantor (1951) in an early longitudinal study. The Army General Classification Test was administered to 23 healthy male recruits who developed MS after their induction into the military. The recruits were retested approximately 4 years later and showed a significant decrease in general intelligence (Cantor 1951). Another longitudinal study of 14 MS patients found significant decrements over a 3-year period on the Vocabulary, Information, and Digit Symbol tests of the Wechsler Adult Intelligence Scale (WAIS) (Ivnik 1978). Studies comparing intelligence test performance of MS patients with normal or neurological control groups usually show no significant group differences (Goldstein and Shelly 1974; Jambor 1969). This discrepancy may result from the greater sensitivity of within-subject experimental designs.

Attention. Several standardized neuropsychological tests of sustained attention and vigilance have been applied to MS patients, with variable findings. Significant impairment has been reported in chronic (primary) progressive MS patients on Wechsler Adult Intelligence Scale—Revised (WAIS-R) Digit Span Forward and Digit Span Backward subtests (Grigsby et al. 1994), but in many studies of other types of MS patients, the Digit Span subtest has not been found to be sensitive to impaired attention (Rao 1990a). More consistently, impaired attention has been detected with the Paced Auditory Serial Addition Test (PASAT; Gronwall 1977), a complex attention and vigilance test that requires subjects to add serial pairs of randomized single digits presented continuously at four different rates of speed. MS patients perform significantly worse on the PASAT than do control subjects (e.g., Litvan et al. 1988). However, the PASAT does not distinguish attentional deficits from poor performance secondary to dysarthria or slowed speech (Lezak 1995). Similarly, motor disturbances may contribute to MS patients' impaired performance on attention tasks that have fine motor demands, which compromises the interpretation of the results (Van der Burg et al. 1987). For example, Kujala et al. (1995) showed that MS patients with mild cognitive impairment had deficits on several tests of sustained attention (PASAT, Stroop, and a computerized vigilance task). Because tests of simple motor abilities were not included in Kujala et al.'s battery, the possibility that a motor performance deficit contributed to these results cannot be excluded.

From these findings we may conclude that many MS patients have greater impairment on tests of complex attention than on simple attentional tasks. This difficulty in complex attention is commonly experienced by MS patients as a decreased ability to function in multitask situations such as work or caring for children (Lezak 1995). However, when interpreting such attentional difficulties, clinicians must consider the effect of other compromised motor functions on test performance.

Learning and memory. Disorders of learning and memory are common in MS. Neuropsychological studies indicate that approximately 50% of MS patients score significantly below control groups on selected tests of memory functioning (Beatty et al. 1988; Fischer 1988; Rao et al. 1984), but not all studies corroborate these findings (Amato et al. 1995; Heaton et al. 1985; Jambor 1969).

Problems with delayed recall of verbal and nonverbal information are well documented and yet somewhat controversial. Memory problems in

MS have not been differentiated adequately from potential problems in learning new information (DeLuca et al. 1994). Specifically, MS patients have demonstrated impaired verbal learning ability (Beatty et al. 1995; DeLuca et al. 1994), yet only one study in the literature attempted to compare MS patients with control subjects on the amount of information learned prior to assessing memory for the material. When MS patients and control subjects were compared for performance on a test of verbal learning, MS patients performed as well as control subjects on measures of delayed free recall and recognition (DeLuca et al. 1994). Whether this finding generalizes to visual learning and memory is not known. Although preliminary in nature, the DeLuca et al. (1994) study indicates that learning and memory problems are common in MS, but the frequency and nature of these impairments are still under investigation.

Memory impairment in MS is independent of problems in attention; however, the interaction between impaired learning and attention has not been well researched. Executive functions such as complex problem solving and abstraction may also play a role in learning and memory impairments. Some evidence indicates that memory functions in MS may deteriorate over time (Feinstein et al. 1992), particularly in the most severely cognitively impaired patients. Observed memory deficits have been correlated with computed tomography (CT), MRI, and positron-emission tomography (PET) findings (Comi et al. 1993; Rao 1990b). However, these findings must be interpreted with caution because of methodological issues such as inconsistencies in brain volumetric measurements and differences in the types of cognitive measurements used.

Complex problem solving.   Neuropsychological tests of executive functions used in the study of MS include the Wisconsin Card Sorting Test (WCST) (Arnette et al. 1994; Heaton et al. 1985), the Category Test (Huber et al. 1992), the Concept Formation test (Rao et al. 1984), and the Block Substitution test (Parsons et al. 1957). In general, MS patients perform more poorly on the WCST than do healthy control subjects (Beatty et al. 1995). MS patients with a high frontal lesion area (quantified using MRI) completed fewer categories and made more errors on the WCST test than did a second group with comparable lesion extent but with a low frontal lesion area (Arnette et al. 1994). Because impairments on the WCST do not correlate well with findings on other tests of frontal-lobe function from the Luria-Nebraska Neuropsychological Battery

(Mendozzi et al. 1993), the specificity of this finding to frontal-lobe dysfunction is unclear.

Interaction With Other Disease Variables

The association between physical and cognitive impairment in MS is not strong. Symptoms common in MS that may adversely affect cognitive functioning include fatigue, depression, distal weakness, loss of dexterity, and visual disturbance. Fatigue is present in 76%–87% of MS patients (Freal et al. 1984; Murray 1985) but does not appear to affect cognitive functioning significantly. When medications are used to treat fatigue in MS, they do not improve cognitive performance (Geisler et al. 1996), and when fatigue has been correlated with cognitive tests in MS the relationship has been weak (Geisler et al. 1996; Rao et al. 1991a). However, fatigue may increase the negative effect of physical and affective problems on neuropsychological functioning (Grossman et al. 1994). Although depression may have a deleterious effect on cognitive abilities, neuropsychological test performance in MS is significantly different from that in control subjects even after controlling for the effects of mood (Krupp et al. 1994; Rao et al. 1991a). Although measurements of physical disability do not correlate strongly with cognitive impairment, these motor problems may limit interpretation of test performance unless appropriate measures are used. For example, although a patient with loss of dexterity would do poorly on the WAIS-R Digit Symbol test, the Symbol Digit Modalities Test (oral version) (Smith 1973) is a more accurate measure of nonmotor visuospatial skill.

Conclusion

Our appreciation of the nature of cognitive problems in MS has grown substantially. It is now well known that a significant number of MS patients experience some type of cognitive impairment. More refined research into the relation between MRI measures and neuropsychological performance will help to improve the understanding of the role CNS white-matter disturbance has on cognitive functions. Table 7–1 summarizes the diagnostic criteria, clinical manifestations, psychiatric manifestations, and neuropsychological deficits in MS. Determining whether newer treatments for MS will help preserve cognitive function will require well-planned clinical trials in which neuropsychological testing is included in the outcome assessment.

Table 7–1. Summary of multiple sclerosis

Diagnostic criteria

  Neurological dysfunction in the central nervous system separated by time
    and location

Clinical manifestations

  Weakness, gait disturbance, visual changes, urinary dysfunction, ataxia,
    paresthesias, dysarthria

  Periventricular abnormalities on magnetic resonance imaging (white matter)

Psychiatric manifestations

  Loss of emotional control

  Euphoria, depression, psychosis

Neuropsychological deficits

  Learning and memory

  Sustained complex attention

  Abstract reasoning

◈ SYSTEMIC LUPUS ERYTHEMATOSUS

Definition

SLE is a chronic multisystemic inflammatory autoimmune disease. It is associated with multiple autoantibodies and is characterized by disorders of the skin, joints, heart, kidneys, blood, immune system, and CNS. The initial diagnosis of SLE is usually based on the accumulation of clinical features consistent with the disorder (Barr and Merchut 1992).

Pathogenesis

SLE results from converging abnormalities in genetic, immunological, hormonal, and environmental pathways (Boumpas et al. 1995). The autoimmune response in SLE patients is extremely diverse (Boumpas et al. 1995). Given the many genetic and environmental factors contributing to the pathogenesis of SLE, it is not surprising that clinical and laboratory findings in these patients are quite heterogeneous.

Diagnosis

The diagnosis of SLE requires the presence of 4 out of 11 clinical features "serially or simultaneously during any interval of observation" (Tan et al.

1982, p. 1272). The clinical features are as follows: malar rash, discoid rash, photosensitivity, oral ulcers, arthritis, serositis, renal disorder, neurological disorder (seizures or psychosis), hematological disorder, immunological disorder, and abnormal antinuclear antibody titer (Barr and Merchut 1992).

Clinical Manifestations

Fatigue, loss of appetite, weight loss, and fever are common problems in SLE (Barr and Merchut 1992; Pisetsky 1986). Other manifestations such as rash, renal failure, and arthralgia may relapse and remit over time. Neuropsychiatric syndromes include focal cerebral dysfunction such as stroke, seizures, and transverse myelitis; diffuse cerebral dysfunction such as dementia, psychosis, or major affective disorders; and movement disorders such as chorea, athetosis, Parkinson's-like disorders, and cerebellar ataxia. Organic brain syndrome, psychosis, and seizures are the most common neuropsychiatric findings (Boumpas et al. 1995). These symptoms typically appear early in the disease course (Ward and Studenski 1991).

Neuroradiological Findings

MRI abnormalities include atrophy and cortical and subcortical microinfarctions (Cauli et al. 1994; Colamussi et al. 1995; Daif et al. 1995; Hanly et al. 1993; McLean et al. 1995; Salmaggi et al. 1994). In one study, abnormal single photon emission computed tomography (SPECT) scans, including both focal and nonfocal lesions, were found in 73% of patients who had mild neuropsychiatric symptoms (e.g., headache or subjective memory problems) and in 90% of patients who had overt neuropsychiatric disease (including motor and sensory deficits) (Rubbert et al. 1993). In contrast, only 10% of patients lacking neuropsychiatric symptoms had abnormalities on SPECT. A combination of focal and diffuse CNS injury likely contributes to the neuropsychiatric complications seen clinically.

Psychiatric Manifestations

Psychiatric disturbance in SLE is characterized by auditory hallucinations, paranoid delusions, schizophreniform psychosis, and depression.

Psychotic symptoms are often accompanied by delirium, seizures, or focal neurological dysfunctions (Bennahum and Messner 1975). These episodes of psychiatric disturbance usually last less than 6 weeks and rarely last more than 6 months (Shannon and Goetz 1989).

Although psychiatric symptomatology is an integral part of the illness, only psychosis is regarded universally as a neuropsychiatric manifestation of SLE (Iverson 1993). However, other psychiatric problems are common (Krupp et al. 1990; Rubbert et al. 1993). Depending on the methodology and the patient sample, the frequency of psychiatric problems in SLE ranges from 17% to 71% (Wekking 1993). Some studies have shown a greater incidence of psychiatric symptoms in SLE compared with chronic illnesses such as rheumatoid arthritis (Wekking 1993).

Studies have revealed that 44% of SLE inpatients had organic mood disorder with depressive symptoms on psychiatric interview (Miguel et al. 1994), and 21% of outpatients had current affective disorders (Hay et al. 1992). Miguel et al. (1994) used the Present State Examination (a semistructured clinical interview) and found psychiatric manifestations in 63% (27/43) of medical inpatients. Diagnosed disorders included depression with delirium or dementia ($n = 7$), hallucinations followed by a depressive episode ($n = 1$), and organic delusions followed by depression ($n = 1$).

The extent to which nonpsychotic psychiatric illness is the result of neurological involvement compared with psychosocial factors is controversial. Cerebrospinal fluid (CSF) measures of antiribosomal P antibodies and ventricular size on CT have been correlated with psychosis but not with nonpsychotic affective disorders (Caminero et al. 1992; Nojima et al. 1992). Nonpsychotic psychiatric disturbance has been variously attributed to direct CNS involvement, psychosocial factors, somatic symptoms (such as pain and fatigue), or a combination of variables (Iverson and Anderson 1994). There is also conflicting evidence for a relation between nonpsychotic psychiatric disorder and cognitive impairment.

Cognitive Manifestations

Cognitive loss, psychiatric illness, pain, and fatigue all may have a deleterious effect on the quality of life for SLE patients. Cognitive problems in SLE patients are most often noted in conjunction with frank CNS involvement (e.g., psychosis, stroke, and seizures) but also occur in patients without these features (Ginsburg et al. 1992; Hanly et al. 1993; Hay et al.

1992; Miguel et al. 1994). Even ambulatory patients who are still working experience cognitive loss and mood disturbance that adversely affect psychosocial functioning (Ginsburg et al. 1992; Hanly et al. 1993; Miguel et al. 1994).

The effect of diffuse cerebral dysfunction on cognition and behavior remains uncertain because most studies have focused on patients with focal neurological deficits such as stroke or seizures (Ginsburg et al. 1992; Hanly et al. 1993; Hay et al. 1992). However, half of the most cognitively impaired patients (9/17) had no other neurological abnormalities (Hay et al. 1992).

General intelligence. Findings have been contradictory regarding the effects of SLE on general intelligence in adults. Hanly et al. (1993) found that SLE outpatients did not differ from patients with rheumatoid arthritis or healthy control subjects in their performance on a short form of the WAIS-R. In contrast, Hay et al. (1992) found that 21% (13/62) of patients demonstrated impaired intellectual functioning on the WAIS. Most of this cognitively impaired group had coexisting psychiatric disorders. Children with SLE appear to have lower-than-average intelligence, academic achievement, reading comprehension, and visual memory (Wyckoff et al. 1995).

Attention and higher cortical functions. SLE patients have significantly more frontal-lobe atrophy than do control subjects (Maeshima et al. 1994). Atrophy was associated with poorer performance on digit span and verbal fluency tasks, suggesting that these cognitive deficits may indicate permanent CNS damage. SLE patients performed poorly on tests of complex attention and simple attention, even in the absence of other neurological or psychiatric SLE manifestations (Ginsburg et al. 1992). Impairments in concentration were associated with increases in current disease activity, indicating that these impairments were transient CNS effects (Fisk et al. 1993). More research on attention in SLE will be needed to determine whether these problems reflect transient disease flare-ups or permanent CNS damage.

Memory. Hanly et al. (1993) found no difference between SLE patients and rheumatoid arthritis patients on the California Verbal Learning Test and the Wechsler Memory Scale—Revised (WMS-R), indicating that verbal and visual memory in SLE patients is no more impaired than in other chronically ill patients.

Hay et al. (1992) used the WMS and the Benton Visual Retention Test (BVRT) to examine verbal and visual memory in SLE patients with and without psychiatric manifestations. SLE patients with psychiatric disorders made significantly more errors on the BVRT than did those without psychiatric problems. Overall, 17% of patients had abnormal results on the WMS, and 23% had impaired performance on the BVRT.

One study examined the relation between memory impairment and disease activity (Fisk et al. 1993). Deficits in immediate memory occurred concurrently with flare-ups of the disease. Impaired delayed recognition memory was associated with overt neurological deficits (past or present). These findings suggest that memory loss in SLE patients is associated with psychiatric or other neurological manifestations of the disease. Nonpsychiatric SLE patients without other neurological signs do not appear to have deficits in memory functions.

Perceptual abilities. In a large series of computerized neuropsychological tests, Ginsburg et al. (1992) found that hand-eye coordination and pattern completion were impaired in SLE compared with rheumatoid arthritis. However, after statistically controlling for multiple comparisons, these differences were no longer significant.

The current findings do not point to a specific memory deficit in SLE because most studies show similar deficits in attention and perceptual processing. A global loss in general intelligence is not generally a feature of SLE and hence would not explain poor performance on measures of memory or perceptual ability.

Interaction With Other Disease Variables

Interpreting the cognitive function of SLE patients requires consideration of potentially confounding factors such as concurrent medication use (e.g., steroids), pain, and fatigue. Some studies suggest that cognitive impairment is associated with psychiatric illness in these patients (Hay et al. 1992; Miguel et al. 1994).

Fatigue is very common in SLE, but its relation to cognitive loss is unclear. Krupp et al. (1990) found no relation between fatigue and laboratory indicators of disease activity. A modest correlation between patients' ratings of their fatigue and physician ratings of disease activity was noted ($r = 0.30$, $P < .05$). Fatigue is correlated with self-reported depressive symptoms (Cardenas and Kutner 1982; Joyce et al. 1989; Krupp et al. 1990).

Steroids are the primary treatment for active SLE (Barr et al. 1992). Steroids may cause psychosis in some SLE patients (Ferstl et al. 1992; Fisk et al. 1993; Iverson and Anderson 1994). However, psychotic symptoms in SLE in the absence of steroid use are well documented (Miguel et al. 1994). In fact, steroids are often helpful in the management of cognitive and psychiatric manifestations of SLE (Barr et al. 1992; Denburg et al. 1994). Most of the other medications used in treating SLE (e.g., anti-inflammatory agents and antimalarial agents) are not known to affect cognitive functioning and only rarely cause psychiatric symptoms.

Conclusion

Table 7–2 summarizes the diagnostic criteria, clinical manifestations, psychiatric manifestations, and neuropsychological deficits in SLE. Some studies have documented a fluctuating course in the cognitive impair-

Table 7–2. Summary of systemic lupus erythematosus

Diagnostic criteria

Malar rash, discoid rash, photosensitivity, oral ulcers, arthritis, serositis, renal disorder, neurological disorder (seizures, psychosis), hematological disorder, immunological disorder, abnormal antinuclear antibody titer

Clinical manifestations

Fatigue, loss of appetite, weight loss, fever

Rash, renal failure, arthralgia

Stroke, seizures, transverse myelitis

Diffuse cerebral dysfunction

Movement disorders

Psychiatric manifestations

Auditory hallucinations

Paranoid delusions

Schizophreniform psychosis

Depression

Neuropsychological deficits

Immediate memory

Delayed recognition

Verbal fluency

Attention

Possible intellectual deterioration

ments associated with SLE (Carbotte et al. 1992; Hanly et al. 1993). Disease flare-ups may be associated with some cognitive problems. SPECT and MRI studies support this hypothesis in that they indicate diffuse cortical and subcortical abnormalities may be transient.

Neuropsychological assessment should be conducted early in the course of SLE so that a baseline can be established. No ideal neuropsychological battery exists for patients with very mild or no CNS involvement. However, assessment of general intellectual functioning, verbal and visual memory, attention, concentration, and visuoperceptual skill is important. Inclusion of a psychiatric status evaluation is critical. Patients with concurrent or past psychiatric disorders (such as psychosis), focal neurological deficits, or peripheral neuropathy are most likely to show cognitive deficits. However, abnormalities may also be present in patients without these neurological features. Neuropsychological assessment is most easily interpreted when information about concurrent fatigue, pain, disease activity (such as recent SLE flare-ups), and medications is taken into account.

◆ LYME DISEASE

Definition

Lyme disease is a tick-borne, multisystemic, infectious disorder caused by the spirochete *Borrelia burgdorferi*. This spirochetal infection is transmitted by a tick whose species varies according to geographic location.

Pathogenesis

Lyme disease is the most rapidly growing vector-borne infection in the United States (Centers for Disease Control 1990; Coyle 1992; Dennis 1993). In North America, Lyme disease is most common in the coastal Northeast, the upper Midwest, the Pacific Northwest, and southeastern Ontario (Coyle 1992). People at greatest risk for contracting Lyme disease work or spend a great deal of leisure time outdoors.

The mechanisms by which *B. burgdorferi* affects the organ systems may be multiple. But the potential effects of subsequent immune activation may be more important. *B. burgdorferi* stimulates the production of interleukin-1, a powerful immune mediator that has a wide range of effects on the body. *B. burgdorferi* also stimulates production of autoantibodies, which may attack nerve axons, myelin, Schwann cells, and cardiac muscles (Coleman and Benach 1994).

Diagnosis

The diagnosis of Lyme disease as determined by the Centers for Disease Control and Prevention (CDC) requires either the pathognomonic skin lesion erythema migrans (EM), a feature of the early infection, or serological evidence of *B. burgdorferi* infection in conjunction with objective late manifestations (e.g., arthritis, neurological signs, or cardiac conduction defects).

Currently, no widely available laboratory tests are sufficiently sensitive and reliable for detecting active *B. burgdorferi* infection. Evidence of intrathecal antibody production is currently required by the CDC for the diagnosis of certain CNS Lyme syndromes. However, intrathecal antibody may be absent in late neurological cases (Coyle 1992; Dattwyler et al. 1988) or may persist after therapy (Hansen and Lebech 1992). Whether CSF markers such as borrelial antigen, DNA, or cytokine disturbances will be helpful in diagnosis, as some studies suggest (Coyle 1992; Coyle et al. 1993; Doscher et al. 1994), will require additional research.

Clinical Manifestations

The common neurological features of Lyme disease include cranial neuropathy, seventh cranial nerve palsy, meningitis, radial nerve palsy, and, less commonly, encephalomyelitis. Neurological disease is common in early and late stages of Lyme disease but is often reported in the chronic form of this illness. Neurobehavioral disability is less common in cases of Lyme disease that are diagnosed and treated rapidly (Halperin et al. 1991). However, in patients in whom diagnosis of Lyme disease is delayed, the long-term neurological sequelae may be disabling.

Nonneurological manifestations include an expanding EM rash, which occurs 3–30 days after acquiring the infection. This rash is the pathognomonic marker of Lyme disease and is present in 65%–90% of cases. The most common late manifestation other than neurological illness is a migratory arthritis.

Neuroradiological Findings

Occasionally Lyme disease patients who have severe neurological complications show abnormalities on neuroimaging, but most patients have normal MRI and CT scans. White-matter abnormalities occur occasionally, but they do not necessarily reflect cognitive dysfunction. SPECT abnormalities have been described in patients who have chronic Lyme disease associated with cognitive loss, but this finding is not universal (Logigian et al. 1990). Unlike SLE or MS, Lyme disease does not show a clear relation between neuroradiological abnormalities and cognitive functioning.

Psychiatric Manifestations

Serious psychopathology, including anxiety disorders (Fallon and Neilds 1994; Fallon et al. 1993), acute psychotic syndromes, severe depression, delirium, and profound chronic fatigue (Sigal 1993), has been reported in cases of Lyme disease (Fallon and Nields 1994; Fallon et al. 1993; Kollikowski et al. 1988; Krupp et al. 1989; Pachner 1986). The relation of these disorders to *B. burgdorferi* infection is unclear (Coyle 1992). This confusion has led to inappropriate diagnosis and treatment (Steere et al. 1993).

Kaplan et al. (1992) compared the psychiatric status of Lyme disease patients with that of nonpsychotic depressed outpatients and a group of patients with chronic pain (from fibromyalgia). Patients with Lyme disease did not differ significantly from patients with fibromyalgia or depression on any scale of the Minnesota Multiphasic Personality Inventory (MMPI), and they scored notably lower than these control groups on scales of depression, anxiety, and somatization. Patients with Lyme disease also scored lower, although not significantly so, on the Beck Depression Inventory. Although this study indicates that Lyme disease patients have less psychopathology than these control groups, it did not include healthy control subjects. Thus all of these groups may show some level of psychopathology.

Fallon et al. (1993) reviewed a series of 85 patients with chronic Lyme disease in which photophobia and other sensory hypersensitivities were reported as psychiatric symptoms. Irritability, emotional lability, word or letter reversals when speaking or writing, and spatial disorientation at some time during the course of the illness were other common symptoms.

In studying psychiatric disorders in Lyme disease, Fallon et al. (1993) reported three case studies of patients who, after disease onset, developed major depression with panic disorder, organic mood syndrome with depression and mania, and panic disorder alone. In our experience with 38 patients who had been treated successfully for Lyme disease, 39% (15/38) had a lifetime history of psychiatric disorder (Gaudino et al. 1994). Current psychiatric disorders were noted in 21% (8/38) and consisted of major depression ($n = 4$), dysthymia ($n = 2$), or anxiety disorder ($n = 2$). Thirty-two percent (12/38) had histories of a past psychiatric disorder including major depression ($n = 7$), anxiety disorder ($n = 3$), and substance abuse ($n = 2$). More than half of these patients developed the psychiatric disorder within 2 years after acquiring Lyme disease. Clearly, mood and anxiety disorders are present in Lyme disease patients and require treatment. The extent to which psychiatric disorders occur in the absence of other symptoms of Lyme disease and the association of psychiatric disorders to direct CNS dysfunction remains unclear.

Cognitive Manifestations

Lyme disease has been associated with deficits in memory, attention, perceptual-motor functions, and problem solving (Bolton and Krupp 1994; Gaudino et al. 1994; Halperin et al. 1988; Kaplan et al. 1992; Krupp et al. 1991a). Greater deficits have been found in Lyme disease patients when compared with patients who have depression or fibromyalgia (Kaplan et al. 1992) and with healthy control subjects (Krupp et al. 1991a; Shadick et al. 1994). Prior studies on cognitive functioning in Lyme disease have also indicated deficits in memory, retrieval, and verbal fluency. One limitation to these studies is the lack of information about whether patients had received adequate treatment for Lyme disease. Future studies should differentiate between patients who have chronic untreated Lyme disease and patients whose Lyme disease treatment failed.

General intelligence. General intelligence does not appear to be compromised in Lyme disease, according to the few studies that assessed patients in this area (Halperin et al. 1988; Krupp et al. 1991a; Logigian et al. 1990).

Verbal and visual memory. Logigian et al. (1990) assessed verbal and visual memory in 27 patients who had chronic Lyme disease. They found that 56% (15/27) had impairment on neuropsychological tests. Shadick et al. (1994) compared 38 patients who had received treatment for chronic Lyme disease with 43 healthy control subjects. Patients with Lyme disease showed more verbal memory deficits than did control subjects. Kaplan et al. (1992) tested 20 patients who had Lyme disease 3 months to 14 years after infection. The Lyme disease patients had more verbal memory loss than did the control group of depressed and fibromyalgia patients.

Bolton and Krupp (1994) used the California Verbal Learning Test (a list-learning test) to study the performance of 20 patients who had received treatment for Lyme disease, and they found verbal retrieval deficits relative to healthy control subjects. Gaudino et al. (1994) found verbal memory problems in Lyme disease patients relative to those in both depressed and healthy control subjects on two separate list-learning tests.

Attention and higher cortical functions. We have found that patients with chronic Lyme disease, compared with healthy control subjects, have deficits in attention as measured by the WAIS-R Digit Span subtest and perform less well on visuomotor search as measured by the Trail Making Test. Gaudino et al. (1994) found that Lyme disease patients had verbal fluency deficits relative to depressed control subjects. In our experience, Lyme disease patients do not perform significantly worse on the WCST, a task involving executive functions (L. B. Krupp, unpublished data, 1994), or on the Booklet Categories test (Krupp et al. 1991a). Patients are significantly slower on the Finger Tapping Test, a test of fine motor dexterity (L. B. Krupp, unpublished data, 1994).

Prognosis for cognitive loss. Halperin et al. (1988) found that abnormalities in attention, psychomotor, and perceptual-motor functions improved after appropriate antibiotic treatment. However, this conclusion must be made with caution because the study lacked a control group. Thus, practice effects could have contributed to improved performance. Nonetheless, various case reports document that most untreated patients with severe encephalopathy or encephalomyelitis improve after antibiotic therapy.

Unfortunately, some patients experience persistent symptoms more than 6 months after therapy. Krupp et al. (1991a) studied cognitive function in patients with chronic Lyme disease who had completed antibiotic therapy but still experienced fatigue, joint pain, and other Lyme disease symptoms. Patients with Lyme disease showed deficits relative to age- and education-matched control subjects in verbal memory and verbal fluency, and they showed a trend for slower performance on the Trail Making Test Parts A and B. These patients were also rated by a clinical neuropsychologist as mild to moderately impaired more frequently than were healthy control subjects (60% vs 0%, respectively) (Krupp et al. 1991a).

Interaction With Other Disease Variables

The evaluation of coexisting fatigue, pain, affective disorder, psychosocial status, and overall health outcome in Lyme disease has been incomplete. Fatigue is elevated significantly in Lyme disease patients compared with healthy control subjects (Krupp et al. 1993b). Patients with chronic Lyme disease also have elevated depressive symptoms relative to healthy control subjects (Krupp et al. 1993b).

Kaplan et al. (1992) found a correlation in Lyme disease patients between the depression subscale of the MMPI and the paired-associate test of the WMS ($r = .67$, $P < .05$). However, the most depressed Lyme disease patients performed only slightly worse than did less depressed patients on most measures of memory function.

Many patients with mild to moderate encephalopathy lack current psychiatric illness but have cognitive problems; however, most severe psychiatric syndromes observed in Lyme disease are associated with encephalopathy. Thus psychiatric and cognitive problems may arise concurrently.

Conclusion

Common deficits associated with chronic Lyme disease are noted in verbal memory, attention, visuomotor search, motor speed, and verbal fluency. The pattern is most consistent with a mild to moderate encephalopathy without clear neuroradiological correlation. Cognitive loss may be a major feature of late or chronic Lyme disease. It may persist even after prolonged antibiotic therapy. For patients with untreated Lyme disease, cognitive loss is a clear indication for antibiotic therapy. For Lyme disease patients who have completed antibiotic therapy, the decision regarding additional antibiotic treatment is more complex. CSF evaluation and documentation of progressive cognitive loss should be completed before considering additional therapy. Table 7–3 summarizes the diagnostic criteria, clinical manifestations, psychiatric manifestations, and neuropsychological deficits in Lyme disease.

◈ CHRONIC FATIGUE SYNDROME

Definition

Patients with severe fatigue that develops in association with flulike symptoms are often defined as having CFS, a condition of severe fatigue, present for at least 6 months and not explained by other medical disorders. CFS is a genuine but poorly understood illness. This disorder has been the subject of much controversy in the lay and medical communities.

Table 7–3. Summary of Lyme disease

Diagnostic criteria

    Pathognomonic skin lesion (erythema migrans rash)

    Serologic evidence of *Borrelia burgdorferi* infection in conjunction with late manifestations (arthritis, neurological signs, cardiac conduction deficits)

Clinical manifestations

    Cranial neuropathy

    Seventh cranial nerve palsy

    Meningitis

    Bell's palsy

    Encephalopathy

    Erythema migrans rash

    Arthritis

Psychiatric manifestations

    Acute psychosis

    Depression

    Delirium (rare)

Neuropsychological deficits

    Verbal fluency

    Verbal memory

    Attention

    Visuomotor search

    Motor speed

Pathogenesis

In the mid-1980s there were reports of patients with chronic fatigue, multiple somatic complaints, and elevated Epstein-Barr Virus (EBV) antibody titers (DuBois et al. 1984; Holmes et al. 1987; Straus et al. 1985; Tobi et al. 1982). Subsequent studies found that EBV was involved only rarely (Hellinger et al. 1988; Sumaya 1991).

Features that suggest infection include abrupt onset of fatigue with flulike symptoms; associated fever, chills, and sore throat; and painful lymphadenopathy. However, no single virus has been identified as the cause of CFS, and many individual agents have been excluded, including retrovirus, HHP-6, enterovirus, and spumavirus (Bode et al. 1992; Khan et al. 1993). Although EBV was once thought to be an etiological agent of CFS, subsequent research has indicated that EBV titers have no bearing on disease course, clinical presentation, or laboratory abnormalities and do not distinguish CFS patients from healthy control subjects (Hellinger et al. 1988).

Despite the lack of a direct link between a specific viral agent and CFS, the finding of increased antibodies to a variety of viruses suggests that a generalized immunological dysfunction might accompany CFS (Klimas et al. 1991). Other implicated factors include immune dysregulation, neuroendocrine disturbance, atopy, physical deconditioning, and psychopathology (Krupp and Pollina 1996). CFS is likely to be heterogeneous, with several different mechanisms leading to a final common pathway.

Diagnosis

The CDC proposed a case definition for CFS in 1987 (Holmes et al. 1987) that was modified in 1991 and further refined in 1994 to acknowledge overlap with fibromyalgia and comorbid psychiatric and behavioral disorders (Fukuda et al. 1994).

The current defining inclusion criterion for a diagnosis of CFS is the recent onset of fatigue that is not associated with physical exertion; does not improve with rest; and has a significant effect on social, occupational, educational, or personal activities. In addition, four of the following symptoms must be persistent or recurrent for at least 6 consecutive months and not predate the fatigue: 1) memory or concentration problems, 2) sore throat, 3) tender cervical or axillary lymph nodes, 4) muscle pain, 5) pain in multiple joints without swelling or redness,

6) headaches that differ from ones experienced in the past, 7) unrefreshing sleep, or 8) malaise that lasts longer than 24 hours after exertion.

Patients are excluded from a diagnosis of CFS if they have a medical or psychiatric disorder in which fatigue may be a symptom or if they have not completely recovered from a medical disorder that could cause fatigue. Patients with a history of alcohol or substance abuse within 2 years of the onset of fatigue are also excluded. CFS may be diagnosed concurrently with the following disorders: fibromyalgia, postinfectious fatigue, nonpsychotic and nonmelancholic depression, somatoform disorders, generalized anxiety disorder, or panic disorder.

Psychiatric Manifestations

The incidence of psychological disturbance in CFS is quite high (Abbey and Garfinkel 1990, 1991). However, a confound to this finding is that the minor symptoms of CFS (generalized headaches, sleep disturbances, and neuropsychological complaints) overlap with symptoms of primary psychiatric diagnoses. Estimates of the frequency of current psychiatric illness in CFS range from 21% to 45% and are as high as 52%–86% for lifetime psychiatric illness (Hickie et al. 1990; Katon and Sullivan 1990; Krupp et al. 1994; Lane et al. 1991; Manu et al. 1988; Pepper et al. 1993). This variability may be partly the result of the clinical setting in which the patients are evaluated (specialty centers versus primary care environments), the criteria for patient selection, and the nature of the psychiatric assessment. In several studies using the Diagnostic Interview Schedule, the majority of 100 patients whose primary complaint was fatigue had psychiatric conditions—in particular, depression or somatization disorder (Manu et al. 1988). Other psychiatric disorders noted in CFS include anxiety disorder and dysthymia. Psychiatric symptoms appear to precede CFS more often than they follow it. This observation suggests either that patients with prior psychiatric illness are vulnerable to developing CFS or that CFS may be a symptom cluster secondary to psychiatric illness. However, one study found no increased premorbid prevalence of depression in CFS patients (Hickie et al. 1990). An alternative explanation for the relation between psychiatric disturbances such as major depression and CFS is that both are secondary to similar immune changes. Mood changes in CFS may be secondary to fatigue, they may be chronic illness factors, or they may relate to the social stigma associated with the disorder and the lack of available treatment.

One way to address these issues is to compare psychiatric illness in CFS with that in other chronic medical disorders, including those associated with severe fatigue. Compared with patients who have rheumatoid arthritis, diabetes, or severe fatigue associated with MS, CFS patients show a higher frequency of current and lifetime psychiatric diagnoses. However, CFS patients compared with patients who have major depression show less psychological distress as measured by self-report inventories. These findings suggest that chronic illness factors alone are probably insufficient to explain the high correlation between psychiatric illness and, in particular, depression in CFS. One way to reconcile these findings is to consider that the etiological factors leading to psychiatric illness and CFS overlap.

It is well established that depression, stress, and psychological vulnerability may predispose patients to prolonged recoveries from viral infection (Imboden et al. 1959, 1961), hypersensitivity reactions to prophylactic inoculation (Canter et al. 1972), and susceptibility to clinical syndromes of several upper respiratory infection viruses after inoculation (Cohen et al. 1991). These findings suggest that psychological factors and stress may predispose patients to the development of CFS. Cope et al. (1994) found that postviral fatigue was associated with increased psychological stress and attributional style. Thus psychological vulnerability, attributional style, and coping are important mechanisms in CFS. One unified approach would suggest that an individual with elevated stress and poor coping skills has associated immune perturbations that, in conjunction with an external insult such as a viral infection, lead to a prolonged illness.

Cognitive Manifestations

Memory. Neuropsychological testing indicates that CFS patients may have mild memory impairment and possible deficits in information-processing speed (DeLuca et al. 1995; Grafman and Johnson 1991; Krupp et al. 1994; McDonald et al. 1993). Mild memory disturbance has been associated with conceptual tasks involving encoding and retrieval (Grafman et al. 1993). Memory problems are not associated with specific measures of disease activity, laboratory abnormalities, or physical findings but were associated with depressive symptoms in one study (Krupp et al. 1994). CFS patients had specific impairments on the Visual Reproduction test of the WMS, relative to healthy (nondepressed) control subjects (Grafman et al. 1993). This finding was in contrast to another study that compared CFS patients with depressed control subjects, in which no group differences were found on tests of memory function, including the Booklet Category Test, the California Verbal Learning Test, and the WMS-R (Ray et al. 1993). Poor test performance on memory measures is likely to be at least partially the result of deficits in other cognitive functions; however, studies that measure more specific constructs of memory (i.e., acquisition versus retrieval) are required to characterize fully the nature of memory deficits in CFS.

Attention. DeLuca et al. (1995) noted that CFS patients had poorer performance on the PASAT than did MS patients. However, CFS patients did not significantly differ from depressed control subjects in their performance on the Trail Making Test, a measure of attention problems (Ray et al. 1993). In our experience, CFS patients perform relatively well on computerized tests of mental speed (D. A. Pollina, unpublished data, 1995) and on standardized neuropsychological batteries, in contrast to patients with chronic medical disorders such as Lyme disease, SLE, or MS (Krupp et al. 1994).

One consistent behavioral finding in CFS is increased variability or mean length of reaction time (DeLuca et al. 1995; Ray et al. 1993). These reaction time changes occur across a relatively wide range of tasks, including a time-estimation task (Grafman et al. 1993), the Stroop Test (Ray et al. 1993; Schmaling et al. 1994), and vigilance tasks (McDonald et al. 1993). Event-related potential (ERP) markers of attention to relevant visual stimuli were normal in CFS patients despite systematic increases in response times to these stimuli (Scheffers et al. 1992). These results suggest that the CFS-related impairments may be limited to response-related processes.

Conclusion

No proven therapy is currently available for CFS. Symptom management includes antidepressants if depression is evident and cognitive-behavioral therapy focusing on restoring illness predictability and control. The course of cognitive problems in CFS is also unclear. Reassessing cognitive functions after symptomatic therapy may help clarify the nature and course of the neuropsychological deficits seen in this disorder. Table 7–4 summarizes the diagnostic criteria, psychiatric manifestations, and neuropsychological deficits in CFS.

Table 7–4.   Summary of chronic fatigue syndrome

Diagnostic criteria

    Recent onset of fatigue that significantly affects daily living and is not associated with physical exertion or rest *and* four of the following:

        Memory or concentration problems

        Sore throat

        Tender lymph nodes

        Muscle pain

        Joint pain without swelling

        Headaches

        Unrefreshing sleep

        Malaise after physical exertion

Psychiatric manifestations

    Depression

    Somatization disorder

    Anxiety disorder

    Dysthymia

Neuropsychological deficits

    Possible mild memory and attentional impairment

    Reaction-time increases

◈ EPILEPSY

Definition

Epilepsy is a neurological disorder in which recurrent, unprovoked disturbances in the brain's electrical activity produce seizures of various types. Seizures involve altered consciousness and may also produce psychiatric and physical symptoms. The prevalence of isolated seizures is quite high, occurring in 0.05% of the population, but the prevalence of epilepsy (recurrent seizures) is much lower, affecting 0.005% of the population (Kolb and Wishaw 1990).

Pathogenesis

Different varieties of epilepsy are associated with distinct abnormal electrical rhythms in the brain. The causes for these abnormalities vary. Symptomatic seizures can be identified with specific causes such as infection, trauma, tumors, vascular malformations, toxin exposure, fever, or other neurological disorders. However, two-thirds of the cases of epilepsy are idiopathic, having no known etiology. The risk is slightly higher within families for some types of epilepsy. For most varieties, environmental influences seem to work in conjunction with a genetic predisposition.

Diagnosis

The usual confirmatory criterion for epilepsy is a history of repetitive unprovoked seizures in association with abnormal spikes in electroencephalographic activity.

Clinical Manifestations

The clinical manifestations of epilepsy vary widely. Epilepsy can be classified broadly into partial (focal) seizures and generalized seizures based on the locus of the abnormal electrical activity within the brain. Partial seizures can be categorized as simple, complex, or partial seizures that generalize secondarily. Simple partial seizures result from abnormal activity in one circumscribed area of the brain. The patient may experience repetitive involuntary movements, abnormal sensations, or autonomic activity. Complex partial seizures most commonly begin with abnormal electrical activity in the temporal lobe (temporal-lobe epilepsy, or TLE), but as many as 20% of patients have complex partial seizures with a frontal-lobe or other focus. Complex partial seizures often involve more than one area of brain tissue. Thus patients may experience automatisms, or repetitive movements, in addition to subjective feelings such as obsessional thoughts, mood changes, déjà vu, or hallucinations. After the seizure, patients may assume a catatonic posture.

Generalized seizures result from abnormal electrical activity with no focal onset. They involve both hemispheres and have a symmetrical distribution. The most common generalized seizures are absence attacks (petit mal) and tonic-clonic (grand mal) seizures. In all generalized seizures, the patient temporarily loses consciousness. Absence attacks are brief (lasting less than 10 seconds) and are characterized by a loss of all motor activity except for blinking, eye rolling, or head turning. Tonic-clonic attacks usually proceed through three stages: 1) the tonic stage, in which the body becomes stiff and breathing stops; 2) the clonic stage, in which rhythmic shaking occurs; and 3) a postictal (postseizure) depression, in which disorientation is common. Tonic-clonic seizures may be relatively brief but can last more than 60 seconds.

The clinical manifestations of epilepsy can be broken down in relation to seizure activity. Psychiatric and cognitive symptoms may occur before seizure activity (prodromal), during it (ictal), or just after it (postictal). Evidence also indicates neuropsychiatric problems during times when there is no seizure activity (interictal).

Psychiatric Manifestations

Although most patients with epilepsy have fairly normal lives, some experience psychiatric problems including depression and anxiety both before and during seizures. Chronic psychosis, affective disorders, and even suicide may occur (Perrine and Congett 1994). During and between seizures, the psychiatric symptoms seen in epileptic patients often represent an atypical form of the psychiatric illness that they mimic.

Before, during, and after seizures, epileptic patients may experience depression, mania, hallucinations, delusions, extreme fear and anxiety, or, in extremely rare cases, violent or explosive behaviors. Anxiety and panic attacks that are similar to but often shorter than psychiatric panic attacks are frequent auras experienced before and during seizures. Patients in status epilepticus (a seizure lasting more than 30 minutes) may have prolonged anxiety symptoms that may not be recognized as epileptiform. Prodromal depression, often accompanied by irritability, is another form of aura. Many patients report that they can predict their seizures days in advance by keeping track of the prodromal depression.

During seizures, depersonalization, derealization, altered consciousness, confusion, hallucinations, and delusions resembling psychotic or psychogenic states may occur. When psychotic symptoms occur during complex-partial status epilepticus without abnormal motor activity, the psychotic behavior may be missed unless an electroencephalogram is done.

These ictal psychiatric syndromes can be distinguished from interictal psychiatric difficulties; however, the distinction between interictal psychiatric illness and symptoms of seizures is not always clear. Whether patients with epilepsy experience interictal psychiatric problems more often than does the normal population is unclear (e.g., Fiordelli et al. 1993; Manchanda et al. 1992). Several studies have found that nonpsychotic interictal psychiatric symptoms occur in 45%–55% of epileptic patients (Kogeorgos et al. 1982; Manchanda et al. 1992; Mendez et al. 1986; Trimble 1991).

Affective disorders, including major depression and dysthymia, are the most commonly reported interictal psychiatric disorders (Mendez et al. 1986). Epileptic individuals have a greater incidence of psychotic and dysthymic symptoms (e.g., hallucinations) and fewer neurotic traits (i.e., somatization) (Mendez et al. 1986), and their depression seems to have a more sudden onset and shorter duration (Blumer 1991) than do other psychiatric cases of depression. Affective disorders may also relate to concurrent antiseizure medications (Fiordelli et al. 1993; Perrine and Congett 1994; Post et al. 1991). Suicidal ideation is more common in epilepsy than in other neurological diseases (Perrine and Congett 1994).

Whether epilepsy is associated with increased interictal psychosis is controversial (Perrine and Congett 1994; Trimble 1991). Epileptic psychosis differs from traditional forms of psychosis mainly in that in the former affect and the ability to maintain interpersonal relationships are preserved. Interictal psychosis may be associated with a long duration of the illness and with a greater frequency of seizures (Fiordelli et al. 1993; Perrine and Congett 1994; Trimble 1991).

Debate exists over whether epileptic individuals exhibit behaviors that could be considered personality disorders. The personality traits most often ascribed to these individuals in general, and to TLE patients in particular, include viscosity, circumstantiality, hyperemotionality, religiosity, hypergraphia, and hyposexuality (Geschwind 1979, 1983; Perrine and Congett 1994). Debate also exists over whether certain constellations of personality variables can distinguish patients with TLE from those with other forms of epilepsy (Perrine and Congett 1994).

Cognitive Manifestations

Most patients with epilepsy lack cognitive impairments (Perrine and Congett 1994); however, given the multiple etiologies for epilepsy, it is not surprising that a variety of cognitive dysfunctions can be associated with this disorder. Approximately 20% of epileptic patients spontaneously report cognitive problems, particularly with memory. Patients with symptomatic epilepsy demonstrate greater cognitive impairment than do those with idiopathic epilepsy, suggesting that the impairment is the result of underlying brain pathology rather than the epilepsy itself (Thompson 1991). Collins and Lennox (1947) found that the IQs of symptomatic epilepsy patients were 10 points lower than were those of idiopathic epilepsy patients (Collins and Lennox 1947). The number of lifetime seizures, brain lesions, multiple antiepileptic drugs, and seizure type may also affect the degree of cognitive impairment (Dodrill 1986). Among subgroups of epileptic patients, those with TLE may show the most consistent patterns of cognitive impairment.

General intelligence. Patients with well-controlled epilepsy have intact global general intelligence. Collins and Lennox (1947) reported that mean IQ scores were normal in 100 children (mean IQ = 104) and 200 adults (mean IQ = 111) in their private practice. Among adults with epilepsy, mean full-scale verbal and performance WAIS scores were normal (Dodrill and Wilensky 1992). Patients with intractable seizures demonstrate below-average performance on the WAIS-R (Gold et al. 1994), and patients with symptomatic epilepsy have lower IQs than do idiopathic epilepsy patients (Collins and Lennox 1947; Perrine and Congett 1994). Children with new-onset epilepsy appear to perform in the average-to-below-average range on tests of intellectual functioning and academic achievement (Hermann 1991). Some evidence indicates that patients with left TLE have lower verbal IQ, but this observation has not been a consistent finding in the literature (Binnie et al. 1991).

Attention and concentration. Attention and concentration problems in epileptic patients have been well documented. Teachers and parents of children with epilepsy report that these children have poorer attention than do other children (Hauser and Hesdorffer 1990).

The presence of epileptic spike waves is associated with decreased attention (Bennett 1992; Binnie 1991; Perrine and Congett 1994). Transitory cognitive impairment (TCI) refers to a momentary cognitive deficit that occurs during subclinical epileptiform activity. Up to 50% of epileptic patients have TCI (Binnie et al. 1991). TCI causes momentary deficits in the neuropsychological functions of the brain regions involved by the discharge. Thus focal seizure activity in the cortex can produce inattentiveness by disrupting selective attention (Bennett 1992). Verbal attention tasks are affected by left-hemisphere discharges, and visual tasks are more disrupted by right-hemisphere discharges (Binnie et al. 1991; Perrine and Congett 1994).

Between seizures, patients with epilepsy may show impaired sustained attention on vigilance tasks (Perrine and Congett 1994), although this finding is not universal (Stores et al. 1992). Generalized seizures tend to be associated with greater impairments in sustained attention and vigilance than are focal seizures (Bennett 1992; Thompson 1991). Patients with focal seizures tend to have greater difficulty with selective attention even between seizures (Perrine and Congett 1994).

Memory. Helmstaedter et al. (1994) studied verbal and nonverbal learning and recognition in patients with right-temporal-, left-temporal-, and frontal-lobe seizures. Patients were tested just before seizures and several times subsequent to postictal reorientation. Patterns of performance differed significantly among the three groups. Patients with frontal seizures did not demonstrate significant deficits on verbal or visual memory. Patients with right-temporal-lobe seizures showed the greatest deficits on visual learning and recognition tasks, whereas patients with left-temporal-lobe seizures showed greater deficits on verbal learning and recognition memory. These patterns have been found in other studies.

Between seizures, patients with complex partial seizures that generalized secondarily have memory impairments relative to control subjects, with long-term memory affected more significantly than short-term memory (Bennett 1992). Among patients with complex partial seizures, verbal memory deficits are greater in left temporal foci, and nonverbal memory deficits may be found in patients with right temporal foci (Thompson 1991). However, the findings for right TLE are less robust than for left TLE (Bennett 1992; Perrine and Congett 1994; Thompson 1991).

Much of the research on memory in epilepsy has been conducted on surgical patients and those seeking treatment in tertiary care units who do not have well-controlled seizures. The nature and extent of memory impairment in individuals with well-controlled seizures is unclear. The deficits would likely vary according to lesion location and severity.

Memory impairment may result from or be compounded by attention problems or naming difficulties, both of which are observed in epilepsy (Bennett 1992; Perrine and Congett 1994). Thus neuropsychological testing should always include tests for naming ability and attention so that memory performance can be interpreted correctly.

Perceptual-motor skills. During seizures, perceptual illusions and hallucinations can be elicited (Gloor 1991). These illusions or hallucinations can be visual, auditory, or olfactory in nature (Bennett 1992; Gloor

1991). Patients may hear voices, but unlike schizophrenic patients, they understand that the voices are misperceptions. Patients may also hear music. Ictal hallucinations are usually experiential phenomena in that affective and memory-like features accompany them. Left and right temporal-lobe seizures may result respectively in verbal and visual disruptions in perception (Perrine and Congett 1994).

Between seizures, epileptic patients show perceptual-motor difficulties on the Tactual Performance Test (Dodrill 1981), particularly on the time needed to complete the form board. Localization of the figures may also be impaired if this score is much lower than the memory score. Children with epilepsy have also demonstrated perceptual-motor difficulties, performing worse than control subjects on the Bender Gestalt Test (Bennett 1992) and the Grooved Pegboard and Digit Symbol coding tasks; however, the disparity between general intellectual deficits (Hermann 1991; Stores 1990) and performance on these perceptual-motor tasks is not reported, making it difficult to interpret these findings. Motor speed and reaction time are also impaired in epileptic individuals (Bennett 1992; Perrine and Congett 1994). Children with focal seizures appear to have the greatest perceptual-motor difficulties.

Higher cortical functions. Complex problem-solving and mental flexibility deficits may arise in association with attention and other cognitive problems, even between seizures (Perrine and Congett 1994). The specific type of executive function that is compromised may be related to seizure type, number of lifetime generalized seizures, or status epilepticus (Perrine and Congett 1994). A few studies have reported impairment on the WCST (Gold et al. 1994; Hermann et al. 1988). Because executive functions are an indication of a person's ability to function effectively in his or her environment, tests of executive functions should always be included in assessments of patients with epilepsy (Dodrill 1981).

Interaction With Other Disease Variables

Psychiatric disturbances may be present in up to 45% of epileptic patients, and cognitive disturbances may be present in approximately 20%–30% of epileptic patients. The nature and extent of these disturbances depends on whether the epilepsy is idiopathic or symptomatic, whether it is focal or generalized, and the frequency and lifetime prevalence of seizures, among other variables. As with other medical disorders, interactions between psychiatric status and cognitive abilities may exist. Psychiatric and cognitive functioning can also be affected by sleep disturbance, fatigue, and medication.

The effects of medication on cognitive and psychiatric functions in epilepsy have been the focus of many investigations (Devinsky 1990). As research methodology has improved, it has become clear that under normal circumstances, with medication levels well controlled, the effects of antiepileptic drugs on mental functioning are negligible. But the side effects experienced by patients can be highly individualized. Thus, patients may respond best either to one drug or to a combination of drugs. Medication regimens should always be developed with close attention paid to the side effects the patient reports. Many studies indicate that when patients change from polytherapy to monotherapy or when they switch to new antiepileptic drugs, their cognitive and psychiatric symptoms improve.

Conclusion

Table 7–5 summarizes the diagnostic criteria, clinical manifestations, psychiatric manifestations, and neuropsychological deficits in epilepsy. The potential cognitive problems in epilepsy depend on a variety of disease factors. These patients may have deficits in intellectual ability, memory, attention, perception, and executive functions. Research that uses uniform, structured epilepsy classification systems and appropriate community samples of epileptic patients will help to clarify the prevalence and nature of psychopathology and cognitive dysfunctions in this illness.

◈ NEUROPSYCHIATRIC DEFICITS IN OTHER MEDICAL ILLNESSES

Neuropsychiatric deficits have been documented in a variety of other medical illnesses. One example is the cluster of symptoms associated with diseases causing chronic airflow obstruction (e.g., bronchitis, emphysema). Hypoxemia caused by chronic airflow obstruction has been related to mild deficits in perceptual-motor learning and problem-solving (Grant et al. 1982). The immobility and tiredness these disorders cause also creates a sense of lack of physical fitness, which may lead to depression and emotional distress (Geddes 1984).

Table 7–5.   Summary of epilepsy

Diagnostic criteria

Repetitive unprovoked seizures with abnormal electroencephalogram findings

Clinical manifestations

Generalized (tonic-clonic, tonic) or partial seizures

Postictal amnesia

Psychiatric manifestations

Depression, hallucinations, delusions, and anxiety during seizures

Interictal depression, anxiety, psychotic symptoms, and personality disorders

Neuropsychological deficits

Deficits in selective attention associated with focal seizures

Long-term memory impairments associated with temporal-lobe epilepsy and generalized epilepsy

Perceptual abnormalities including misperception of size, motion, color, loudness

Deficits in executive functions such as abstract reasoning and mental flexibility

Impairments in emotional and intellectual function have also been reported in patients with disorders of the pancreas, including pancreatitis and diabetes mellitus (Rovet et al. 1987). In one study, adolescents with early-onset diabetes were significantly more impaired on tests of motor dexterity, memory for verbal and nonverbal materials, and general intelligence than were later-onset diabetic patients (those diagnosed after age 5 years) (Ryan 1988). Psychiatric symptomatology in children and adolescents with type I diabetes includes poor self-esteem and heightened anxiety (Fälström 1974; Grey et al. 1980). Diabetic patients must monitor their disorder and their diet constantly, and they must worry about possible complications related to their illness. Over time, these rigors may contribute to their emotional anxiety (Grey et al. 1980). Cognitive deficits have also been reported in people with type II diabetes, but these deficits may partly reflect the effects of other risk factors such as hypertension (Lowe et al. 1994).

Several studies have documented the association between disturbances in cognitive function and essential hypertension, especially on tests of attention and visuomotor ability (Kuusisto et al. 1993; Schmidt et al. 1995). The mechanisms thought to underlie this association in-

clude increased risk for stroke and brain infarcts caused by arterial occlusion. Cardiovascular risk factors are also associated with white-matter
lesions seen on brain MRI (Breteler et al. 1994). Hyperinsulinemia cou-
pled with hypertension can lead to deficits in several cognitive domains,
including attention, semantic memory, and problem-solving (Kuusisto et
al. 1993). However, the few studies that have explored the complex relationship between cognition, hypertension, and diseases such as diabetes
mellitus have not specifically controlled for psychiatric variables such as
depression. Some authors believe that the neuropsychological impairments reported in these studies are called into question until more is
known about these patients' psychiatric profiles (Atiea et al. 1995).

◆ POTENTIAL CONFOUNDS IN NEUROPSYCHOLOGICAL ASSESSMENT OF CHRONIC MEDICAL ILLNESS

The diseases we covered in this chapter are each associated with clinical
problems that can confound the interpretation of cognitive performance.
Psychiatric problems such as depression or psychosis are present to some
degree in all of these diseases. In SLE and MS, psychiatric symptoms are
most likely a primary reflection of the disease pathology. However, in any
of these diseases psychiatric disturbance may also be a coincidental occurrence or a functional reaction to the disease. Several different guidelines for assessing psychiatric problems in the setting of medical illness
have been proposed (Caine 1984; Cameron 1990; Cavanaugh et al.
1983). Recommendations include the following: considering a psychiatric diagnosis only if symptoms such as dysphoria or anhedonia are present that do not respond to treatment of the primary medical illness,
assessing past and family history for affective disorder, and evaluating
psychosocial risk factors preceding onset of the medical condition. Another approach is to substitute psychiatric symptoms that overlap with
medical symptoms with alternative criteria for diagnosing psychopathology (Endicott 1983). For example, "loss of energy" can be replaced with
"brooding, self-pity, or pessimism" and "difficulty concentrating" can be
replaced with "mood not reactive to outside influences."

The effect of chronic pain on cognitive functioning is not fully known.
We have found that pain shows little association with cognitive perfor-

mance in eosinophilia myalgia syndrome, a chronic, painful rheumatological condition that develops in association with L-tryptophan ingestion (Pollina et al., in press). However, the effect of chronic pain in medical illness on functions such as attention or vigilance has not been well studied. One would expect an adverse effect. Pain often leads to the use of narcotics or other analgesics that can interfere with cognitive functioning.

Fatigue is a feature of all of these neurological and medical conditions. It is defined as an overwhelming sense of tiredness, lack of energy, or feeling of exhaustion. It is distinguished from depression, feelings of hopelessness, or limb weakness, and it is most easily conceptualized as a feeling of exhaustion that, in healthy individuals, accompanies mild flulike illness.

In isolation, fatigue does not appear to have a severe effect on cognitive functioning. For example, in a treatment study of fatigue in which fatigue was improved, cognitive functioning did not change (Geisler et al. 1996). In addition, the correlation of cognitive functioning and fatigue measures is not significant. However, studies of chronically fatigued patients (e.g., those with MS or CFS) have found slowed reaction times (Sandroni et al. 1992; Scheffers et al. 1992), which may contribute to perceived cognitive deficits. Further, fatigue is often associated with pain, depression, and concurrent medication use, which can adversely affect cognitive performance.

Sleep disturbance is a feature of many of these disorders. In some cases, sleep deprivation clearly affects cognitive functioning adversely. Primary sleep disorders are also associated with a variety of neurobehavioral deficits. As a result, neuropsychological evaluations in these settings should include inquiry regarding the patient's previous night's sleep.

Concurrent medication use can be an important potential confounding factor. Patients with each of these disorders are often prescribed medications with potential CNS effects to help alleviate their neurological symptoms. Many patients taking these medications complain of impairments in attention, concentration, and memory. Whether these perceived impairments are directly the result of their neurological disorders, their functional reactions to the disorders, or their medications is not always clear. Little is known about the side effects of CNS-active medications on nonpsychiatric patients with mild brain dysfunction. (See Jaeger and Berns, Chapter 10, in this volume for a review of the effects of these and other medications.)

◈ CONCLUSION

As summarized in Table 7–6, varying degrees of problems with memory, attention, executive functions, and perceptual and motor abilities occur in MS, SLE, Lyme disease, CFS, and epilepsy. The patterns of cognitive impairment within each of these diseases vary widely from one individual to the next, with patients ranging from those who are completely cognitively intact to those who have dementia. Therefore, no one pattern of cognitive impairment can be applied to any of these disorders. Cognitive dysfunction may result from the disease process itself, as a secondary reaction to disease symptoms or treatment, or as a reaction to the life-altering nature of the disease. Accurate neuropsychological assessment in chronically ill patients must take into account the potential effects of all of these variables. Our knowledge in this field of inquiry will be greatly enhanced by more comprehensive medication and symptom inventories, accurate classifications of psychopathology, and improved design and analysis of neuropsychological an neuroradiological investigations.

◈ REFERENCES

Abbey SE, Garfinkel PE: Chronic fatigue syndrome and the psychiatrist. Can J Psychiatry 35:625–633, 1990

Abbey SE, Garfinkel PE: Chronic fatigue syndrome and depression: cause, effect or covariate. Rev Infect Dis 13 (suppl 1):S73–S83, 1991

Amato M, Ponziani G, Pracucci G, et al: Cognitive impairment in early onset multiple sclerosis. Arch Neurol 52:168–172, 1995

Arnette P, Rao S, Bernardin L, et al: Relationship between frontal lobe lesion and Wisconsin Card Sorting Test performance in patients with multiple sclerosis. Neurology 44:420–425, 1994

Atiea J, Moses J, Sinclair A: Neuropsychological function in older subjects with non-insulin-dependent diabetes mellitus. Diabet Med 12:679–685, 1995

Barr W, Merchut M: Systemic lupus erythematosus with central nervous system involvement. Psychiatr Clin North Am 15:439–454, 1992

Beatty WW, Goodkin DE, Monson N, et al: Anterograde and retrograde amnesia in patients with chronic progressive multiple sclerosis. Arch Neurol 45:611–619, 1988

Beatty WW, Paul RH, Wilbanks SL, et al: Identifying multiple sclerosis patients with mild or global cognitive impairment using the Screening Examination for Cognitive Impairment (SEFCI). Neurology 45:718–723, 1995

Table 7–6. Summary of neuropsychological function impairment in chronic medical illnesses						
Disorder	General intelligence	Memory	Attention	Perceptual-motor	Abstract reasoning	Language
Multiple sclerosis	EE	SE	SE	SE	SE	SE
Systemic lupus erythematosus	EE	SE	SE	NA	NA	SE
Lyme disease	NI	SE	SE	SE	NA	SE
Chronic fatigue syndrome	NI	EE	EE	SE	NA	NA
Epilepsy	EE	SE	SE	SE	SE	SE

Note. SE = strong evidence for impairment, EE = equivocal evidence for impairment, NI = evidence for no impairment, NA = evidence of no impairment, NA = evidence for presence or absence of impairment is not available currently.

Beatty WW, Wilbanks SL, Blanco CR, et al: Memory disturbance in multiple sclerosis: reconsideration of patterns of performance on the Selective Reminding Test. J Clin Exp Neuropsychol 18:56–62, 1996

Bennahum D, Messner R: Recent observations on central nervous system lupus erythematosus. Semin Arthritis Rheum 4:253–266, 1975

Bennett TL: Cognitive and emotional consequences of epilepsy, in The Neuropsychology of Epilepsy. Edited by Bennett TL. New York, Plenum, 1992, pp 73–87

Binnie CD: Methods of detecting transitory cognitive impairment during epileptiform EEG discharges, in The Assessment of Cognitive Function in Epilepsy. Edited by Dodson WE, Kinsbourne W, Hiltbrunner B. New York, Demos Publications, 1991, pp 127–136

Binnie CD, Channon S, Marston DL: Behavioral correlates of interictal spikes, in Advances in Neurology, Vol 55. Edited by Smith DB, Treiman DM, Trimble MR. New York, Raven, 1991, pp 113–126

Blumer D: Epilepsy and disorders of mood, in Advances in Neurology, Vol 55. Edited by Smith DB, Treiman DM, Trimble MR. New York, Raven, 1991, pp 185–196

Bode L, Komaroff AL, Ludwig N: No serologic evidence of Borna disease virus in patients with CFS. Clin Infect Dis 15:1049–1052, 1992

Bolton AK, Krupp LB: Learning and memory processes in Lyme disease and multiple sclerosis. Paper presented at the annual meeting of the International Neuropsychology Society, 1994

Boumpas D, Fessler B, Austin H, et al: Systemic lupus erythematosus: emerging concepts. Ann Intern Med 123:42–53, 1995

Breteler M, van Swieten J, Bots M, et al: Cerebral white matter lesions, vascular risk factors, and cognitive function in a population-based study. Neurology 44:1246–1252, 1994

Caine ED: The neuropsychology of depression: the pseudodementia syndrome, in Neuropsychological Assessment of Neuropsychiatric Disorders. Edited by Grant I, Adams KM. New York, Oxford University Press, 1984, pp 221–243

Cameron OG: Guidelines for diagnosis and treatment of depression in patients with medical illness. J Clin Psychiatry 51 (suppl 7):49–54, 1990

Caminero AB, Vivancos F, Diez-Tejedor E: Atypical neuroradiologic manifestation of systemic lupus erythematosus. Arch Neurobiol 55:270–275, 1992

Canter A, Cluff LE, Imboden JB: Hypersensitive reactions to immunization inoculations and antecedent psychological vulnerability. J Psychosom Res 16:99–101, 1972

Cantor AH: Direct and indirect measures of psychological deficit in multiple sclerosis. J Gen Psychol 44:3–50, 1951

Carbotte RM, Denburg SD, Denburg JA, et al: Fluctuating cognitive abnormalities and cerebral glucose metabolism in neuropsychiatric systemic lupus erythematosus. J Neurol Neurosurg Psychiatry 55:1054–1059, 1992

Cardenas DD, Kutner NG: The problem of fatigue in dialysis patients. Nephron 30:336–340, 1982

Cauli A, Montaldo C, Peltz MT, et al: Abnormalities of magnetic resonance imaging of the central nervous system in patients with systemic lupus erythematosus correlate with disease severity. Clin Rheumatol 13:615–618, 1994

Cavanaugh S, Clark D, Gibbons R: Diagnosing depression in the hospitalized medically ill. Psychosomatics 24:809–815, 1983

Centers for Disease Control: Case definitions for public health surveillance. MMWR 39:19–22, 1990

Cohen S, Tyrrell AJ, Smith AP: Psychological stress and susceptibility to the common cold. N Engl J Med 325:606–612, 1991

Colamussi P, Giganti M, Cittanti C, et al: Brain single-photon emission tomography with 99mTc-HMPAO in neuropsychiatric systemic lupus erythematosus: relations with EEG and MRI findings and clinical manifestations. Eur J Nucl Med 22:17–24, 1995

Coleman JL, Benach JL: Pathogenesis of Lyme disease, in Lyme Disease. St. Louis, MO, Mosby Year Book, 1994, pp 179–183

Collins AL, Lennox WG: The intelligence of 300 private epileptic patients. Assoc Res Nerv Ment Dis 26:586–603, 1947

Comi G, Filippi M, Martinelli V, et al: Brain magnetic resonance imaging correlates of cognitive impairment in multiple sclerosis. J Neurol Sci 115 (suppl): S66–S73, 1993

Cope H, David A, Pelosi A, et al: Prediction of chronic "postviral" fatigue. Lancet 344:864–868, 1994

Coyle PK: Neurologic Lyme disease. Semin Neurol 12:200–208, 1992

Coyle PK, Deng Z, Scheutzer SE, et al: Detection of Borrelia burgdorferi antigens in cerebrospinal fluid. Neurology 43:1093–1097, 1993

Daif A, Awada A, al-Rajeh S, et al: Cerebral venous thrombosis in adults: a study of 40 cases from Saudi Arabia. Stroke 26:1193–1195, 1995

Dattwyler RJ, Volkman DJ, Luft BJ, et al: Seronegative Lyme disease. N Engl J Med 319:1441–1446, 1988

DeLuca J, Barbieri-Berger S, Johnson SK: The nature of memory impairments in multiple sclerosis: acquisition versus retrieval. J Clin Exp Neuropsychol 16: 183–189, 1994

DeLuca J, Johnson SK, Beldowicz D, et al: Neuropsychological impairments in chronic fatigue syndrome, multiple sclerosis, and depression. J Neurol Neurosurg Psychiatry 58:38–43, 1995

Denburg SD, Carbotte RM, Denburg JA: Corticosteroids and neuropsychological functioning in patients with systemic lupus erythematosus. Arthritis Rheum 37:1311–1320, 1994

Dennis RT: Epidemiology, in Lyme Disease. Edited by Coyle PK. St. Louis, MO, Mosby Year Book, 1993, pp 27–37

Devinsky O: The differential diagnosis of epilepsy. Semin Neurol 10:321–327, 1990

Dodrill CB: Neuropsychology of epilepsy, in Handbook of Clinical Neuropsychology. Edited by Fiskov SB. New York, Wiley, 1981, pp 366–395

Dodrill CB: Correlates of generalized tonic-clonic seizures with social factors in patients with epilepsy. Epilepsia 27:399–411, 1986

Dodrill CB, Wilensky AJ: Neuropsychological abilities before and after 5 years of stable antiepileptic drugs. Epilepsia 33:327–334, 1992

Doscher C, Coyle PK, Krupp LB, et al: Cytokine levels in treated Lyme patients with persistent fatigue and encephalopathy. Neurology 44 (suppl):A186, 1994

DuBois R, Seeley JK, Brus I, et al: Chronic mononucleosis syndrome. South Med J 77:1376–1382, 1984

Endicott J: Use of DSM-III criteria. Arch Gen Psychiatry 40:700, 1983

Fallon BA, Nields JA: Lyme disease: a neuropsychiatric illness. Am J Psychiatry 151:1571–1583, 1994

Fallon BA, Nields JA, Parsons B, et al: Psychiatric manifestations of Lyme borreliosis. J Clin Psychiatry 54:263–268, 1993

Fälström K: On the personality structure of diabetic children aged 7–15 years. Acta Paediatr Scand 63 (suppl 251):1–70, 1974

Feinstein A, Kartsounis LD, Miller D, et al: Clinically isolated lesions of the type seen in multiple sclerosis: a cognitive, psychiatric, and MRI follow-up study. J Neurol Neurosurg Psychiatry 55:869–876, 1992

Ferstl R, Niemann T, Biehl G, et al: Neuropsychological impairment in auto-immune disease. Eur J Clin Invest 22 (suppl 1):16–20, 1992

Fiordelli E, Beghi E, Bogliun G, et al: Epilepsy and psychiatric disturbance: a cross-sectional study. Br J Psychiatry 163:446–450, 1993

Fischer JS: Using the Wechsler Memory Scale–Revised to detect and characterize memory deficits in multiple sclerosis. Clin Neuropsychol 2:149–172, 1988

Fisk JD, Eastwood B, Sherwood G, et al: Patterns of cognitive impairment in patients with systemic lupus erythematosus. Br J Rheumatol 32:458–462, 1993

Fontaine B, Seihean D, Tourbah A, et al: Dementia in two histologically confirmed cases of multiple sclerosis: one case with isolated dementia and one case associated with psychiatric symptoms. J Neurol Neurosurg Psychiatry 57:353–359, 1994

Franklin GM, Nelson LM, Filley CM, et al: Cognitive loss in multiple sclerosis: case reports and review of the literature. Arch Neurol 46:162–167, 1989

Freal JE, Kraft GH, Coryell SK: Symptomatic fatigue in multiple sclerosis. Arch Phys Med Rehabil 65:135–138, 1984

Fukuda K, Straus SE, Hickie I, et al: The chronic fatigue syndrome, a comprehensive approach to this definition and study. Ann Intern Med 121:953–959, 1994

Garland E, Zis A: Multiple sclerosis and affective disorders. Can J Psychiatry 36: 112–117, 1991

Gaudino E, Coyle PK, Doscher C, et al: Neuropsychiatric profile of post-Lyme syndrome. Neurology 44 (suppl 2):A376, 1994

Geddes D: Chronic airflow obstruction. Postgrad Med J 60:194–200, 1984

Geisler MW, Sliwinski M, Coyle PK, et al: The cognitive effects of fatigue treatment in multiple sclerosis. Arch Neurol 53:185–188, 1996

Geschwind N: Behavioral changes in temporal lobe epilepsy. Psychol Med 9: 217–219, 1979

Geschwind N: Interictal behavioral changes in epilepsy. Epilepsia 24 (suppl 1): S23–S30, 1983

Ginsburg K, Wright E, Larson M, et al: A controlled study of the prevalence of cognitive dysfunction in randomly selected patients with systemic lupus erythematosus. Arthritis Rheum 35:776–782, 1992

Gloor P: Neurobiological substrates of ictal behavior, in Advances in Neurology, Vol 55. Edited by Smith DB, Treiman DM, Trimble MR. New York, Raven, 1991, pp 1–34

Gold JM, Hermann BP, Randolf C, et al: Schizophrenia and temporal lobe epilepsy: a neuropsychological analysis. Arch Gen Psychiatry 51:265–272, 1994

Goldstein G, Shelly CH: Neuropsychological diagnosis of multiple sclerosis in a neuropsychiatric setting. J Nerv Ment Dis 158:280–289, 1974

Goodstein R, Ferrell R: Multiple sclerosis—presenting as depressive illness. Diseases of the Nervous System 38:127–131, 1977

Grafman J, Johnson R: Cognitive and mood-state changes in patients with chronic fatigue syndrome. Rev Infect Dis 13 (suppl 1):S45–S52, 1991

Grafman J, Schwartz V, Dale JK, et al: Analysis of neuropsychological functioning in patients with chronic fatigue syndrome. J Neurol Neurosurg Psychiatry 56:684–689, 1993

Grant I, Heaton R, McSweeny A, et al: Neuropsychologic findings in hypoxemic chronic obstructive pulmonary disease. Arch Intern Med 142:1470–1476, 1982

Grey M, Genel M, Tamborlane W: Psychosocial adjustment of latency-aged diabetics: determinants and relationship to control. Pediatrics 65:69–73, 1980

Grigsby J, Ayarbe S, Kraveisin N, et al: Working memory impairment among persons with chronic progressive multiple sclerosis. J Neurol 241:125–131, 1994

Gronwall DM: Paced auditory serial-addition task: a measure of recovery from concussion. Percept Mot Skills 44:367–373, 1977

Grossman M, Armstrong C, Onishi K, et al: Patterns of cognitive impairment in relapsing-remitting and chronic progressive multiple sclerosis. Neuropsychology, Neuropsychiatry, and Behavioral Neurology 7:194–210, 1994

Halperin JJ, Pass HL, Anand AK, et al: Nervous system abnormalities in Lyme disease. Ann N Y Acad Sci 539:24–34, 1988

Halperin JJ, Volkman DJ, Wu P: Central nervous system abnormalities in Lyme neuroborreliosis. Neurology 41:1581–1582, 1991

Hanly JG, Walsh NM, Fisk JD, et al: Cognitive impairment and autoantibodies in systemic lupus erythematosus. Br J Rheumatol 32:291–296, 1993

Hansen K, Lebech AM: The clinical and epidemiologic profile of Lyme neuroborreliosis in Denmark. Brain 115:399–423, 1992

Hauser WA, Hesdorffer DC: Epilepsy: Frequency, Causes and Consequences. New York, Epilepsy Foundation of America, 1990, pp 245–272

Hay E, Black D, Huddy A, et al: Psychiatric disorder and cognitive impairment in systemic lupus erythematosus. Arthritis Rheum 35:411–416, 1992

Heaton RK, Nelson LM, Thompson DS, et al: Neuropsychological findings in relapsing-remitting and chronic-progressive multiple sclerosis. J Consult Clin Psychol 53:103–110, 1985

Hellinger WC, Smith TF, Van Scoy RE, et al: Chronic fatigue syndrome and the diagnostic utility of antibody to Epstein-Barr virus early antigen. JAMA 260: 971–973, 1988

Helmstaedter C, Elger CE, Lendt M: Postical courses of cognitive deficits in focal epilepsies. Epilepsia 35:1073–1078, 1994

Hermann BP: Contributions of traditional assessment procedures to an understanding of the neuropsychology of epilepsy, in The Assessment of Cognitive Function in Epilepsy. Edited by Dodson WE, Kinsbourne M, Hiltbrunner B. New York, Demos Publications, 1991, pp 1–22

Hermann BP, Wyler AR, Richey ET: Wisconsin Card Sorting Test performance in patients with complex partial seizures of temporal-lobe origin. J Clin Exp Neuropsychol 10:467–476, 1988

Hickie I, Lloyd A, Wakefield D, et al: The psychiatric status of patients with the CFS. Br J Psychiatry 156:534–540, 1990

Holmes GP, Kaplan JE, Stewart JA, et al: A cluster of patients with chronic mononucleosis-like symptoms. JAMA 257:2297–2302, 1987

Huber SJ, Bornstein RA, Rammohan KW, et al: Magnetic resonance imaging correlates of neuropsychological impairment in multiple sclerosis. J Neuropsychiatry Clin Neurosci 4:152–158, 1992

Imboden JB, Canter A, Cluff LE, et al: Brucellosis: psychologic aspects of delayed convalescence. Arch Intern Med 103:406–444, 1959

Imboden JB, Canter A, Cluff LE: Convalescence from influenza: a study of the psychological and clinical determinants. Arch Intern Med 108:393–399, 1961

Iverson G: Psychopathology associated with systemic lupus erythematosus: a methodological review. Semin Arthritis Rheum 22:242–251, 1993

Iverson G, Anderson K: The etiology of psychiatric symptoms in patients with systemic lupus erythematosus. Scand J Rheumatol 23:277–282, 1994

Ivnik RJ: Neuropsychological stability in multiple sclerosis. J Consult Clin Psychol 46:913–923, 1978

Jambor KL: Cognitive functioning in multiple sclerosis. Br J Psychiatry 115: 765–775, 1969

Joyce K, Berkebile C, Hastings C, et al: Health status and disease activity in systemic lupus erythematosus. Arthritis Care and Research 2:65–69, 1989

Kaplan RF, Meadows ME, Vincent LC: Memory impairment and depression in patients with Lyme encephalopathy: comparison with fibromyalgia and nonpsychotically depressed patients. Neurology 42:1263–1267, 1992

Katon W, Sullivan MD: Depression and chronic medical illness. J Clin Psychiatry 51 (suppl 6):3–14, 1990

Khan AS, Heneine WM, Chapman LE, et al: Assessment of a retrovirus sequence and other possible risk factors for the chronic fatigue syndrome in adults. Ann Intern Med 118:241–245, 1993

Klimas NG, Salvato FR, Morgan R, et al: Immunologic abnormalities in CFS. J Clin Microbiol 28:1403–1410, 1991

Kogeorgos J, Foragy P, Scott DF: Psychiatric symptom patterns of chronic epileptics attending a neurologic clinic, a controlled investigation. Br J Psychiatry 140:236–243, 1982

Kolb B, Wishaw IQ: Fundamentals of Human Neuropsychology. New York, WH Freeman, 1990, pp 139–143

Kollikowski HH, Schwendemann G, Schulz M, et al: Chronic borrelia encephalomyeloradiculitis with severe mental disturbance: immunosuppressive versus antibiotic therapy. J Neurology 235:140–142, 1988

Krupp LB, Pollina DA: Neuroimmune and neuropsychiatric aspects of chronic fatigue syndrome. Advances in Neuroimmunology 6:155–167, 1996

Krupp LB, LaRocca NG, Luft BJ, et al: Comparison of neurologic and psychologic findings in patients with Lyme disease and chronic fatigue syndrome (abstract). Neurology 39:144, 1989

Krupp LB, LaRocca NG, Muir J, et al: A study of fatigue in systemic lupus erythematosus. J Rheumatol 17:1450–1452, 1990

Krupp LB, Masur DM, Schwartz D, et al: Cognitive functioning in late Lyme borreliosis. Arch Neurol 48:1125–1129, 1991a

Krupp LB, Mendelson WB, Friedman R: An overview of chronic fatigue syndrome. J Clin Psychiatry 52:403–410, 1991b

Krupp LB, Masur DM, Kaufman LD: Neurocognitive dysfunction in the eosinophilia-myalgia syndrome. Neurology 43:931–936, 1993a

Krupp LB, Schwartz JE, Jandorf L: Fatigue, in Lyme Disease. Edited by Coyle PK. St. Louis, MO, Mosby Year Book, 1993b, pp 196–203

Krupp LB, Sliwinski M, Masur D, et al: Cognitive functioning and depression in patients with chronic fatigue syndrome and multiple sclerosis. Arch Neurol 51:705–710, 1994

Kujala P, Portin R, Revonsuo A, et al: Attention related performance in two cognitively different subgroups of patients with multiple sclerosis. J Neurol Neurosurg Psychiatry 59:77–82, 1995

Kuusisto J, Koivisto K, Mykkänen L, et al: Essential hypertension and cognitive function. Hypertension 22:771–779, 1993

Lane TJ, Manu P, Matthews DA: Depression and somatization in the chronic fatigue syndrome. Am J Med 91:335–344, 1991

Lezak M: Neuropsychological Assessment. New York, Oxford University Press, 1995

Litvan I, Grafman J, Vendrell P, et al: Slowed information processing in multiple sclerosis. Arch Neurol 45:281–285, 1988

Logigian EL, Kaplan RF, Steere AC: Chronic neurologic manifestations of Lyme disease. N Engl J Med 21:1433–1437, 1990

Lowe L, Tranel D, Wallace R, et al: Type II diabetes and cognitive function. Diabetes Care 17:891–896, 1994

Maeshima E, Maeshima S, Yamada Y, et al: Cortical atrophy and higher cortical dysfunction in systemic lupus erythematosus. Ryumachi 34:30–33, 1994

Manchanda R, Schaefer B, McLachlan RS, et al: Interictal psychiatric morbidity and focus of epilepsy in treatment-refractory patients admitted to an epilepsy unit. Am J Psychiatry 149:1096–1098, 1992

Manu P, Matthews DA, Lane TJ: The mental health of patients with a chief complaint of chronic fatigue. Arch Intern Med 148:2213–2217, 1988

McDonald E, Cope H, David A: Cognitive impairment in patients with chronic fatigue, a preliminary study. J Neurol Neurosurg Psychiatry 56:812–815, 1993

McLean BN, Miller D, Thompson EJ: Oligoclonal banding of IgG in CSF, blood-brain barrier function, and MRI findings in patients with sarcoidosis, systemic lupus erythematosus, and Behcet's disease involving the nervous system. J Neurol Neurosurg Psychiatry 58:548–554, 1995

Mendez MF, Cummings JL, Benson DF: Depression in epilepsy: significance and phenomenology. Arch Neurol 43:766–770, 1986

Mendozzi L, Pugnetti L, Saccani M, et al: Frontal lobe dysfunction in multiple sclerosis as assessed by means of Lurian tasks: effect of age at onset. J Neurol Sci 115 (suppl):S42–S50, 1993

Miguel E, Pereira R, Pereira C, et al: Psychiatric manifestations of systemic lupus erythematosus: clinical features, symptoms, and signs of central nervous system activity in 43 patients. Medicine 73:224–232, 1994

Möller A, Wiedermann G, Rohde U, et al: Correlates of cognitive impairment and depressive mood disorder in multiple sclerosis. Acta Psychiatr Scand 89:117–121, 1994

Murray TS: Amantadine therapy for fatigue in multiple sclerosis. Can J Neurol Sci 12:251–254, 1985

Nojima Y, Minota S, Yamada A, et al: Correlation of antibodies to ribosomal P protein with psychosis in patients with systemic lupus erythematosus. Ann Rheum Dis 51:1053–1055, 1992

O'Connor MG: Neuropsychological investigations of multiple sclerosis: a clinical perspective. Clin Neurosci 2:225–228, 1994

Pachner AR: Spirochetal diseases of the CNS. Neurologic Clinics of North America 4:207–222, 1986

Parsons OA, Stewart KD, Arenberg D: Impairment of abstracting ability in multiple sclerosis. J Nerv Ment Dis 125:221–225, 1957

Pepper C, Krupp LB, Friedberg F, et al: Comparison of psychiatric characteristics in chronic fatigue syndrome, multiple sclerosis, and depression. J Neuropsychiatry Clin Neurosci 5:1–7, 1993

Perrine K, Congett S: Neurobehavioral problems in epilepsy, in Neurologic Clinics, Epilepsy II: Special Issues, Vol 12. Edited by Devinsky O. Philadelphia, PA, WB Saunders, 1994, pp 129–152

Peyser JM, Poser CM: Neuropsychological correlates of multiple sclerosis, in Handbook of Clinical Neuropsychology, Vol 2. Edited by Filskov SB, Boll TJ. New York, Wiley, 1986, pp 364–397

Pine D, Douglas C, Charles E, et al: Patients with multiple sclerosis presenting to psychiatric hospitals. J Clin Psychiatry 56:297–306, 1995

Pisetsky D: Systemic lupus erythematosus. Med Clin North Am 70:337–353, 1986

Pollina DA, Kaufman LD, Masur DM, et al: Pain, fatigue, and sleep in eosinophilia-myalgia syndrome: relationship to neuropsychological performance. J Neuropsychiatry Clin Neurosci (in press)

Post RM, Altshuler LL, Ketter TA, et al: Anti-epileptic drugs in affective illness, clinical and theoretical implications, in Advances in Neurology, Vol 55. Edited by Smith DB, Treiman DM, Trimble MR. New York, Raven, 1991, pp 239–278

Pozzilli C, Gasperini C, Anzini A, et al: Anatomical and functional correlates of cognitive deficits in multiple sclerosis. J Neurol Sci 115 (suppl):S53–S58, 1993

Pugnetti L, Mendozzi L, Motta A, et al: MRI and cognitive patterns in relapsing-remitting multiple sclerosis. J Neurol Sci 115 (suppl):S59–S65, 1993

Rao SM: Neuropsychology of multiple sclerosis: a critical review. J Clin Exp Neuropsychol 8:503–542, 1986

Rao SM (ed): Neurobehavioral Aspects of Multiple Sclerosis. New York, Oxford University Press, 1990a

Rao SM: Neuroimaging correlates of cognitive dysfunction, in Neurobehavioral Aspects of Multiple Sclerosis. Edited by Rao SM. New York, Oxford University Press, 1990b, pp 118–135

Rao SM, Hammeke TA, McQuillen MP, et al: Memory disturbance in chronic progressive multiple sclerosis. Arch Neurol 41:625–631, 1984

Rao SM, Leo GJ, Bernardin L, et al: Cognitive dysfunction in multiple sclerosis, I: frequency, patterns, and prediction. Neurology 41:685–691, 1991a

Rao SM, Leo GJ, Ellington L, et al: Cognitive dysfunction in multiple sclerosis, II: impact on employment and social functioning. Neurology 41:692–696, 1991b

Ray C, Phillips L, Weir W: Quality of attention in chronic fatigue syndrome: subjective reports of everyday attention and cognitive difficulty, and performance on tasks of focused attention. J Clin Psychol 32:357–364, 1993

Rovet J, Ehrlich R, Hoppe M: Specific intellectual deficits associated with the early onset of insulin-dependent diabetes mellitus in children. Diabetes Care 10:510–515, 1987

Rubbert A, Marienhagen J, Pirner K, et al: Single-photon emission computed tomography analysis of cerebral blood flow in the evaluation of central nervous system involvement in patients with systemic lupus erythematosus. Arthritis Rheum 9:1253–1262, 1993

Ryan C: Neurobehavioral disturbances associated with disorders of the pancreas, in Medical Neuropsychology. Edited by Tarter R, Van Thiel D, Edwards K. New York, Plenum, 1988, pp 121–158

Salmaggi A, Lamperti E, Eoli M, et al: Spinal cord involvement and systemic lupus erythematosus: clinical and magnetic resonance findings in 5 patients. Clin Exp Rheumatol 12:389–394, 1994

Sandroni P, Walker C, Starr A: "Fatigue" in patients with MS. Arch Neurol 49:517–524, 1992

Scheffers MK, Johnson R Jr, Grafman J, et al: Attention and short-term memory in CFS patients. Neurology 42:1667–1675, 1992

Schiffer RB, Wineman N, Weitkamp L: Association between bipolar affective disorder and multiple sclerosis. Am J Psychiatry 143:94–95, 1986

Schmaling KB, DiClementi JD, Cullum CM, et al: Cognitive functioning in chronic fatigue syndrome and depression: a preliminary comparison. Psychosom Med 56:383–388, 1994

Schmidt R, Fazekas F, Koch M, et al: Magnetic resonance imaging cerebral abnormalities and neuropsychological test performance in elderly hypertensive subjects. Arch Neurol 52:905–910, 1995

Shadick NA, Phillips CB, Logigian EL, et al: The long-term clinical outcomes of Lyme disease. Ann Intern Med 121:560–567, 1994

Shannon KM, Goetz CG: Connective tissue diseases and the nervous system, in Neurology and General Medicine. Edited by Aminoff MJ. New York, Churchill Livingstone, 1989, pp 389–411

Sigal LH: Persisting symptoms, in Lyme Disease. Edited by Coyle PK. St. Louis, MO, Mosby Year Book, 1993, pp 187–191

Skegg K: Multiple sclerosis presenting as a pure psychiatric disorder. Psychol Med 23:909–914, 1993

Smith A: Symbol Digital Modalities Test. Los Angeles, CA, Western Psychological Services, 1973

Steere AC, Taylor E, McHugh GL, et al: The overdiagnosis of Lyme disease. JAMA 269:1812–1816, 1993

Stores G: A clinical approach to poorly controlled seizures in children. Br J Hosp Med 48:93–98, 1990

Straus SE, Tosato G, Armstrong G, et al: Persisting illness and fatigue in adults with evidence of Epstein-Barr virus infection. Ann Intern Med 102:7–16, 1985

Sumaya CV: Serologic and virologic epidemiology of Epstein-Barr virus: relevance to CFS. Rev Infect Dis 13 (suppl):S19–S25, 1991

Tan E, Cohen A, Fries J, et al: The 1982 revised criteria for the classification of systemic lupus erythematosus. Arthritis Rheum 25:1271–1277, 1982

Thompson PJ: Memory function in patients with epilepsy, in Advances in Neurology, Vol 55. Edited by Smith DB, Treiman DM, Trimble MR. New York, Raven, 1991, pp 369–384

Tobi M, Morag A, Ravid Z, et al: Prolonged atypical illness associated with serological evidence of persistent Epstein-Barr virus infection. Lancet 1:61–64, 1982

Trimble MR: Interictal psychoses of epilepsy, in Advances in Neurology, Vol 55. Edited by Smith DB, Treiman DM, Trimble MR. New York, Raven, 1991, pp 143–152

Van der Burg W, Van Zomeren AH, Minderhoud JM, et al: Cognitive impairment in patients with multiple sclerosis and mild physical disability. Arch Neurol 44:494–501, 1987

Ward M, Studenski S: The time course of acute psychiatric episodes in systemic lupus erythematosus. J Rheumatol 18:535–539, 1991

Wekking E: Psychiatric symptoms in systemic lupus erythematosus: an update. Psychosom Med 55:219–228, 1993

Whitlock F, Siskind M: Depression as a major symptom of multiple sclerosis. J Neurol Neurosurg Psychiatry 43:861–865, 1980

Wyckoff P, Miller L, Tucker L, et al: Neuropsychological assessment of children and adolescents with systemic lupus erythematosus. Lupus 4:217–220, 1995

8

NEUROPSYCHOLOGICAL ASSESSMENT IN DEMENTING CONDITIONS

Philip D. Harvey, Ph.D., and Karen L. Dahlman, Ph.D.

DEMENTIA IS A major public health problem, with an estimated 6 million cases in the United States at present and more cases expected as the population ages. Neuropsychological assessment is a crucial component of any dementia evaluation. Both American (McKhann et al. 1984) and European Community (CPMP Working Party 1992) standards require neuropsychological assessment as a component of the diagnostic workup. The neuropsychological assessment of dementia is also crucial for the evaluation of progression (Katzman 1986), a major component in the course of most dementing conditions.

◆ DEFINITION OF DEMENTIA

Dementia is defined similarly in several different diagnostic systems (e.g., DSM-IV, ICD-10) (American Psychiatric Association 1994; World

Health Organization 1992): a condition marked by the loss of memory functions; deterioration in adaptive functioning from a higher, better level; and the presence of at least one additional sign of major cognitive deficit. These additional deficits include aphasia (loss of language function), apraxia (loss of skilled motor actions), agnosia (inability to recognize familiar objects), and loss of executive functions (i.e., conceptual skills, planning, and control over component skill areas). The definition of dementia *does not necessarily require a progressive course of illness, although many dementing conditions have progressive degeneration as a clinical feature. The definition of dementia also differentiates the condition from others in which the loss of cognitive function is limited to a single function, such as amnesia or aphasia wherein loss of memory or loss of language competence is the principal change in cognitive functioning. Dementia has multiple causes, and whenever possible the etiological factor is coded during the diagnostic process.*

In this chapter, our discussion of dementia is limited in scope and describes the key aspects of a neuropsychological evaluation aimed at the assessment of dementia. In addition, the typical neuropsychological profiles of the most commonly seen dementias are compared with one another. Only those aspects of neuropsychological assessment that are crucial to the evaluation of dementia are presented in this chapter.

◈ Varieties of Dementia

Many different conditions can cause dementia, including viral conditions and their consequences, vascular disorders, and several different neurodegenerative processes. Some of these conditions are progressive, such as Alzheimer's disease (AD), Parkinson's disease, and dementia of the frontal type, whereas others are apparently static after initial diagnosis, such as dementia associated with head trauma. Some other dementing conditions are associated with deterioration in cognitive functioning only if the etiological agent is still operative, such as continued infarctions in vascular dementia.

We have focused on the most common types of dementing conditions, including Alzheimer's, Huntington's, and Parkinson's diseases, dementia of the frontal type, HIV/AIDS dementia, and vascular dementia. In so doing, we have excluded on the basis of space constraints some important but less common conditions, such as progressive supranuclear palsy, and have not discussed dementia associated with head trauma or brain tumors. In the discussion of each of the selected dementing conditions we provide brief descriptions of etiological factors and neuropathology and cite sources that provide a detailed description of these important factors.

◈ CORTICAL VERSUS SUBCORTICAL DEMENTIA

The constellation of impairments seen in Parkinson's disease and Huntington's disease, combined with the neuropathology of these disorders, which is limited to subcortical regions, has led to an ongoing distinction between cortical and subcortical dementias (Cummings 1986; Cummings and Benson 1990; Rebok and Folstein 1993). In this conception, dementias such as Alzheimer's disease that affect the cortex (and, eventually, all of the cognitive functions dependent on the intact cortex) can be discriminated from dementing conditions that have their principal effect on the subcortical regions. Recent studies have suggested that subcortical (e.g., Huntington's disease) and cortical (e.g., Alzheimer's disease) dementias can be discriminated even at the later stages of illness (Paulsen et al. 1995b). Although there is some controversy about this distinction, in line with findings of certain types of language and other "cortical" abnormalities in Parkinson's disease (see Rebok and Folstein 1993 for a discussion), most dementias that affect subcortical regions (e.g., HIV-related dementia, Huntington's disease, and Parkinson's disease) have similar features. The question of the validity of this distinction will continue to be debated, but there are some clear differences between the group of "subcortical" dementias and Alzheimer's disease in the breadth and magnitude of impairments, especially in terms of early impairments in attention in subcortical dementia, global slowing processes in subcortical dementias even in their early stages, very salient signs of depression, and sparing of recognition memory. Accordingly, we organize our discussion of these conditions in line with this distinction.

◈ AGING AND COGNITIVE CHANGE

No discussion of dementing conditions would be complete without mentioning that aging itself is associated with changes in many different cognitive functions. In fact, most of the cognitive impairments seen in dementing conditions occur with normal aging, but to a much more limited extent. In fact, in most dementias the functions that are preserved late in the illness, such as word recognition and vocabulary, are the functions most resistant to decline with normal aging. Thus, to be effective, any neuropsychological assessment must include careful comparison of performance with age- and education-corrected normative standards.

Although the domain of aging-related changes is beyond the scope of this chapter, several general points can be made. Major aging-related changes occur in motor speed and in memory functions, whereas the level of change in long-term memory and ability to access and use previously learned material is much more modest. As a consequence, baseline functioning can be estimated from performance on tests of prior learning such as reading and vocabulary, because of the minimal aging-related changes in these areas. For a complete review of aging and neuropsychology, the reader is referred to Albert and Moss (1988). All cognitive impairments identified in dementia must be referenced to age-corrected norms and to the patient's previous levels of functioning. Because raw scores on memory tests universally decline with age, a raw score that is lower than what would have been obtained when the individual was younger means very little without reference to age norms. In addition, an individual's baseline level of cognitive functioning establishes parameters of possible cognitive decline. Individuals whose best score ever on a memory test was in the age-corrected 20th percentile will not be showing exaggerated memory deficits if they obtain a score in this same range when assessed in late life. In contrast, an individual who would have achieved a score in the 95th percentile when younger and who receives an age-corrected score in the 20th percentile in late life is experiencing cognitive decline. Thus, changes possibly associated with dementing conditions must be discriminated from change associated with normal aging and with performance associated with low baseline levels of cognitive functioning.

Baseline cognitive functions have often been estimated with tests of word recognition (i.e., reading) performance. This particular measure is selected because it measures old learning, acquired before the onset of any cognitive changes associated with dementia. It is strongly associated with overall intellectual functioning in nonimpaired populations (Crawford et al. 1988b, 1989). Furthermore, reading scores have been shown to decline only modestly in the early stages of Alzheimer's disease (O'Carroll et al. 1987), although the late stages are associated with more profound impairments. There are some indications, however, that in Huntington's disease, reading scores decline from premorbid levels (Crawford et al. 1988a). Thus, reading scores are probably best used as an estimate of premorbid function in Alzheimer's disease, which is the most common dementing condition in any case. This discussion is complicated somewhat by the fact that low baseline functioning is apparently in itself a risk factor for dementia and that low baseline scores predict more rapid or more profound decline in several conditions we discuss. These issues are addressed in detail below.

Cognitive Change With Aging in Psychiatric Disorders

Many psychiatric conditions are associated with compromised cognitive performance early in the course of the illness. Rarely, however, is the cognitive impairment so profound as to be consistent with a diagnosis of dementia. With advanced age, however, some evidence shows greater than normal aging effects on cognitive functions. Although studies of cognitive impairment in late-life psychiatric conditions are in their infancy, the results of some of these studies are presented below and are compared with accepted standards for dementing conditions and evaluated.

◈ DEMENTIAS AND THEIR ASSESSMENT

Alzheimer's Disease

Alzheimer's disease, first reported by Alzheimer at the beginning of the twentieth century, is the most common of the dementing conditions. As many as half of all patients with dementia who are older than 65 will have symptoms that meet criteria for Alzheimer's disease at a postmortem assessment (Arriagada et al. 1992), and the proportion of cases of Alzheimer's disease compared with other dementias increases as the age of the patients increases (Rebok and Folstein 1993). It has an age at onset ranging from the late 30s (rarely) to the end of life and a prevalence of as high as 6% of the current living population (Terry and Katzman 1992). These figures are greatly increased in old age, with as much as 50% of the population older than 85 meeting criteria for Alzheimer's disease (Evans et al. 1989). Most studies note that the course of the illness is around 10 years from the first identifiable symptom, unless the patient does not survive this period (Katzman 1976). Risk factors for the illness are age, family history of Alzheimer's disease, reduced educational attainment, Down's syndrome, head trauma, and female gender (Cummings and

Benson 1983). The neuropathological signature of the illness includes amyloid plaques and neurofibrillary tangles, localized initially in the medial temporal cortex and hippocampus and found later in the illness in the more lateral structures of the temporal lobe, parietal cortex, and perisylvian region (Huff et al. 1987; Khachaturian 1985). Plaques are irregularly shaped deposits of amyloid, and tangles are neurofibrillary masses that are irregularly distributed in the same general regions as plaques. The presence of these neuropathological stigmata is required for the postmortem diagnosis of Alzheimer's disease according to all current criteria.

The clinical hallmark of Alzheimer's disease is its progressive course. When measured with a global clinical rating scale, such as the Mini-Mental State Exam (MMSE; M. F. Folstein et al. 1975) or the Alzheimer's Disease Assessment Scale (ADAS; W. G. Rosen et al. 1984), the average deterioration is about 10% per year (G. Berg et al. 1987; Huff et al. 1987; Salmon et al. 1990). Thus, the expected decline in the MMSE is about 3 points per year on average. This decline is not, however, linear. In the early and later stages of the illness, the annual decline is considerably less than in the middle, leading to a curvilinear course (J. C. Morris et al. 1993). As a result, the expected annual loss of functioning measured globally depends considerably on the severity of illness at the time of first assessment.

There are multiple aspects of cognitive impairment seen in Alzheimer's disease, but the presence and severity of each cognitive impairment also depend on the stage of illness. In fact, as the illness progresses, eventually every cognitive function of the cerebral cortex becomes impaired. Some of the cognitive impairments are seen very early in the course of the illness, and others appear later (Welsh et al. 1992). Of these cognitive impairments, some become progressively worse during the course of the illness, and others appear to be static after their appearance (J. C. Morris et al. 1993). The first measurable cognitive sign of Alzheimer's disease is profound deficits in exposure-related learning and delayed recall, either with or without intervening distracting information. This empirical finding is not surprising, because the first subjective sign of the illness is forgetfulness and problems in learning new information. This deficit is substantial, in that patients with "mild" Alzheimer's disease (MMSE score > 23) have been found to learn as few as 3 words after three exposures to a 10-item serial word list, whereas control subjects (without Alzheimer's disease) matched in age and education to these patients learned 8 words. On testing of delayed recall, the patients with Alzheimer's disease recalled fewer than 1 word on average, whereas the control subjects retained 7 of 8 words that they learned (Welsh et al. 1991). Deficits in delayed recall do not progress with continued overall worsening of the illness, whereas exposure-related learning appears to worsen steadily with increases in the overall severity of impairment.

After the impairments in learning and memory appear at the earliest stages of the illness, verbal skills such as confrontation naming and verbal fluency appear to worsen next, and these deficits progress with a roughly linear course. The next aspects of functioning to deteriorate are praxis and spatial-perceptual operations. These declines appear to be linear as well (J. C. Morris et al. 1993; Welsh et al. 1992). Thus, the curvilinear course of Alzheimer's disease, as measured by global scales such as the MMSE, may be determined by the scaling properties of the assessment instruments as well as by the actual course of the illness. The "accelerated" pace of cognitive decline in the middle of the illness may be a function of the fact that more of the cognitive functions measured by the instrument are in decline in the middle of the illness than at the very early stages (when only delayed recall and verbal learning are impaired) and the late stages (at which most cognitive tests are now manifesting floor effects). It must be noted that Alzheimer's disease does not follow the same course in every patient, and these descriptions are based on average statements about large samples of patients.

Many other aspects of cognitive assessment in Alzheimer's disease merit attention. Impairment in executive functioning appears early in the illness. Deficits in executive functioning may be exacerbated, or possibly even caused, by deficits in the cognitive components controlled by executive functions. For instance, a profound deficit in working memory would make adequate performance on an executive functioning test such as the Wisconsin Card Sorting Test (WCST; Heaton et al. 1993) essentially impossible. As in many amnestic conditions, procedural learning (i.e., learning of motor skills) appears to be more intact than declarative learning. Similarly, implicit memory functions (i.e., memory aided by prompts or cues) appear more intact than explicit memory, although they are still impaired (Zec 1993). Recognition memory (i.e., the ability to identify previously presented information) is not spared, in contrast to findings in specific frontal-lobe damage (Freedman 1990) or Parkinson's disease (see below). Finally, several studies have suggested that interventions designed to augment memory functioning, including provision of practice and alteration of encodability of information, do not benefit patients with Alzheimer's disease to the same extent that they do age-matched control subjects, patients with affective disorders, or patients with other dementing conditions (Weingartner et al. 1993).

Another important aspect of the study of Alzheimer's disease is that of motor speed and visuomotor performance. Both motor speed and visuomotor performance are impaired quite early in the course of the illness, and some evidence indicates that these are also progressive deficits (Nebes and Brady 1992; Nebes and Madden 1988). The issue of attentional impairment in Alzheimer's disease is a complex one. As a general statement, attentional impairment is a less salient feature of Alzheimer's disease than deficits in learning and memory. That said, there is still considerable evidence that concentration impairment is present in the illness, especially with continued progression (Kaszniak et al. 1986). In the area of deficient verbal skills, some evidence suggests that letter fluency is less impaired than category fluency until the very late stages of the illness, possibly because of the greater dependence of category fluency on the intactness of the temporal and parietal cortices (Randolph et al. 1993).

As Alzheimer's disease progresses, function is lost to the point that by the time of death, performance on all tests is so poor that all scores are essentially zero (see Zec 1993 for a comprehensive review of this issue). This is in contrast to some other cortical and subcortical dementias in which many functions are preserved until the very latest stages. Behavioral disturbances in Alzheimer's disease, including delusions, hallucinations, agitation, and depression, can also interfere with the assessment of cognitive functions in the illness, and special care must be taken to ensure that low scores are based on cognitive impairments and not behavioral abnormalities (Teri et al. 1992). Alzheimer's disease is one of the dementing conditions in which a low baseline level of intellectual functioning is a risk factor for the illness. Several studies have indicated that using an estimate of premorbid functions such as a reading level obtained from the Wide Range Achievement Test (Wilkinson 1993) or the National Adult Reading Test (Nelson 1982) is valid up until the severe stages of Alzheimer's disease (e.g., O'Carroll et al. 1987). Thus, relative decline can be assessed against a reasonable measure of premorbid functioning.

Cognitive assessment of Alzheimer's disease. A focused assessment battery would include a serial word list learning test with delayed recall; measures of verbal skills, including fluency and naming; a measure of constructional praxis; assessment of motor speed; and some estimate of premorbid functioning. Assessment with a global scale such as the MMSE or ADAS is also useful to gauge the general level of the patient's cognitive intactness. A neuropsychological assessment alone is inadequate for the differential diagnosis of Alzheimer's disease because of the very large overlap between the cognitive impairments seen in Alzheimer's disease and those seen in other dementing conditions such as vascular dementia. As demonstrated by Thal et al. (1988), the only aspect of cognitive-behavioral functioning that was a clear discriminator of the illnesses was abnormalities in gait, in which patients with a vascular dementia were more likely to be impaired. A prospective approach is required, as are laboratory tests and neurological assessment. Reexamination after 6–12 months to document a progressive course in addition to the presence of the prototypical cognitive impairments is required to diagnose the condition correctly. Some skill in interpretation is required. Because delayed recall deficits are not progressive, evidence of progression in this type of memory function is clearly not to be expected. Furthermore, because praxic deficits are often absent in mild Alzheimer's disease, a finding of no impairment in this area does not rule out the presence of the illness. Cognitive assessment is a crucial component of treatment trials in Alzheimer's disease, because cognitive-enhancing drugs should have a detectable effect on many different aspects of the illness. A full discussion of this issue is contained in Mohs (1995).

Structured rating scales for Alzheimer's disease. An alternative approach to the use of a neuropsychological battery to assess the severity of Alzheimer's disease is the use of a structured rating scale. Several of these instruments are available and in common use, and all have high reliability. The main difference between these scales is their level of comprehensiveness.

- ◆ *Alzheimer's Disease Assessment Scale (ADAS):* The ADAS (W. G. Rosen et al. 1984), a 21-item scale, is designed to assess the severity of cognitive and behavioral impairments in Alzheimer's disease. The cognitive component includes both a short neuropsychological assessment and items rated by the interviewer on the basis of interaction with the patient and caregiver. Scores on the cognitive subscale range from 0 to 70, and scores on the noncognitive subscale range from 0 to 50.
- ◆ *Mini-Mental State Exam (MMSE):* The MMSE (M. F. Folstein et al. 1975) is a widely used assessment instrument designed to screen the cognitive impairments seen in a variety of dementing conditions, al-

though the content areas focus on those associated with Alzheimer's disease. The examination has 21 different items in 11 different tests, with scores ranging from 0 to a perfect score of 30. Scores of 23 or less are typically seen as reflecting dementia and meriting more detailed assessment. In patients with high levels of premorbid functioning, this cutoff should be raised to any score less than 30. Note that the MMSE may be insensitive to subcortical dementia, as one study (Rothlind and Brandt 1993) found that patients with confirmed Parkinson's disease and Huntington's disease were indistinguishable from subjects without dementia on the MMSE.

◆ *Clinical Dementia Rating (CDR):* The CDR (L. Berg 1988) is a global summary measure designed to identify the overall severity of dementia. Six content areas (memory, orientation, judgment and problem solving, community affairs, home and hobbies, and personal care) are rated individually. Ratings are assigned on a scale of 0–5 (0 = absent; 0.5 = questionable; 1 = present but mild; 2 = moderate; 3 = severe; 4 = profound; 5 = terminal). A global summary score is obtained, which has led to the CDR being used for grouping patients according to severity of dementia.

◆ *Mattis Dementia Rating Scale (DRS):* The DRS (Mattis 1976) is more comprehensive and longer than the MMSE and the CDR and is also more informative. Similar to the ADAS, the DRS assesses a number of cognitive functions associated with dementia. Scores range from 0 to 144, with the cutoff for normal performance at 140. The cutoff for "severe" dementia is a score of less than 100.

All of these instruments have a role, particularly in research that requires large-scale screening. For purposes of research-oriented assessment, the use of the ADAS or the DRS is likely to be more efficient than use of a full neuropsychological battery.

Dementia Involving the Frontal Lobe

The prototypical progressive dementing condition is Alzheimer's disease, with an insidious decline across cognitive functions as described above. The classic dementia involving the frontal lobes is Pick's disease (see Cummings and Benson 1983 for a discussion and description). In this illness, which is quite rare, the age at onset is typically in the 40s or 50s, and the patients manifest the classic signs of frontal-lobe impairment described below. At autopsy, Pick's bodies are found in the frontal and temporal lobes, and bilateral atrophy of the frontal and temporal cortices is noted. Pick's bodies occur intracytoplasmically, in swollen (i.e., achromasic) neurons. This illness is well understood and described, with clearly delineated cognitive impairments (see Knopman et al. 1989 for a description). However, there are many recent reports of another progressive dementing condition that superficially resembles Alzheimer's disease, but with a focus of degeneration localized to the frontal lobes. This disorder has been called dementia of the frontal type (DFT). Behaviorally, this condition is marked by the typical functional changes seen in damage to the frontal lobes. In this way, DFT is similar to Pick's disease. Changes in personality are quite salient, including explosiveness, emotional lability, and impaired self-care. Individuals may engage in behaviors that are extremely uncharacteristic of them in their lifetime, including acts of violence oriented at family members, substance abuse, and poor financial decisions. This personality change has been described as "pseudo-psychopathic," in contrast to the "pseudo-depressed" character seen in other types of frontal-lobe impairment. At autopsy, evidence of neuronal loss, gliosis, and spongiosis is seen, but no discrete neuropathological entities such as Pick's bodies, Lewy bodies, or amyloid plaques and neurofibrillary tangles are found (Brun 1987). Cell loss and gliosis are limited to the frontal lobes and the cingulate cortex, with no evidence of these processes in posterior regions or major portions of the temporal lobes (Gustafson 1987).

This condition was extensively described by a research group in Sweden (Gustafson et al. 1990), who have prospectively followed up a large sample of individuals and identified their specific characteristics. The average age at onset was approximately 56 years, with a course of illness that averaged 8.1 years. These data suggest an earlier age at onset and a briefer course to mortality than in Alzheimer's disease. Thus, the illness differs in course as well as behavioral presentation from Alzheimer's disease (Brun 1987; Gustafson 1987; Knopman et al. 1990). Neuroimaging studies of this condition have revealed a gross and focal loss of cortical activity in the regions of the lateral frontal lobes. For instance, studies have found that patients with this condition manifest highly selective deficits when examined with a single photon emission computed tomography (SPECT) study. In contrast to patients with Alzheimer's disease, who show generalized underactivity of the temporoparietal aspects of the cortex, patients with this disease manifest nearly complete inactivity in the dorsolateral prefrontal region. Longitudinal images reveal that the region of reduced cortical activation spreads to encompass the entire frontal lobe but does not extend to more posterior regions (B. L. Miller et al. 1991).

As would be expected in an illness that manifests itself by progressive loss of functions of the frontal lobes, the cognitive deficits seen are in the areas of executive functioning and verbal skills, with a highly specific pattern of memory impairment. Patients with this condition manifest significant inability to perform the WCST and are also impaired in selective attention performance. Deficits in confrontation naming and verbal fluency are commonly seen. Memory impairments do not have the total anterograde amnesia characteristics seen in Alzheimer's disease, but rather are marked by reductions in the ability to use encoding strategies. For example, patients with DFT do not appear to benefit from the categorizability of information in lists presented to them for recall (Neary and Snowden 1991; Neary et al. 1988). They also manifest signs of confabulation in memory performance, wherein they produce unrelated information as responses when they are unable to perform correctly on a memory assessment. There are no signs of visuospatial deficits and only modest signs of formal apraxia.

One additional feature seen in DFT that is also common to other localized impairments of the prefrontal cortex is interindividual variability in affective and cognitive impairment (Gustafson et al. 1990). No single pattern of impairment can be described in a generalized manner, as can be attempted in Alzheimer's disease. In fact, given the role of the frontal cortex in the organization of behavior, the variability of presentation among patients with degeneration of the frontal lobe is probably a direct sign of loss of organization. A further contributor to this situation is that the cell death seen in DFT is quite widespread and variable among patients. This wide variation may itself contribute to the relatively variable presentation seen in DFT and may in fact raise questions about its status as a distinct syndromal entity. Although this concept is still new, recent advances in neuroimaging technology will allow for a considerable expansion of the possibilities of studying DFT, and we expect that research in the next few years will lead to a considerable expansion of information about this condition and determine whether it is truly distinct from Alzheimer's disease.

Assessment of frontal-type dementias. Assessment of executive functioning (e.g., with the WCST) is clearly crucial in this illness, as is an assessment of recall and recognition memory. Tests of verbal skills (fluency and naming) are recommended, as is an assessment of attentional functioning under complex task conditions (e.g., Trail Making Test Part B [Army Individual Test Battery 1944] or Symbol Digit Modalities Test

[Smith 1982]). Patients with DFT often present with poorly controlled behavior that is accompanied by modest overall intellectual decline. As is commonly seen in cases of frontal-lobe damage, behavioral abnormalities are often out of line with the very subtle cognitive changes seen (Stuss and Benson 1986). DFT can be discriminated from Alzheimer's disease by early signs of affective and behavioral impairment and personality change, profound executive functioning impairments relative to estimated intelligence, preserved recognition memory, and much less impairment in recall memory than is seen in Alzheimer's disease. DFT is distinguished from Pick's disease by its greater prevalence and by the absence of Pick's bodies at autopsy.

Parkinson's Disease

Although Parkinson's disease is primarily identified by marked impairments in motor control, cognitive deficits are associated with the disorder. The particular pattern of cognitive deficits has now been clearly enough described that DSM-IV identifies Parkinson's disease as a discrete cause of dementia. Parkinson's disease is caused by deficits in dopamine transmission, particularly in the pathways that link the substantia nigra and striatum. Connections with areas in the cortex, including prefrontal and other association regions, are implicated on the basis of cognitive changes apparent in neuropsychological test results. Other neurotransmitter systems in addition to dopamine have been identified as contributing to cognitive deficits in Parkinson's disease. Irregularities in these systems—including acetylcholine, serotonin, glutamate, γ-aminobutyric acid (GABA), and various neuropeptides—have also been identified as contributing to cognitive deficits in Parkinson's disease (Agid 1991), but their exact role remains unclear. When assessing cognitive performance in Parkinson's disease, it is important to take into account the medications being used, which may affect intellectual functioning on neuropsychological tests.

Parkinson's disease occurs in the elderly population with a prevalence of about 1% among those older than 60 (Schoenberg 1987). It is marked by tremor in resting musculature: a somewhat rapid and rhythmical shaking of the limbs, jaw, and tongue, which diminishes and even disappears with voluntary movement; muscular rigidity; difficulty initiating movement (akinesia); and slowed movement (bradykinesia). In most cases, patients have a hunched posture, loss of facial expressiveness (known as masked facies, a characteristic unblinking, blank stare), and some instability as well as loss of agility and fine coordination. Onset is usually in the 50s or 60s, although early-onset Parkinson's disease may begin after age 20 years. Motor impairment in Parkinson's disease is the result of decreasing dopamine (along with other neurotransmitters) and the interruption of its effects on neuronal pathways that control motor activity. Neurons actually decrease in number, and the level of dopamine continues to diminish in the substantia nigra as the disease progresses (McGeer et al. 1977), although notable physical symptoms do not appear until dopamine is reduced to 80% of its original level.

Originally Parkinson's disease was thought to have mainly physical manifestations; in James Parkinson's (1817) original article describing the syndrome ("The Shaking Palsy"), he stated that cognition was unaffected. Research has shown, however, that cognitive impairment is clearly and often a major part of Parkinson's disease, with the presence of an actual dementia in as many as 50% of all patients with Parkinson's disease. It may be possible to have Parkinson's disease for many years and die without having experienced symptoms of dementia, and it is unclear whether without interruption of the illness by the patient's death, dementia would eventually occur in all Parkinson's disease patients. Deficits associated with Parkinson's disease include visual construction impairments, verbal and nonverbal short-term memory impairment (especially in the area of recall memory), reduction in verbal fluency, executive dysfunction, disruption of new learning, reduced ability to use advance information, and visuoperceptive problems. Most patients experience some or many of these symptoms, but few patients have them all. Once a dementing process begins in Parkinson's disease, its course is likely to be progressive.

Attentional problems are common in Parkinson's disease and are more marked on complex tasks that require shifting or sustaining attention (Cummings 1986; Horne 1973; Huber et al. 1989b; Pirozzolo et al. 1982; Stern et al. 1987; Wright et al. 1990). Researchers who have administered simple primary memory tests such as the Digit Span subtest of the Wechsler Adult Intelligence Scale—3rd Edition (WAIS-III; Wechsler 1997a) to patients with Parkinson's disease have mixed opinions about whether those with Parkinson's disease are impaired. Some find that performance is within normal limits (Brown and Marsden 1988; Huber and Shuttleworth 1990; Koller 1984a, 1984b), whereas others have found that patients with Parkinson's disease are impaired (Pirozzolo et al. 1982; Sullivan and Sagar 1988). One explanation for these contradictory findings may be the considerable variation in cognitive status among different subject groups used in studies of patients with Parkinson's disease, yielding large variances in test results (Lezak 1995).

In the area of formal memory functions, as in other areas of cognitive functioning studied in patients with Parkinson's disease, findings are contradictory regarding the impairments associated with the disease. Many of the apparent contradictions in findings, both between and within studies, can be explained by variations within the patient group, with large interindividual variation often obscuring the deficit that exists in a general way among patients with Parkinson's disease. Most investigations point to deficits in both verbal and nonverbal episodic memory. Some studies find equal impairments in recent memory for Parkinson's disease and Alzheimer's disease (Gainotti et al. 1980; Huber et al. 1989a; Pillon et al. 1986), but most studies find that when groups are matched for age, current MMSE score, and premorbid cognitive ability, patients with Parkinson's disease have less memory impairment than those with Alzheimer's disease. In particular, Parkinson's disease patients have been found to have superior delayed recognition in a verbal selective-reminding task. In delayed story recall, patients with Parkinson's disease also benefited more from cues and rehearsal than Alzheimer's disease patients, suggesting either better encoding of material (Helkala et al. 1988) or more intact retrieval processes.

Recent research indicates that short-term memory (STM) is more impaired than long-term memory (LTM) in Parkinson's disease (e.g., Huber et al. 1989b; Levin et al. 1989; Massman et al. 1990). The underlying causes of the STM deficit in Parkinson's disease include basal ganglia dysfunction and consequential disruption of corticostriatal connections, or deafferentation of basal ganglia cortical projections (e.g., Bowen et al. 1975). These inferences must be tempered with the knowledge that patients with Parkinson's disease in those studies were treated with antiparkinsonian medication, which can itself disrupt new learning and memory. A study of untreated patients with Parkinson's disease (Sullivan et al. 1993) found that STM impairment occurred for both verbal and nonverbal material, suggesting that memory impairments are tied directly to the disease itself rather than to antiparkinsonian medication.

Results of investigations of new learning in Parkinson's disease are mixed. Grossman et al. (1994) found that 55% of patients with Parkinson's disease had significant impairment in their recall of some aspect of a new verb. Most of these patients demonstrated a language-sensitive deficit in understanding the grammatical information in the new verb, and some patients responded randomly to prompting. These authors concluded that difficulty in assimilating grammatical information contributes to the language impairments of patients with Parkinson's disease. Vocabulary, grammar, and syntax have long been thought to be unimpaired in Parkinson's disease (Bayles 1988; Brown and Marsden 1988; Sullivan et al. 1989), although some note that utterance length and overall output are reduced (Bayles et al. 1985; Cummings and Benson 1989). Even in Parkinson's disease patients who appear to have no pronounced signs of dementia, a verbal fluency deficit has been documented, albeit of lesser severity and with a less drastic deteriorating course than the verbal fluency deficit that is characteristic of Alzheimer's disease. Studies indicate that patients with Parkinson's disease are better able to use cues than are those with Alzheimer's disease and Huntington's disease (Randolph et al. 1993). Confrontation naming deficits have been found in some studies and not in others, with the likely explanation that naming disorders appear later than other verbal dysfunctions in the course of Parkinson's disease (Bayles and Tomoeda 1983; El-Awar et al. 1987; Gurd and Ward 1989). Another important feature of Parkinson's disease patients that cannot be overlooked in the assessment of verbal functions is their characteristic impairment of the mechanical operation of speech (hypokinetic dysarthria): the articulation aspects of language production. Difficulties in written language are usually on a par with deficits in speech and are affected by motor disturbance typical of Parkinson's disease. Writing can be cramped and jerky, with written samples reduced in size (micrographia).

Visual construction impairment has been well documented in patients with Parkinson's disease but may not be specific to dementia (Boller et al. 1984; Levin 1990; Levin et al. 1991; Pirozzolo et al. 1982; Ransmayr et al. 1986; Stern et al. 1984; Villardita et al. 1982). In a study of 24 patients with Parkinson's disease who were identified as nondemented (MMSE scores were greater than 26 in all subjects), Grossman et al. (1993) asked their subjects to copy and then recall the Rey-Osterrieth Complex Figure (Rey 1941), dividing the units of the figure into "main structural" and "detail" components. Patients with Parkinson's disease consistently omitted some of the main structural units from their recall of the figure. When the main structures were produced, Parkinson's disease patients were impaired at drawing the features in any organized way, and they produced the main units late in the process of making the drawing. Patients with Parkinson's disease also omitted a greater proportion of the details than did the control group—in the copy as well as in the

1-minute recall and 5-minute recall sessions—although it was notable that their detail recall pattern resembled that of control subjects, whereas their pattern of producing main units was different. The analysis provided support for the hypothesis that patients with Parkinson's disease have difficulty chunking main structural units because of a failure to recognize the main units as coherent and organizing features of the figure.

In a study of executive system impairment in memory and perceptual abilities in Parkinson's disease, Bondi et al. (1993) found that learning, memory, visuoperceptual, and visuoconstructive skills were not significantly impaired, once performance on the frontal-related tasks such as the WCST was covaried. Deficits in areas sensitive to the well-being of the frontal lobes among patients with Parkinson's disease are thought to reflect impairment in the ability to generate efficient strategies when engaged in self-directed and task-specific planning (Brown and Marsden 1988; St-Cyr et al. 1988; Taylor et al. 1988).

Assessment of Parkinson's disease. An adequate assessment battery for Parkinson's disease would include measures of learning and memory that allow for discrimination of differences between recall and recognition, an assessment of complex attentional functioning (e.g., Trail Making Test Parts A and B), the Rey-Osterrieth Complex Figure, an assessment of primary memory in both verbal and spatial modalities (e.g., the Wechsler Memory Scale—3rd Edition [WMS-III; Wechsler 1997b] Digit Span and Spatial Span tests), and a test of verbal fluency. To capture the possible contribution of the subcortical pathology to linked cortical regions, the WCST is recommended as well. This assessment battery is reminiscent of that seen in frontal-lobe dementias, with good reason. Many of the signs of subcortical dementias are possibly due to the deterioration of prefrontal-subcortical connections, with a resulting effect on the functions that are dependent on the frontal lobe. Although this battery is not exhaustive, a patient with Parkinson's disease who had normal performance on all of these tests would not meet the criteria for Parkinson's dementia. Assessment of motor speed with finger tapping may prove informative but contributes little to the diagnosis of dementia, because bradykinesia is a common feature of the illness even in cases with no overt cognitive impairment.

Huntington's Disease

Huntington's disease is a neuropsychiatric disorder marked by choreoathetosis, caudate atrophy, and an autosomal dominant inheritance.

Equally common in men and women, Huntington's disease affects 3–10 per 100,000 people (Martin 1984). Age at onset is typically in the early 40s, although this is quite variable. The typical course is 13–17 years, with death usually resulting from pneumonia, choking, nutritional deficiencies, skin ulcers, or suicide or other self-destructive behavior (Lanska et al. 1988).

A diagnosis of Huntington's disease is usually based on identification of choreoathetosis, the hallmark movement disorder associated with the disease. Choreoathetosis is a combination of jerky movements and slower, twisting movements that often result in dystonic posturing. Early in the course of the disease, these movements occur on initiation of action and include "piano-playing" movements of the fingers, ulnar deviation of the hands, and facial tics. Later in the course, choreoathetosis includes a virtually constant stream of movement, including severe grimacing, head bobbing and rolling, and a "dancing gait." These movements, even when severe, cease during sleep. With time, choreoathetosis decreases, and dystonia, with akinesis and rigidity, becomes more salient.

Huntington's disease is now known to result from a gene on the terminal short arm of chromosome 4 (Mendez 1994). The Huntington's disease gene causes delayed atrophy and gliosis of the caudate nuclei, with dendritic abnormalities in small to medium spiny cells. The basal ganglia have decreased concentrations of the inhibitory neurotransmitter GABA and the enzymes required for GABA synthesis. Other neurotransmitters are relatively preserved. There is also early cell loss in the putamen and, later on, in the globus pallidus and the prefrontal cortex. Unlike Alzheimer's disease, Huntington's disease does not involve significant loss of neurons from the nucleus basalis of Meynert or loss of choline acetyl transferase activity in the cortex. As Huntington's disease progresses, however, neuropathological changes in the caudate nucleus show up consistently in neuroimaging studies.

Dementia in Huntington's disease is a prototypical subcortical dementia. Cognitive impairments include reduced motor speed; decreased selective and sustained attention; decreased behavioral initiation, spontaneity, and engagement; decreased Performance Scale IQ with verbal performance discrepancy; executive deficits; faulty encoding with poor storage; faulty retrieval strategies in the context of unimpaired recognition; deficient memory requiring effortful processing; decreased motor skill and procedural learning; decreased verbal fluency and output; abnormal egocentric spatial orientation; and abnormal visuomotor integration (Mendez 1994). Unlike those with Alzheimer's disease, patients with Huntington's disease have insight into their neuropsychiatric disorder, despite undergoing personality changes.

About 50% of patients with Huntington's disease have non-dementia-related psychiatric disorders, with a range of about 35%–73% (S. E. Folstein 1989; M. Morris 1991; Saugstad and Odegard 1986). Included in these disorders are depression, personality changes, and anxiety disorders that often precede the onset of choreoathetosis by as long as 10 years or longer (Dewhurst et al. 1970). Patients with Huntington's disease complain early in their illness of difficulty with attention and concentration. They do particularly poorly on the WAIS-III subtests that gauge attentional capacity, as well as on measures of visuomotor skills such as the Trail Making Test. Patients with Huntington's disease have been shown to have greater attentional and concentration problems than patients with Alzheimer's disease, Parkinson's disease, and progressive supranuclear palsy (Pillon et al. 1993; Rothlind et al. 1993).

Patients with Huntington's disease have significant executive functioning deficits, with dysfunction in the areas of maintaining and changing a cognitive set, abstraction, judgment, and reasoning, as well as difficulty with planning and organization and impaired mental flexibility (Brandt and Butters 1986; S. E. Folstein 1989; Paulsen et al. 1995b; Rothlind et al. 1993). Patients with Huntington's disease usually have verbal and visual memory deficits early in their disease. Although the deficit is not as severe as that found in patients with Alzheimer's disease (Paulsen et al. 1995a) or amnesia, memory problems in Huntington's disease are well documented. Huntington's disease patients have flawed encoding strategies that result in poor storage (Lundervold et al. 1994b). Patients have diminished ability to benefit from cuing in recall (Lyle and Gottesman 1977), difficulty with free learning of new material (Pillon et al. 1993), and impaired ability to learn items in a sequence (Caine et al. 1977; Massman et al. 1990). However, unlike those with Alzheimer's disease, patients with Huntington's disease can benefit from interventions targeting their encoding strategies (Bylsma et al. 1990; Kramer et al. 1988; Lyle and Gottesman 1977), as well as from priming or partial cues from prior exposure (Heindel et al. 1990). The importance of testing that is focused specifically on discriminating the ability of a patient with Huntington's disease to benefit from modification of input strategies, as opposed to simply establishing that a memory impairment exists, has been noted in the literature (Paulsen et al. 1995b).

Language in Huntington's disease is relatively intact insofar as the ability to complete verbally mediated tasks is concerned. Confrontation naming is stronger than in Alzheimer's disease patients. Although aphasia is not part of the cognitive picture in Huntington's disease, early in the disease verbal fluency is somewhat impaired. Fluency changes include more single-word and short-phrase responses and more pauses in conversation; the absolute numbers of words in speech samples have been shown to be lower than in those of control subjects without Huntington's disease (Gordon and Illes 1987). Ability to understand verbal intonation (prosody) is also impaired (Speedie et al. 1990), as is written expression (Podoll et al. 1988). Impairments in visuospatial functioning have been noted in terms of lowered scores on constructional tasks, both building and drawing (Fedio et al. 1979; Mohr et al. 1991), as well as in spatial orientation (Bylsma et al. 1992).

Neuropsychological assessment of Huntington's disease.   The assessment of Huntington's disease is essentially similar to that recommended in Parkinson's disease and HIV dementia. Similar patterns of results are expected, with several exceptions. Some evidence indicates that patients with Huntington's disease have more severe semantic memory deficits than those with Parkinson's disease (reviewed in Rebok and Folstein 1993). In addition, patients with Huntington's disease have also been reported to manifest severe impairments in personal space perception (i.e., the ability identify the location of an object or direction of movement in terms of their own location), a deficit not noted in Parkinson's disease or Alzheimer's disease (Brouwers et al. 1984). Rebok and Folstein (1993) argued that Huntington's disease is a better exemplar of subcortical dementia than Parkinson's disease. This assertion is now being studied.

Human Immunodeficiency Virus–Related Dementia

HIV-associated dementia complex or AIDS dementia complex (ADC) is now recognized as a distinct complication of HIV infection. ADC presents as a progressive dementia that includes cognitive, motor, and behavioral dysfunction. It is thought to involve pathology of the basal ganglia, thalamus, and brain stem, given the subcortical nature of many of the deficits that appear early in the course. Onset is usually insidious, with signs of mental and verbal slowness, inattention, loss of concentration, and recent memory loss. Evidence suggests that as many as one-third of patients with AIDS have neurological complications at the time of diagnosis (Denning et al. 1987; Ho et al. 1985; Levy et al. 1985; Ruutu et al.

1987), indicating that HIV crosses the blood-brain barrier and reaches the central nervous system very soon after infection. In fact, as many as 28% of HIV-positive individuals who are medically asymptomatic show some signs of cognitive decline on psychometric testing (Rosci et al. 1992). The impairment attributed to ADC is generally thought to increase linearly with the severity of other HIV-related disease (Grant et al. 1987).

Studies (e.g., Maruff et al. 1994) have found that patients with mild ADC were markedly worse in the areas of executive function, memory, and complex attention than were both neurologically intact AIDS patients and HIV-negative control subjects. No impairments were found in affect, simple motor function, orientation, language, or visuospatial construction. This pattern of deficits is more comparable with the cognitive performance of patients with "subcortical" dementias such as Huntington's disease, Parkinson's disease, and progressive supranuclear palsy than of those with "cortical" dementia, such as Alzheimer's disease (Lundervold et al. 1994a).

Visuomotor and attentional performance deficits have been clearly documented among HIV-seropositive subjects on the Trail Making Test Parts A and B and the Symbol Digit Modalities Test, as well as on an extended version of the Mental Control subtest of the WMS-III. However, no differences were found in performance between HIV-positive and HIV-seronegative subjects on the arithmetic subtest of the WAIS-R (Franzblau et al. 1991; Wechsler 1981) or results of Golden's (1978) Stroop Color and Word Test (Stern et al. 1991), the Seashore Rhythm Test of the Halstead-Reitan (Reitan and Wolfson 1993) Battery (Claypoole et al. 1990), or various cancellation tests (Perry et al. 1989; Rubinow et al. 1988).

A review of the literature shows that the mixed results described above stem at least in part from disagreement about what tests are appropriate measures of attention. For example, Maruff et al. (1994) used the Digit Span subtest of the WMS-R (Wechsler 1987) to measure "memory," whereas a large group of studies used this subtest to assess attention and found no difference in performance between HIV-positive and HIV-negative subjects (Grant et al. 1987; E. Miller et al. 1990; Ollo and Pass 1988; Ollo et al. 1991; Saykin et al. 1988; Tross et al. 1988; van Gorp et al. 1989). In addition, patients who are experiencing more severe medical problems would be expected to have attentional complications secondary to affective disturbance, fatigue, and physical discomfort, independent of any aspects of impaired concentration directly related to infection (van Gorp et al. 1993).

Investigations of language function among HIV-seropositive individuals have generally demonstrated normal language abilities. Confrontation naming, as measured by the Boston Naming Test (Goodglass and Kaplan 1983), is unimpaired (Janssen et al. 1989; Maruff et al. 1994; Stern et al. 1989; Tross et al. 1988; van Gorp et al. 1989). On tests of verbal fluency, again, most studies find no differences between HIV-seronegative and HIV-seropositive individuals (e.g., Goethe et al. 1989; Maruff et al. 1994; E. Miller et al. 1990). Vocabulary has also been found to be unimpaired, according to results of the WAIS-R. Except for one or two studies (e.g., Saykin et al. 1988), the data largely support the conclusion that language function is for the most part unimpaired by ADC, even in later stages of medical illness.

Mixed results have been reported in terms of the visuoconstructive and visuoperceptive abilities of seropositive versus seronegative individuals. Several investigations (Maruff et al. 1994; Poutiainen et al. 1988; van Gorp et al. 1989) report no differences on either drawing or copying tasks using both simple and complex figures. Block design is reported to be unimpaired among HIV-seropositive individuals (Poutiainen et al. 1988), although some impairment in cube drawing has been noted. Object assembly and picture completion, assessed in the above-mentioned studies, failed to discriminate between groups, as did Benton et al.'s (1983) Line Orientation Test (Stern et al. 1989), the Tactual Performance Test (see Reitan and Wolfson 1993; Saykin et al. 1988), and a mental rotation test (Wilkie et al. 1990). Differences that have been found on block design between HIV-seropositive patients with and without ADC are possibly problematic because the tests are timed. Psychomotor slowing and reduced processing speed have been noted in ADC patients in a variety of studies (Reinvang et al. 1991). Overall, it seems that visuospatial functioning is relatively unaffected by ADC when response speed is not a factor.

Memory functioning has been found to discriminate successfully between patients with AIDS and other diagnostic groups; in particular, verbal memory deficits have been seen in many studies (Maruff et al. 1994; E. Miller et al. 1991; Reinvang et al. 1991). Deficiencies have been documented primarily in delayed recall, with sparing of encoding processes, similar to the pattern of decline found in normal aging and dissimilar to the pattern found in Alzheimer's disease, in which encoding is impaired (Mitrushina et al. 1994; Pajeau and Roman 1992). HIV-seropositive subjects consistently have psychomotor slowing on computerized choice reaction time tests and tests of motor speed (Kokkevi et al. 1991;

Lundervold et al. 1994a; E. Miller et al. 1991). This slowing of responses seems to be pervasive and contributes to confusion in the findings of HIV-related deficits in other areas of cognitive functioning, such as verbal fluency, memory, and attention and concentration.

One of the major problems associated with HIV dementia is the psychological consequences of HIV infection, in terms of both anxiety and depression. Many of the cognitive tests described above are affected by those dysphoric states. Intravenous drug users who have contracted HIV often have comorbid affective disorders or personality disorders, also confounding the results. Many cases of mild cognitive impairments in HIV-related conditions either may be caused by concurrent affective syndromes or may be a function of low levels of premorbid functioning. Special care should be taken to avoid a dementia diagnosis when functioning has not declined.

Assessment of HIV dementia. As noted above, deficits in motor speed, attention, and recall memory are most salient in this illness. Thus, an adequate assessment battery would include measures of motor speed (Purdue Pegboard [Tiffin 1968] or Finger Tapping Tests [Reitan and Wolfson 1993]), visuomotor tests (Trail Making Test or the WAIS-R Digit Symbol test), and a differential assessment of serial learning, recall, and recognition memory, such as would be found in the California Verbal Learning Test (Delis et al. 1986). A patient who meets the criteria for ADC would often perform the Trail Making Test at about the 5th percentile (age corrected) or manifest an age-corrected scaled score on the Digit Symbol test of 4 or less. If this is significantly less than the current age-corrected vocabulary score as evidenced by scatter analysis, then decline would be supported. Preserved recognition memory would be expected, but impaired delayed recall might be found.

Vascular Dementias

After Alzheimer's disease, various forms of vascular disease are the most common cause of dementia. The typical cause of dementia associated with vascular disease is multiple cerebral infarctions, hence the term formerly used to describe this set of dementing conditions, *multi-infarct dementia* (Hachinski et al. 1974). A stroke is the consequence of a blockage (occlusion) or hemorrhage of a cerebral blood vessel, which leads to cell death in the areas directly served by that vessel as well as death of cells that are exposed to significant amounts of blood from the ruptured vessel (in the case of hemorrhagic stroke). Although dementia may result from a single cerebral infarction, multiple vascular events are much more typical. Criteria for a diagnosis of vascular dementia include 1) substantial cognitive impairments meeting diagnostic criteria for dementia; 2) evidence of vascular events, generally from neuroimaging; and 3) a close temporal relation between the vascular events and the cognitive impairments (American Psychiatric Association 1994).

Because nearly all cortical regions are vulnerable to being affected by infarction, the cognitive deficits seen in vascular dementia are very wide ranging. In fact, there is no "common profile" of cognitive impairments seen in vascular dementias (Metter and Wilson 1993). For instance, in a comprehensive study by Thal et al. (1988), impairments in memory, orientation, language, and concentration and attention were noted in patients with vascular dementia, as well as in patients with a combination of vascular and Alzheimer's disease neuropathology. In fact, in that study, the only aspects of functioning that discriminated patients with Alzheimer's disease alone from those with vascular dementia alone were an increase in gait disturbances in vascular dementia patients and the absence of profound agnosia and apraxia in patients with pure vascular disease.

Some intrinsic definitional confusion exists in the area of vascular dementia. For example, should a patient who has a single devastating stroke and manifests several cognitive impairments be given a diagnosis of vascular dementia, but not a patient who experiences a single cerebrovascular accident that causes profound and permanent aphasia (Metter and Wilson 1993)? One of the classic clinical presentations of vascular dementia is "patchy deficits," meaning that individual patients have varied patterns of cognitive impairment. Some may have principally anterograde memory impairments and aphasia signs, whereas others manifest retrograde memory loss and disorientation. Although it has not yet been clearly proven with prospective studies, it is likely that these patchy deficits are linked to infarctions that affect either localized brain regions and their respective cognitive functions or networks of functions. Since single infarctions have been clearly demonstrated to have specific consequences, multiple infarctions may induce multiple independent deficits or cause a cascade of insults to the same system, leading to gross impairments (Fisher 1982).

Because vascular dementia is quite heterogeneous, the location of the infarctions is probably related, in general, to the specific types of cognitive impairment seen. For instance, a dementia with prominent deficits in language functions would implicate strokes in the left hemisphere, including the temporal and frontal lobes, whereas increasing impairments in memory would implicate the hippocampus, medial temporal lobe, or entorhinal cortex. Many strokes affect the middle cerebral artery, which is particularly vulnerable because of its large size and high blood volume. This type of stroke causes the classic presentation of initial fluent and nonfluent aphasia, hemiparesis resolving to hemiplegia, and limited deficits in attention and memory. In contrast, prominent deficits in spatial-constructional functions would implicate a largely posterior focus of stroke, and a stroke with depression and reductions in performance of motor tests would implicate a subcortical focus (Erkinjuntti 1987). Infarctions can be concentrated in subcortical regions or in cortical regions, leading to syndromes that are marked primarily by deficits in cortical or subcortical functions. For instance, cortical syndromes may be marked by aphasia or disorientation, and subcortical syndromes marked by pseudo-parkinsonian features such as slow thinking (bradyphrenia) and slow movements (bradykinesia).

One of the assessment concerns involved is the progression of impairment from initial focused syndromes involving single deficits (typically aphasia from a single infarction) to a more generalized syndrome involving memory impairments and global dementia (Chui 1989). Most research suggests that a steadily progressive course is the best discriminator of Alzheimer's disease from vascular dementia and that identifiable vascular events are present at the time of development of additional cognitive impairments after initial diagnosis (Meyer et al. 1986; Molsa et al. 1982, 1985). The classic definition of multi-infarct dementia involved a "stepwise progression" (Hachinski et al. 1974). In fact, some studies note slight improvement in cognitive functions after the development of dementia, if the underlying vascular pathology is brought under control (Hershey et al. 1986). Thus, progression in vascular dementia is actually a function of the underlying vascular pathology and is often eliminated by aggressive treatment of the underlying pathology, often hypertension, after the patient comes to clinical attention (Cummings 1987).

A final issue in vascular dementia is whether a subtype of vascular dementia that is not related to discrete cerebral infarction can exist. Early conceptions of vascular contributions to dementia focused on "hardening of the arteries," meaning that narrowing (i.e., stenosis) of arteries caused by atherosclerosis was believed to reduce cerebral blood flow, causing chronic hypoxia and hence dementia. There appears to be little reason to believe that this type of process is actually a potential cause of dementia. Thus, vascular dementia is associated with a variety of cognitive impairments that are probably linked to the locations of multiple infarctions (Liston and LaRue 1983).

Binswanger's disease.   The basal ganglia and thalamus (deep gray matter nuclei) and deep white matter of the brain are fed by small vessels that stem from larger arteries. These small vessels are vulnerable to the effects of arteriosclerosis, which can produce ischemia, or hypoperfusion, leading to dementia. Such small-vessel disease is generally referred to as Binswanger's disease. Relatively little is known about the neuropsychological profile of this condition, which has been defined as numerous lacunae in the basal ganglia, pons, and white matter of the brain. Most studies have focused on overall impairments characterized by frontal-lobe-localized functions (e.g., Corbett et al. 1994).

Binswanger's disease is a gradually progressive syndrome characterized clinically by dementia and motor system abnormalities and pathologically by ischemic demyelination in the deep white matter of the cerebral hemispheres. The dementia syndrome produced by Binswanger's disease results from injury to subcortical hemispheric structures and has the clinical presentation of a subcortical dementia. Binswanger's disease is characterized by markedly enlarged ventricles with diffuse subcortical white matter lesions. Dementia results when demyelination and infarction occur in multiple areas of the cerebral white matter, as well as in the basal ganglia and thalamus in many cases.

Although Binswanger's disease was long believed to be a relatively rare condition, this perception has changed with the introduction of magnetic resonance imaging (MRI) as a principal imaging modality in many medical centers. Hyperintensities in the periventricular white matter have been seen in healthy individuals but are more common in older individuals with cardiovascular risk factors (see Rao 1996 for a comprehensive reference list). These lesions, or hyperintensities, have been called UBOs (unidentified bright objects) or leukoaraiosis (thinning of the white matter)(Hachinski et al. 1987). Roman (1987) suggested that these lesions occur in the initial stages of Binswanger's disease and that the severity of cognitive impairment depends on the extent of the leukoaraiosis.

Neuropsychological findings in Binswanger's disease are not clearly delineated in the literature. Generally, Binswanger's disease has been presumed to be most similar to a subcortical dementing picture, with relative sparing of memory functioning (Bennett et al. 1994). Several studies reported by Bennett et al. (1994) found that patients with Alzheimer's disease had greater impairment in episodic memory than patients with Binswanger's disease, who in turn had greater impairment than control subjects without Binswanger's disease. Alzheimer's disease and Binswanger's disease patients showed equal impairment on semantic memory tasks. Bernard et al. (1992) reached similar conclusions, confirming that Alzheimer's disease and Binswanger's disease patients show comparable impairment on memory tests, whereas patients with Binswanger's disease show less impairment on verbal recognition memory tests than do Alzheimer's disease patients. Another study revealed that Binswanger's disease patients performed worse than patients with Alzheimer's disease on a measure of abstraction and conceptual problem solving, consistent with a frontal-deficit, subcortical dementia picture (Bernard et al. 1990). Libon et al. (1997) reported similar findings in their paper on dementia associated with periventricular and deep white matter alterations, such as that found in Binswanger's disease. Their research also confirmed differences in performance on memory tests between patients with Alzheimer's disease and those with Binswanger's disease, with the Binswanger's disease patients more likely to benefit from saturation cuing than Alzheimer's disease patients.

In summary, Binswanger's disease is diagnosed when criteria for vascular dementia are met: dementia, cerebrovascular disease manifested by focal neurological signs and abnormalities on computed tomography (CT) or MRI and a relation between the dementia and the cerebrovascular disease marked by onset within 3 months of a recognized stroke or abrupt onset, and fluctuation or stepwise progression of cognitive deficits (Roman et al. 1993). Relative to Alzheimer's disease, Binswanger's disease is associated with less profound deficits in memory, more impairment in executive functioning, more depressive psychopathology, more apathy, and a more variable course of decline (Bennett et al. 1994).

Assessment of vascular dementias.   In contrast to other dementias, vascular dementia is expected to be extremely heterogeneous. No common assessment battery exists for vascular dementias. Two options include either use of a full neuropsychological assessment battery, with the risk of not being able to finish the assessment on certain patients, or use of neuroimaging, subjective complaints, and observations of the patient to examine the level of magnitude of various noted cognitive impairments with selected tests. The risk of the second approach is the possibility of missing deficits that cannot be reported by the patient or that have simply not yet been noted. Neither approach is optimal, but our general tendency, despite our general bias in the direction of selective assessment, is to use a broad-ranging assessment battery.

As noted above, the course of illness may be the best discriminator between vascular dementia and Alzheimer's disease. Consistent progression argues against vascular dementia, unless additional vascular events occur. As noted above, the absence of agnosia can be an indicator of vascular dementia, as can be the presence of gait disturbance. In general, however, a presentation with clear vascular events and patchy cognitive deficits within an individual may be the best "single-case indicator." Follow-up assessment, with evaluation of intervening vascular events, is the best strategy for differential diagnosis.

Aging in Psychiatric Conditions

Many recent studies of late-life psychiatric conditions have focused on illness that has its onset in late life (see Jeste 1993). These illnesses are of considerable interest, because they affect individuals who have no lifelong history of psychiatric disturbance. Most individuals with late-onset serious psychiatric conditions manifest depressive disorders, but significant numbers of individuals manifest psychotic disorders with late-life onset (Harris and Jeste 1988). Because many progressive dementing conditions have both psychotic and depressive symptoms (Greenwald et al. 1989), a crucial question is whether the psychiatric syndrome seen is actually a component of the presentation of some dementing condition, such as DFT, Huntington's disease, or some atypical variant of Alzheimer's disease or Parkinson's disease. As noted above, all of these dementias may have a prominent psychiatric component. Because several studies have suggested that late-onset psychiatric conditions are not typically accompanied by profound cognitive impairments, a cognitive assessment is a crucial differential diagnostic procedure in these cases. This is an important issue, and readers are referred to two studies that address this issue in some detail (Greenwald et al. 1989; J. Rosen and Zubenko 1991).

Based on anecdotal reports and studies of highly selected populations, the belief has been propagated that early-onset psychiatric conditions are generally "burned out" in the later stages of life (e.g., Harding et al.

1987). In contrast, several recent studies have indicated that geriatric psychiatric patients who have had a particularly chronic course of illness manifest continued positive and negative symptoms of schizophrenia, as well as manifesting severe cognitive impairments and meeting diagnostic criteria for dementia (Arnold et al. 1994; Davidson et al. 1995). These severe cognitive impairments have largely been reported in patients with chronic schizophrenia, although a recent study suggested that a substantial proportion of patients who have a lifelong history of cyclical bipolar disorder also show signs of gross cognitive impairment in later life (McKay et al. 1995).

A natural question that arises is whether the severe cognitive impairment seen in inpatients with a chronic course of schizophrenia or affective psychosis is "simply" a manifestation of the development of a degenerative condition such as Alzheimer's disease or the onset of symptoms from vascular pathology. An initial report indicated that the prevalence of Alzheimer's disease–like pathology in brains of individuals with schizophrenia was increased (Prohovnik et al. 1993). Later studies with prospective methodology indicated that the presence of either vascular pathology or Alzheimer's disease–like neuropathological changes cannot be the sole cause of these gross cognitive impairments in these chronically ill psychiatric patients (Arnold et al. 1993; Powchik et al. 1993; Purohit et al. 1993). In addition, several other studies examining cognitive functioning have found that the presentation of geriatric chronically institutionalized patients 1) does not resemble the cognitive impairments seen in typical dementing conditions such as Alzheimer's disease (Davidson et al. 1996; Harvey et al. 1996; Heaton et al. 1994) and 2) resembles an exaggerated version of the cognitive impairments seen in younger patients with schizophrenia (Harvey et al. 1993, 1995).

For example, in a study examining the classic cognitive impairments seen in Alzheimer's disease, 302 schizophrenic patients ranging in age from 26 to 98 were tested, and their performance on the indicators of dementia was compared across subgroups of patients formed on the basis of MMSE scores (Harvey et al. 1996). In contrast to the pattern of impairments in memory seen in Alzheimer's disease, in which delayed recall performance is impaired early in the illness and is not correlated with MMSE scores, MMSE scores were linearly associated with delayed recall in the patients with schizophrenia. No patterns of differential progression were noted for any of the cognitive impairments, suggesting a roughly linear course. In a study directly comparing the performance of patients with Alzheimer's disease with the performance of younger and older patients with schizophrenia, deficits in delayed recall were considerably more severe in those with Alzheimer's disease (Heaton et al. 1994). This finding was replicated in a study in which patients with Alzheimer's disease and patients with schizophrenia were matched on MMSE scores and compared across the various cognitive skill areas that are affected by Alzheimer's disease (Davidson et al. 1996). Despite the groups' being matched on MMSE, the patients with Alzheimer's disease were more impaired in delayed recall, the patients with schizophrenia were more impaired in naming and praxic performance, and the groups did not differ in their rate of learning. These data highlight both the profound recall memory deficits in Alzheimer's disease and the high level of cognitive impairment seen in many geriatric chronically hospitalized schizophrenic patients. These patterns of differential cognitive impairment demonstrate that global cognitive impairment on the part of patients with schizophrenia cannot be used to explain these results.

In terms of the characteristics of the cognitive impairments in geriatric patients with chronic schizophrenia, two recent studies suggested that the deficits in geriatric patients who have low MMSE scores are exacerbated versions of the cognitive impairment seen in less impaired geriatric patients and in younger schizophrenic patients. Two studies specifically examined the memory performance of geriatric patients with schizophrenia. In the first study, patients with CDR scores of 2.0 (moderate) were compared with patients with CDR scores in the mild to unimpaired range on a battery of memory tests that had been found to identify memory impairments in younger patients with schizophrenia (Harvey et al. 1995). Deficits in spatial working memory and in practice-related learning independently discriminated between the more impaired and the less impaired patients, with the less impaired patients performing no more poorly than younger patients studied in previous investigations. In a study comparing geriatric and nongeriatric patients on procedural learning (Schwartz et al. 1996), no age-related changes were found in aspects of performance that are generally considered to be modestly impaired in schizophrenia. Thus, aging in schizophrenia is not associated with the development of new memory impairments not seen in younger patients, but rather with an increase in the severity of the type of impairment seen in patients with chronic schizophrenia much earlier in life.

The study of cognitive functioning in late-life schizophrenia is still developing. As a result, this is an area in which considerable advances should be expected in the future, on the basis of the work of several different investigative teams focusing on this topic. Perhaps the most important finding to date, however, is that cognitive impairments in schizophrenia can progress late in life in a manner above and beyond that seen in normal aging. Whether this is simply the interactive result of normal age-related changes in a compromised brain system or whether it reflects some yet unidentified neurodegenerative process is the principal question to be addressed by this research area. Although it is too early to recommend a specific assessment battery for these conditions, the bulk of the evidence suggests that assessment of memory functions is crucial, as is an assessment of the prototypical cognitive impairments seen in younger patients with schizophrenia (e.g., executive functions, fluency, concentration, and attention). Profound deficits in delayed recall were previously absent in geriatric patients with chronic schizophrenia, in both outpatient (Heaton et al. 1994) and inpatient (Harvey et al. 1995) samples.

◈ COMPARISON ACROSS DEMENTING CONDITIONS

Table 8–1 presents the type of performance profiles seen across the different dementing conditions described in this chapter. Note that in some cases these characterizations may be imprecise, such as in the case of vascular dementia, in which variability in performance is the norm. For other conditions, the comparisons are based on patients with moderate-severity global dementia, because in severe cortical dementia, profound impairments exist in essentially every domain of cognitive functioning, and the causes may be nonspecific.

◈ CONCLUSION

Cognitive assessment has a crucial role in the diagnosis and treatment of dementia. In the current care climate, neuropsychological assessment should be focused and selective. We have adopted this perspective in preparing this chapter. The study of dementia has expanded considerably in the past few years, and the level of new findings is reflected in the length of this chapter despite our goal of providing a simple overview. Clinicians must carefully monitor new developments in the treatment of dementia and its biological substrates and should adjust their assessment strategies accordingly. When assessing rare dementias or cognitive impair-

Table 8–1. Comparative profiles of cognitive impairment across the dementias

Cognitive area	Alzheimer's disease	Frontal type dementia	Huntington's disease	Parkinson's disease	HIV dementia	Vascular dementia
Attention	+	++	++	+	+	Variable
Primary memory	++	+	+	–	–	Variable
Learning/encoding	++	++	++	+	–	+
Recall memory (retrieval)	++	+	+	+	+	+
Recognition memory	++	–	–	–	–	Variable
Executive functions	++	++	++	+	+	Variable
Psychomotor speed	++	–	++	++	++	Variable
Visuomotor performance	++	+	++	++	++	Variable
Verbal fluency	++	+	+	+/?	+	Variable
Confrontation naming	++	+	–	–/?	–	Variable
Spatial functions	++	–	–	+/?	–/?	Variable

Note. ++ = very impaired; + = impaired; – = not impaired; ? = questionable or inconsistent.

ment of unknown origin, clinicians are encouraged to use a broader assessment than when simply evaluating the severity of impairment in patients with known dementia. In these cases, clinicians must determine the patient's premorbid level of functioning to avoid misdiagnosing dementia in cases of lifelong low achievement.

◈ REFERENCES

Agid Y: Parkinson's disease: pathophysiology. Lancet 337:1321–1324, 1991

Albert MS, Moss MB: Geriatric Neuropsychology. New York, Guilford, 1988

American Psychiatric Association: Diagnostic and Statistical Manual of Mental Disorders, 4th Edition. Washington, DC, American Psychiatric Association, 1994

Army Individual Test Battery: Manual of Directions and Scoring. Washington, DC, War Department, Adjutant General's Office, 1944

Arnold SE, Franz BR, Trojanowski JQ: Lack of neuropathological findings in elderly patients with schizophrenia and dementia. Neuroscience Abstracts 19: 349–350, 1993

Arnold SE, Franz BR, Trojanowski JQ: Elderly patients with schizophrenia exhibit infrequent neurodegenerative lesions. Neurobiol Aging 15:299–303, 1994

Arriagada PV, Marzloff K, Hyman BT: Distribution of Alzheimer-type pathologic changes in nondemented elderly individuals matches the pattern in Alzheimer's disease. Neurology 42:1681–1688, 1992

Bayles KA: Dementia: the clinical perspective. Semin Speech Lang 9:149–165, 1988

Bayles KA, Tomoeda CK: Confrontation naming impairment in dementia. Brain Lang 19:98–114, 1983

Bayles KA, Tomoeda CK, Kaszniak AW, et al: Verbal perseveration of dementia patients. Brain Lang 25:102–116, 1985

Bennett DA, Gilley DW, Lee S, et al: White matter changes: neurobehavioral manifestations of Binswanger's disease and clinical correlates in Alzheimer's disease. Dementia 5:148–152, 1994

Benton AL, Hamsher K des, Varney NR, et al: Contributions to Neuropsychological Assessment. New York, Oxford University Press, 1983

Berg G, Edwards DF, Danzinger WL, et al: Longitudinal change in three brief assessments of SDAT. J Am Geriatr Soc 35:205–212, 1987

Berg L: Clinical dementia rating (CDR). Psychopharmacol Bull 24:637–639, 1988

Bernard BA, Wilson RS, Gilley DW, et al: Performance of patients with BD and AD on the Mattis Dementia Rating Scale (abstract). J Clin Exp Neuropsychol 12:22, 1990

Bernard BA, Wilson RS, Gilley DW, et al: Memory failure in Binswanger's disease and Alzheimer's disease. The Clinical Neuropsychologist 6:230–240, 1992

Boller F, Passafiume D, Keefe NC, et al: Visuospatial impairments in Parkinson's disease: role of perceptual and motor factors. Arch Neurol 41:485–490, 1984

Bondi MW, Kaszniak AW, Bayles KA, et al: Contributions of frontal system dysfunction to memory and perceptual abilities in Parkinson's disease. Neuropsychology 1:89–102, 1993

Bowen FP, Kamienny RS, Burns MM, et al: Parkinsonism: effects of levodopa treatment on concept formation. Neurology 25:701–704, 1975

Brandt J, Butters N: The neuropsychology of Huntington's disease. Trends Neurosci 9:118–120, 1986

Brouwers P, Cox C, Martin A, et al: Differential spatial-perceptual impairments in Huntington's and Alzheimer's dementias. Arch Neurol 41:1073–1076, 1984

Brown RG, Marsden CD: Internal versus external cues and the control of attention in Parkinson's disease. Brain 111:323–345, 1988

Brun A: Frontal lobe degeneration of non-Alzheimer type, I: neuropathology. Archives of Gerontology and Geriatrics 6:193–208, 1987

Bylsma FW, Brandt J, Strauss ME: Aspects of procedural memory are differentially impaired in Huntington's disease. Archives of Clinical Neuropsychology 5:287–297, 1990

Bylsma FW, Brandt J, Strauss ME: Personal and extrapersonal orientation in Huntington's disease patients and those at risk. Cortex 28:113–122, 1992

Caine ED, Ebert MH, Weingartner H: An outline for the analysis of dementia: the memory disorder of Huntington's disease. Neurology 27:1087–1092, 1977

Center for Public Management and Policy Working Party on Efficacy of Medicinal Products: Antidementia Medicinal Products. Brussels, Commission of the European Communities, November 1992

Chui HC: Dementia: a review emphasizing clinicopathological correlation and brain-behavior relationship. Arch Neurol 46:806–814, 1989

Claypoole K, Townes B, Collier A, et al: Neuropsychological aspects of early HIV infection. Presented at the 18th annual International Neuropsychological Society Conference, Orlando, FL, February 1990

Corbett AJ, Bennett H, Kos S: Cognitive dysfunction following subcortical infarction. Arch Neurol 51:999–1007, 1994

Crawford JR, Besson JAO, Parker DM: Estimation of premorbid intelligence in organic conditions. Br J Psychiatry 153:178–181, 1988a

Crawford JR, Stewart LE, Garthwaite PH, et al: The relationship between demographic variables and NART performance in normal subjects. Br J Clin Psychol 27:181–182, 1988b

Crawford JR, Parker DM, Stewart LE, et al: Prediction of WAIS IQ with the NART: a cross-validation and extension. Br J Clin Psychol 28:267–273, 1989

Cummings JL: Subcortical dementia: neuropsychology, neuropsychiatry, and pathophysiology. Br J Psychiatry 149:682–697, 1986

Cummings JL: Multi-infarct dementia: diagnosis and management. Psychosomatics 28:117–126, 1987

Cummings JL, Benson DF: Dementia: A Clinical Approach. 2nd Edition. Boston, MA, Butterworths-Heinemann, 1983

Cummings JL, Benson DF: Speech and language alterations in dementia syndromes, in Brain Organization of Language and Cognitive Processes. Edited by Ardila A, Ostrosky-Solis F. New York, Plenum, 1989, pp 107–120

Cummings JL, Benson DF: Subcortical mechanisms and human thought, in Subcortical Dementia. Edited by Cummings JL. New York, Oxford University Press, 1990, pp 251–259

Davidson M, Harvey PD, Powchik P, et al: Severity of symptoms in geriatric schizophrenic patients. Am J Psychiatry 152:197–207, 1995

Davidson M, Harvey P, Welsh KA, et al: Cognitive functioning in late-life schizophrenia: a comparison of elderly schizophrenic patients and patients with Alzheimer's disease. Am J Psychiatry 153:1274–1279, 1996

Delis D, Kramer J, Fridlund A, et al: California Verbal Learning Test. San Antonio, TX, Psychological Corporation, 1986

Denning DW, Anderson J, Rudge P, et al: Acute myelopathy associated with primary infection with human immunodeficiency virus. BMJ 294:143–144, 1987

Dewhurst K, Oliver JE, McKnight AL: Sociopsychiatric consequences of Huntington's disease. Br J Psychiatry 116:255–258, 1970

El-Awar M, Becker JT, Hammond KM, et al: Learning deficit in Parkinson's disease: comparison with Alzheimer's disease and normal aging. Arch Neurol 44:180–184, 1987

Erkinjuntti T: Types of multi-infarct dementia. Acta Neurol Scand 75:391–399, 1987

Evans DA, Funkenstein HH, Albert MS, et al: Prevalence of Alzheimer's disease in a community population of older persons. JAMA 262:2551–2556, 1989

Fedio P, Cox CS, Neophytides A, et al: Neuropsychological profile of Huntington's disease, in Advances in Neurology, Vol 23: Huntington's Disease. Edited by Chase TN, Wexler NS, Barbeau A. New York, Raven, 1979, pp 239–255

Fisher CM: Lacunar strokes and infarcts: a review. Neurology 32:871–876, 1982

Folstein MF, Folstein SE, McHugh PR: Mini-Mental State: a practical method for grading the cognitive state of patients for the clinician. J Psychiatr Res 12: 189–198, 1975

Folstein SE: Huntington's Disease: A Disorder of Families. Baltimore, MD, Johns Hopkins University Press, 1989

Franzblau A, Letz R, Hershman D, et al: Quantitative neurologic and neurobehavioral testing of persons infected with human immunodeficiency virus type 1. Arch Neurol 48:263–268, 1991

Freedman M: Object alternation and orbitofrontal system dysfunction in Alzheimer's and Parkinson's disease. Brain Cogn 14:134–143, 1990

Gainotti G, Caltagirone C, Massullo C, et al: Patterns of neuropsychologic impairment in various diagnostic groups of dementia, in Aging of Brain and Dementia. Edited by Amaducci L, Davison AN, Antvono P. New York, Raven, 1980, pp 245–250

Goethe KE, Mitchell JE, Marshall DW, et al: Neuropsychological and neurological function of human immunodeficiency virus seropositive asymptomatic individuals. Arch Neurol 46:129–133, 1989

Golden JC: Stroop Color and Word Test. Chicago, IL, Stoelting, 1978

Goodglass H, Kaplan E: Boston Naming Test. Boston, MA, Lea & Febiger, 1983a

Gordon WP, Illes J: Neurolinguistic characteristics of language production in Huntington's disease: a preliminary report. Brain Lang 31:1–10, 1987

Grant I, Atkinson J, Hesselink J, et al: Evidence of early central nervous system involvement in the acquired immunodeficiency syndrome (AIDS) and other human immunodeficiency virus (HIV) infections. Ann Intern Med 107:828–836, 1987

Greenwald BS, Kramer-Ginzberg E, Marin DB, et al: Dementia with coexistent depression. Am J Psychiatry 146:1472–1478, 1989

Grossman M, Carvell S, Peltzer L, et al: Visual construction impairments in Parkinson's disease. Neuropsychology 4:536–547, 1993

Grossman M, Stern MB, Gollomp S, et al: Verb learning in Parkinson's disease. Neuropsychology 3:413–423, 1994

Gurd JM, Ward DD: Retrieval from semantic and letter-initial categories in patients with Parkinson's disease. Neuropsychologia 27:743–746, 1989

Gustafson L: Frontal lobe degeneration of non-Alzheimer type, II: clinical picture and differential diagnosis. Archives of Gerontology and Geriatrics 6:209–223, 1987

Gustafson L, Brun A, Risberg J: Frontal lobe dementia of the non-Alzheimer type, in Advances in Neurology, Vol 51: Alzheimer's Disease. Edited by Wurtman RJ. New York, Raven, 1990, pp 65–71

Hachinski VC, Lassen NA, Marshall J: Multi-infarct dementia: a cause of mental deterioration in the elderly. Lancet 2:207–209, 1974

Hachinski VC, Potter P, Merskey H: Leuko-araiosis. Arch Neurol 44:21–23, 1987

Harding CM, Brooks GW, Ashikaga T, et al: The Vermont longitudinal study of persons with severe mental illness, II: long term outcome of subjects who retrospectively met DSM-III criteria for schizophrenia. Am J Psychiatry 144:727–735, 1987

Harris MJ, Jeste DV: Late-onset schizophrenia: an overview. Schizophr Bull 14:39–55, 1988

Harvey PD, Davidson M, Mohs RC: Leukotomy and aging in chronic schizophrenia: a followup study 40 years after psychosurgery. Schizophr Bull 12:723–732, 1993

Harvey PD, Powchik P, Mohs RC, et al: Memory functions in geriatric schizophrenic inpatients: a neuropsychological Study. J Neuropsychiatry Clin Neurosci 7:207–212, 1995

Harvey PD, Lombardi J, Leibman M, et al: Performance of geriatric chronic schizophrenic patients on cognitive neuropsychological measures sensitive to dementia. Int J Geriatr Psychiatry 11:621–627, 1996

Heaton RK, Chelune GJ, Talley JL, et al: Wisconsin Card Sorting Test (WCST) Manual—Revised and Expanded. Odessa, FL, Psychological Assessment Resources, 1993

Heaton RK, Paulsen JS, McAdams LA, et al: Neuropsychological deficits in schizophrenics: relationship to age, chronicity, and dementia. Arch Gen Psychiatry 51:469–476, 1994

Heindel WC, Salmon DP, Butters N: Pictorial priming and cued recall in Alzheimer's and Huntington's disease. Brain Cogn 13:282–295, 1990

Helkala EL, Laulumaa V, Soininen H, et al: Recall and recognition memory in patients with Alzheimer's and Parkinson's diseases. Ann Neurol 24:214–217, 1988

Hershey LA, Modic MT, Jaffe DF, et al: Natural history of the vascular dementias: a prospective study of seven cases. Can J Neurol Sci 13:559–565, 1986

Ho D, Rota D, Schooley R, et al: Isolation of HTLV-III from cerebrospinal fluid and neural tissue of patients with neurologic syndromes related to the acquired immunodeficiency syndrome. N Engl J Med 313:1493–1497, 1985

Horne DJ: Sensorimotor control in parkinsonism. J Neurol Neurosurg Psychiatry 36:742–746, 1973

Huber SJ, Shuttleworth EC: Neuropsychological assessment of subcortical dementia, in Subcortical Dementia. Edited by Cummings JL. New York, Oxford University Press, 1990, pp 71–86

Huber SJ, Shuttleworth EC, Christy JA, et al: Magnetic resonance imaging in dementia of Parkinson's disease. J Neurol Neurosurg Psychiatry 52:1221–1227, 1989a

Huber SJ, Shuttleworth EC, Freidenberg DL: Neuropsychological differences between the dementias of Alzheimer's and Parkinson's diseases. Arch Neurol 46:1287–1291, 1989b

Huff FJ, Growdon JH, Corkin S, Rosen TJ: Age at onset and rate of progression of Alzheimer's disease. J Am Geriatr Soc 35:27–30, 1987

Janssen R, Saykin J, Cannon L, et al: Neurologic and neuropsychologic manifestations of human immunodeficiency virus (HIV-1) infection: association with AIDS-related complex but not asymptomatic HIV-1 infection. Ann Neurol 26:592–600, 1989

Jeste DV: Late life schizophrenia: editor's introduction. Schizophr Bull 19: 687–689, 1993

Kaszniak AW, Poon LW, Riege WL: Assessing memory deficits: an information-processing approach, in Clinical Memory Assessment of Older Adults. Edited by Poon LW. Washington, DC, American Psychological Association, 1986, pp 277–284

Katzman R: The prevalence and malignancy of Alzheimer's disease: a major killer. Arch Neurol 33:217–218, 1976

Katzman R: Alzheimer's disease. N Engl J Med 314:964–973, 1986

Khachaturian ZS: Diagnosis of Alzheimer's disease. Arch Neurol 42:1097–1105, 1985

Knopman DS, Christensen KJ, Schut LJ, et al: The spectrum of neuroimaging and neuropsychological functions in Pick's disease. Neurology 39:362–368, 1989

Knopman DS, Mastri AR, Frey WH, et al: Dementia lacking distinctive histologic features: a common non-Alzheimer degenerative dementia. Neurology 40: 251–256, 1990

Kokkevi A, Hatzakis A, Maillis A, et al: Neuropsychological assessment of HIV-seropositive haemophiliacs. AIDS 5:1223–1229, 1991

Koller WC: Disturbance of recent memory function in Parkinsonian patients on anticholinergic therapy. Cortex 20:307–311, 1984a

Koller WC: Sensory symptoms in Parkinson's disease. Neurology 34:957–959, 1984b

Kramer JH, Delis DC, Blusewicz MJ, et al: Verbal memory errors in Alzheimer's and Huntington's dementias. Developmental Neuropsychology 4:1–15, 1988

Lanska DJ, Lanska MJ, Lavine L, et al: Conditions associated with Huntington's disease at death, a case-control study. Arch Neurol 45:878–880, 1988

Levin BE: Spatial cognition in Parkinson's disease. Alzheimer Dis Assoc Disord 4: 161–170, 1990

Levin BE, Llabre MM, Weiner WJ: Cognitive impairments associated with early Parkinson's disease. Neurology 39:557–561, 1989

Levin BE, Llabre MM, Reisman S, et al: Visuospatial impairment in Parkinson's disease. Neurology 41:365–369, 1991

Levy RM, Bredesen DE, Rosenblum ML: Neurological manifestations of the acquired immunodeficiency syndrome (AIDS): experience at UCSF and review of the literature. J Neurosurg 62:475–495, 1985

Lezak MD: Neuropsychological Assessment, 3rd Edition. New York, Oxford University Press, 1995

Libon DJ, Bogdanoff B, Bonavita J, et al: Dementia associated with periventricular and deep white matter alterations: a subtype of subcortical dementia. Archives of Clinical Neuropsychology 12:239–250, 1997

Liston EH, LaRue A: Clinical differentiation of primary degenerative and multi-infarct dementia: a critical review of the evidence, part II: pathological studies. Biol Psychiatry 18:1467–1484, 1983

Lundervold AJ, Karlsen NR, Reinvang I: Assessment of subcortical dementia in patients with Huntington's disease, Parkinson's disease, multiple sclerosis and AIDS by a neuropsychological screening battery. Scand J Psychol 35:48–55, 1994a

Lundervold AJ, Reinvang I, Lundervold A: Characteristic patterns of verbal memory function in patients with Huntington's disease. Scand J Psychol 35:38–47, 1994b

Lyle OE, Gottesman II: Premorbid psychometric indicators of the gene for Huntington's disease. J Consult Clin Psychol 45:1011–1022, 1977

Martin JB: Huntington's disease: new approaches to an old problem. Neurology 34:1059–1072, 1984

Maruff P, Currie J, Malone V, et al: Neuropsychological characterization of the AIDS dementia complex and rationalization of a test battery. Arch Neurol 51:689–695, 1994

Massman PJ, Delis DC, Butters N, et al: Are all subcortical dementias alike? Verbal learning and memory in Parkinson's and Huntington's disease patients. J Clin Exp Neuropsychol 12:729–744, 1990

Mattis S: Mental status exam for organic mental syndrome in the elderly patient, in Geriatric Psychiatry. Edited by Bellack L, Karasu TB. New York, Grune & Stratton, 1976, pp 77–121

McGeer PL, McGeer EG, Suzuki JS: Aging and extrapyramidal function. Arch Neurol 34:33–35, 1977

McKay AP, Tarbuck AF, Spapleske J, et al: Neuropsychological functions in manic-depressive psychosis: evidence of chronic persistent deficits in patients with chronic, severe illness. Br J Psychiatry 167:51–57, 1995

McKhann G, Drachman D, Folstein M, et al: Clinical diagnosis of Alzheimer's disease: report of the NINCDS-ADRDA Work Group under the auspices of Department of Health and Human Services Task Force on Alzheimer's disease. Neurology 34:939–944, 1984

Mendez MF: Huntington's disease: update and review of neuropsychiatric aspects. Int J Psychiatry Med 24:189–208, 1994

Metter EJ, Wilson RS: Vascular dementia, in Neuropsychology of Alzheimer's Disease and Related Disorders. Edited by Parks RW, Zec RF, Wilson RS. New York, Oxford University Press, 1993, pp 416–437

Meyer JS, Judd BW, Tawaklna T, et al: Improved cognition after control of risk factors for multi-infarct dementia. JAMA 256:2203–2209, 1986

Miller BL, Cummings JL, Villaneuve-Meyer J, et al: Frontal lobe degeneration: clinical neuropsychological, and SPECT characteristics. Neurology 41:1374–1382, 1991

Miller E, Selnes O, McArthur J, et al: Neuropsychological performance in HIV-1 infected homosexual men: the Multicenter AIDS Cohort Study (MACS). Neurology 40:197–203, 1990

Miller E, Satz P, Visscher B: Computerized and conventional neuropsychological assessment of HIV-1-infected homosexual men. Neurology 41:1608–1616, 1991

Mitrushina M, Satz P, Drebing C, et al: The differential pattern of memory deficit in normal aging and dementias of different etiology. J Clin Psychol 50:246–252, 1994

Mohr E, Brouwers P, Claus JJ, et al: Visuospatial cognition in Huntington's disease. Mov Disord 6:127–132, 1991

Mohs RC: Neuropsychological assessment of patients with Alzheimer's disease, in Psychopharmacology: The Fourth Generation of Progress. Edited by Bloom FE, Kupfer DJ. New York, Raven, 1995, pp 1377–1388

Molsa PK, Marttila RJ, Rinne UK: Epidemiology of dementia in a Finnish population. Acta Neurol Scand 86:541–552, 1982

Molsa PK, Paljarvi L, Rinne JO, et al: Validity of clinical diagnosis in dementia: a prospective clinicopathological study. J Neurol Neurosurg Psychiatry 48:1085–1090, 1985

Morris JC, Edland S, Clark C, et al: The Consortium to Establish a Registry for Alzheimer's Disease (CERAD), Part IV: Rates of cognitive change in the longitudinal assessment of probable Alzheimer's disease. Neurology 43:2457–2465, 1993

Morris M: Psychiatric aspects of Huntington's disease, in Huntington's Disease: Major Problems in Neurology. Edited by Harper PS. London, WB Saunders, 1991, pp 81–126

Neary D, Snowden JS: Dementia of the frontal lobe type, in Frontal Lobe Function and Dysfunction. Edited by Levin HS, Eisenberg HM, Benton AL. New York, Oxford University Press, 1991, pp 304–317

Neary D, Snowden JS, Northen B, et al: Dementia of the frontal lobe type. J Neurol Neurosurg Psychiatry 51:353–361, 1988

Nebes RD, Brady CB: Generalized cognitive slowing and severity of dementia in Alzheimer's disease: implications for the interpretation of response-time data. J Clin Exp Neuropsychol 14:317–326, 1992

Nebes RD, Madden DJ: Different patterns of cognitive slowing produced by Alzheimer's disease and normal aging. Psychol Aging 3:102–104, 1988

Nelson HE: NART: National Adult Reading Test: Test Manual. Windsor, Berks, UK, NFER-Nelson, 1982

O'Carroll RE, Baikie EM, Whittick JE: Does the NART hold in dementia? Br J Clin Psychol 26:315–316, 1987

Ollo C, Pass H: Neuropsychological performance in HIV disease: effect of depression and chronic CNS infection. Presented at the 16th annual meeting of the International Neuropsychological Society, New Orleans, LA, February 1988

Ollo C, Johnson R, Grafman J: Signs of cognitive change in HIV disease: an event-related brain potential study. Neurology 41:209–215, 1991

Pajeau AK, Roman GC: HIV encephalopathy and dementia. Psychiatr Clin North Am 15:455–466, 1992

Parkinson J: An Essay on the Shaking Palsy. London, Sherwood, Nely, and Jones, 1817

Paulsen JS, Salmon DP, Monsch A, et al: Discrimination of cortical from subcortical dementias on the basis of memory and problem-solving tests. J Clin Psychol 51:48–58, 1995a

Paulsen JS, Butters N, Sadek JR, et al: Distinct cognitive profiles of cortical and subcortical dementia in advanced illness. Neurology 45:951–956, 1995b

Perry S, Belsky-Barr D, Barr W, et al: Neuropsychological performance in physically asymptomatic, HIV seropositive men. J Neuropsychiatry Clin Neurosci 1:296–302, 1989

Pillon B, Dubois B, Lhermitte F, et al: Heterogeneity of cognitive impairment in progressive supranuclear palsy, Parkinson's disease, and Alzheimer's disease. Neurology 36:1179–1185, 1986

Pillon B, Deweer B, Agid Y, et al: Explicit memory in Alzheimer's, Huntington's, and Parkinson's disease. Arch Neurol 50:374–379, 1993

Pirozzolo FJ, Hansch EC, Mortimer JA, et al: Dementia in Parkinson's disease: a neuropsychological analysis. Brain Cogn 1:71–83, 1982

Podoll K, Caspary P, Lange HW, et al: Language functions in Huntington's disease. Brain 111:1475–1503, 1988

Poutiainen E, Iivanainen M, Elovaara I, et al: Cognitive changes as early signs of HIV infection. Acta Neurol Scand 78:49–52, 1988

Powchik P, Davidson M, Nemeroff CB, et al: Alzheimer's disease related protein in geriatric, cognitively impaired schizophrenic patients. Am J Psychiatry 50:1726–1727, 1993

Prohovnik I, Dwork AJ, Kaufman MA, et al: Alzheimer-type neuropathology in elderly schizophrenia. Schizophr Bull 19:805–816, 1993

Purohit DP, Davidson M, Perl DP, et al: Severe cognitive impairments in elderly schizophrenic patients: clinicopathologic study. Biol Psychiatry 33:255–260, 1993

Randolph C, Braun AR, Goldberg TE, et al: Semantic fluency in Alzheimer's, Parkinson's, and Huntington's disease: dissociation of storage and retrieval failures. Neuropsychology 1:82–88, 1993

Ransmayr G, Poewe W, Ploerer S, et al: Psychometric findings in clinical subtypes of Parkinson's disease. Adv Neurol 45:409–411, 1986

Rao SM: White matter disease and dementia. Brain Cogn 31:250–268, 1996

Rebok GW, Folstein MF: Dementia. J Neuropsychiatry Clin Neurosci 5:265–276, 1993

Reinvang I, Froland SS, Skripeland V: Prevalence of neuropsychological deficit in HIV infection: incipient signs of AIDS dementia complex in patients with AIDS. Acta Neurol Scand 83:289–293, 1991

Reitan RM, Wolfson D: The Halstead Reitan Neuropsychological Test Battery: Theory and Clinical Interpretation. Tucson, AZ, Neuropsychology Press, 1993

Rey A: L'examen psychologique dans les cas d'encephalopathie tramatique [The psychological exam in the cases of traumatic encephalopathy]. Archives de Psychologie 28:286–340, 1941

Roman GC: Senile dementia of the Binswanger type: a vascular form of dementia in the elderly. JAMA 258:1782–1788, 1987

Roman CG, Tatemichi TK, Erkinjuntti T, et al: Vascular dementia: diagnostic criteria for research studies: report of the NINDS-AIREN International Workshop. Neurology 43:250–260, 1993

Rosci MA, Pigorini F, Bernabei A, et al: Methods for detecting early signs of AIDS dementia complex in asymptomatic HIV-1-infected subjects. AIDS 6: 1309–1316, 1992

Rosen J, Zubenko GS: Emergence of psychosis and depression in the longitudinal evaluation of Alzheimer's disease. Biol Psychiatry 29:224–232, 1991

Rosen WG, Mohs RC, Davis KL: A new rating scale for Alzheimer's disease. Am J Psychiatry 141:1356–1364, 1984

Rothlind J, Brandt J: A brief assessment of frontal and subcortical functions in dementia. J Neuropsychiatry Clin Neurosci 5:73–77, 1993

Rothlind JC, Bylsma FW, Peyser C, et al: Cognitive and motor correlates of everyday functioning in early Huntington's disease. J Nerv Ment Dis 181:194–199, 1993

Rubinow D, Berettini C, Brouwers P, et al: Neuropsychiatric consequences of AIDS. Ann Neurol 23:S24–S26, 1988

Ruutu P, Suni J, Oksanen K, et al: Primary infection with HIV in a severely immunosuppressed patient with acute leukemia. Scand J Infect Dis 19:369–372, 1987

Salmon DP, Thal LJ, Butters N, et al: Longitudinal evaluation of dementia of the Alzheimer type: a comparison of 3 standardized mental status examinations. Neurology 40:1225–1230, 1990

Saugstad L, Odegard O: Huntington's chorea in Norway. Psychol Med 16:39–48, 1986

Saykin A, Janssen R, Sprehn G, et al: Neuropsychological dysfunction in HIV-infection: characterization in a lymphadenopathy cohort. International Journal of Clinical Neuropsychology 10:81–95, 1988

Schoenberg BS: Epidemiology of movement disorders, in Movement Disorders. Edited by Mardsen CD, Fahn S. Boston, MA, Butterworth Scientific, 1987, pp 17–32

Schwartz BL, Rosse RB, Veazey C, et al: Impaired motor skill learning in schizophrenia: implications for corticostriatal dysfunction. Biol Psychiatry 39: 234–240, 1996

Smith A: Symbol Digit Modalities Test: Manual. Los Angeles, CA, Western Psychological Services, 1982

Speedie LJ, Brake N, Folstein SE, et al: Comprehension of prosody in Huntington's disease. J Neurol Neurosurg Psychiatry 53:607–610, 1990

St-Cyr JA, Taylor AE, Lang AE: Procedural learning and neostriatal dysfunction in man. Brain 111:941–959, 1988

Stern Y, Mayeux R, Rosen J: Contribution of perceptual motor dysfunction to construction and tracing disturbances in Parkinson's disease. J Neurol Neurosurg Psychiatry 47:983–989, 1984

Stern Y, Sano M, Mayeux R: Comparisons of dementia and intellectual change in Parkinson's and Alzheimer's disease (abstract). J Clin Exp Neuropsychol 9: 66, 1987

Stern Y, Sano M, Williams J, et al: Neuropsychological consequences of HIV infection (abstract). J Clin Exp Neuropsychol 11:78, 1989

Stern Y, Marder K, Bell K, et al: Multidisciplinary baseline assessment of homosexual men with and without human immunodeficiency virus infection, III: neurologic and neuropsychological findings. Arch Gen Psychiatry 48:131–138, 1991

Stuss DT, Benson DF: The Frontal Lobes. New York, Raven, 1986

Sullivan EV, Sagar HJ: Nonverbal short-term memory impairment in Parkinson's disease (abstract). J Clin Exp Neuropsychol 10:34, 1988

Sullivan EV, Sagar HJ, Gabrieli JDE, et al: Different cognitive profiles on standard behavioral tests in Parkinson's disease and Alzheimer's disease. J Clin Exp Neuropsychol 11:799–820, 1989

Sullivan EV, Sagar HJ, Cooper JA, et al: Verbal and nonverbal short-term memory impairment in untreated Parkinson's disease. Neuropsychology 3:396–405, 1993

Taylor AE, Saint-Cyr JA, Lang AE: Idiopathic Parkinson's disease: revised concepts of cognitive and affective status. Can J Neurol Sci 15:106–113, 1988

Teri L, Rabins P, Whitehouse P, et al: Management of behavior disturbance in Alzheimer's disease: current knowledge and future directions. Alzheimer Dis Assoc Disord 6:77–88, 1992

Terry R, Katzman R: Alzheimer's disease and cognitive loss, in Principles of Geriatric Neurology. Edited by Katzman R, Rowe JW. Philadelphia, PA, FA Davis, 1992, pp 207–265

Thal LJ, Grundman M, Klauber MR: Dementia: characteristics of a referral population and factors associated with progression. Neurology 38:1083–1090, 1988

Tiffin J: Purdue Pegboard Examiner's Manual. Rosemont, IL, London House, 1968

Tross S, Price R, Navia B, et al: Neuropsychological characterization of the AIDS dementia complex: a preliminary report. AIDS 2:81–88, 1988

Van Gorp W, Miller EN, Satz P, et al: Neuropsychological performance in HIV-1 immunocompromised patients: a preliminary report. J Clin Exp Neuropsychol 11:763–773, 1989

Van Gorp W, Hinkin C, Satz P, et al: Neuropsychological findings in HIV infection, encephalopathy, and dementia, in Neuropsychology of Alzheimer's Disease and Other Dementias. Edited by Parks RW, Zec RF, Wilson RS. New York, Oxford University Press, 1993, pp 153–185

Villardita C, Smirni P, LePira F, et al: Mental deterioration, visuoperceptive disabilities and constructional praxis in Parkinson's disease. Acta Neurol Scand 66:112–120, 1982

Wechsler D: Wechsler Adult Intelligence Scale—Revised. San Antonio, TX, Psychological Corporation, 1981

Wechsler D: Wechsler Memory Scale—Revised. San Antonio, TX, Psychological Corporation, 1987

Wechsler D: Wechsler Adult Intelligence Scale—3rd Edition (WAIS-III). New York, Psychological Corporation, 1997a

Wechsler D: Wechsler Memory Scale—3rd Edition. New York, Psychological Corporation, 1997b

Weingartner HR, Eckart M, Grafman J, et al: The effects of repetition on memory performance in cognitively impaired patients. Neuropsychology 7:385–395, 1993

Welsh KA, Butters N, Hughes J, et al: Detection of abnormal memory decline in mild cases of Alzheimer's disease using CERAD neuropsychological measures. Arch Neurol 48:278–281, 1991

Welsh KA, Butters N, Hughes J, et al: Detection and staging of dementia in Alzheimer s disease: use of the neuropsychological measures developed for the Consortium to Establish a Registry for Alzheimer's disease (CERAD). Arch Neurol 49:448–452, 1992

Wilkie FL, Eisdorfer C, Morgan R, et al: Neuropsychological performance in asymptomatic HIV infection. Arch Neurol 147:433–440, 1990

Wilkinson GS: Wide Range Achievement Test—3rd Edition (WRAT-3). Wilmington, DE, Jastak Associates, 1993

World Health Organization: International Classification of Diseases, 10th Edition. Geneva, World Health Organization, 1992

Wright MJ, Burns RJ, Geffen GM, et al: Covert orientation of visual attention in Parkinson's disease: an impairment in the maintenance of attention. Neuropsychologia 28:151–159, 1990

Zec RF: Neuropsychological functioning in Alzheimer's disease, in Neuropsychology of Alzheimer's Disease and Related Disorders. Edited by Parks RW, Zec RF, Wilson RS. New York, Oxford University Press, 1993, pp 3–80

9

Neuropsychology and Neuroimaging of Alcohol and Illicit Drug Abuse

Marsha E. Bates, Ph.D., and Antonio Convit, M.D.

IN THIS CHAPTER, we review research aimed at determining whether and to what extent the chronic excessive use of alcohol and illicit psychoactive drugs is associated with neuropsychological impairment at behavioral, functional, and anatomical levels. Our aim is to provide an overview of the kinds of neuropsychological impairments found in persons with substance use disorders (compared with control subjects or normative data) and, whenever possible, to relate these abnormalities to findings from functional and structural brain imaging studies.

Preparation of this chapter was supported by grants AA 08747 and AA11594 from the National Institute on Alcohol Abuse and Alcoholism and grant DA/AA 03395 from the National Institute on Drug Abuse.

In the first section of the chapter, we outline the influence of subject characteristics on neuropsychological functioning and describe the methodological concerns common to studies of users of alcohol and other drugs. In the second section, we review the major neuropsychological impairments associated with the chronic excessive use of alcohol, cocaine, inhalants, opiates, phencyclidine, and marijuana, as well as polydrug use. We describe methodological issues peculiar to the study of specific drugs, as well as evidence for the recovery of brain and behavioral functioning with abstinence or reduced use. In the third section, we discuss the various risk factors that have been purported to increase vulnerability to use-related deficits. In the fourth section, we describe the relative merits of tests and assessment approaches used to delineate neurocognitive impairment in this population. In the final section, we discuss the relationship of neurocognitive impairment to treatment outcome and the implications for treatment planning with patients with substance use disorders. Research needs are identified, and new research directions are suggested within each section.

The literature on the chronic effects of alcohol is much more extensive than comparable literature on other drugs, partly because alcohol has a greater prevalence of use and it is used exclusively more often than other psychoactive drugs. Our review emphasizes the more extensive knowledge base on alcohol while also attempting to provide a comprehensive overview of the growing literature on other drugs of abuse. Methodological problems and knowledge gaps are identified.

The importance of increasing our understanding of the cognitive and neuropsychological deficits secondary to psychoactive substance use—as well as the brain substrate of substance users as seen through functional and structural imaging—is fourfold: 1) to tailor behavioral intervention strategies to the cognitive capacity of the individuals (see "Neurocognitive Deficit, Treatment Process, and Treatment Outcome" below); 2) to serve as an educational tool in treatment to impress upon individuals the need for discontinuation of use; 3) to monitor improvement and ascertain compliance with treatment; and 4) to improve our understanding of how associated behavior, such as violence, may be related to the use of drugs or be the result of the brain sequelae of use. Substance use and violence are clearly linked in different populations. Apart from the violence associated with the business of drug use, these associations are probably caused by both the pharmacological properties of psychoactive substances and the neurotoxic effects of chronic use on brain structure and function. By increasing our understanding of these functional alterations and their brain substrates, we may be in a better position to intervene and prevent other antisocial behavior.

Specific understanding of the brain sequelae of substance use disorders will provide clinicians with a powerful educational tool. When shared appropriately and sensitively, this knowledge will provide concrete reasons for some individuals in treatment to attempt to modify their use behavior. Moreover, as our understanding grows through further research, it may be possible to use such assessments to evaluate and reinforce compliance with treatment. At present, we know that brain damage secondary to substance abuse is at least partially reversible. New technologies, such as magnetic resonance diffusion imaging (which provides an estimate of the ability of water to move in tissues and thus measures "swelling" or "shrinking"), may be useful tools in the assessment of compliance with alcohol treatment. Although at present these technologies are not generally available clinically, this situation is likely to change in a few years.

◆ METHODOLOGICAL LIMITATIONS AND CONCERNS

Variance across studies in the control of relevant subject variables known to affect neurocognitive performance obscures understanding of the etiology of neuropsychological impairments and of individual differences in vulnerability to impairment. Most of these subject factors are not specific to the study of drug effects per se, but some have unique implications in this area.

Control of Subject Characteristics

Age. Performance levels on many behavioral tests (Lezak 1995), as well as brain structure (Convit et al. 1995) and function (De Santi et al. 1995), are substantially influenced by age. The behavioral consequences of brain damage typically increase with increasing age (Lezak 1995). Furthermore, the association between aging and brain atrophy may be stronger in chronic heavy drinkers than in the general population (Di Sciafani et al. 1995). Chronic heavy users of alcohol alone tend to be older than those who abuse other psychoactive drugs and to have longer use histories than other drug users. These "naturally" occurring and interrelated age and chronicity differences add to the difficulty in interpreting differences between the damage caused by alcohol and that caused by other drugs. The extent to which structural and functional resiliency may mask use-associated deficits in youthful substance abusers is unknown.

Gender.   Until recently, most studies of individuals with substance use disorders included only male subjects or had sample sizes too small to examine the performance of men and women separately. More attention has recently been focused on women, especially in alcohol research. Sample sizes often remain small, however, and both sexes are seldom tested in the same study. Recent study has begun to interpret sex differences in alcohol-related impairment within the context of gender-related differences in brain structure and function, although differences between individuals tend to be much larger than the average differences between genders (Lezak 1995).

Few studies have taken into account the lower rate of alcohol metabolism at the stomach lining in women (Yoshida 1993). For a given dose, more alcohol enters the blood of women, who thus achieve higher blood alcohol levels (BALs) more quickly than men. Women's increased rate of absorption and the higher BALs achieved may contribute to increased toxicity. Women develop liver disease with lower daily alcohol intake and shorter drinking histories than do men (Lancaster 1994). As a rule, women have smaller body mass than men, which contributes to sex differences in BALs and may increase overall burden on the target organs. Lack of attention to these gender-related differences when combining or contrasting data from men and women perhaps contributes to the unresolved literature on gender differences in neuropsychological vulnerability to alcohol effects and to the relation between duration of drinking and degree of damage.

Racial and ethnic group.   Performance on standardized tests may also be affected by cultural differences between racial groups (R. L. Adams et al. 1982; Helms 1992). Normative data on neuropsychological impairment rates in different racial groups are lacking (Drebing et al. 1994). In addition, different modes of use of various illicit drugs may not be distributed equally across different racial and sociodemographic groups, especially in circumscribed geographical regions proximal to active research laboratories (e.g., Beatty et al. 1995). To further complicate the issues related to race, there are well-known ethnic differences in the metabolism of alcohol (Yoshida 1993). Although no published studies show ethnic differences in the pharmacokinetics of other substances of abuse, an emerging body of literature indicates such differences in the handling of psychiatric medications (Lin et al. 1993), many of which share metabolic pathways with substances of abuse. Current National Institutes of Health (NIH) guidelines for the inclusion of women and ethnic minorities in federally funded research in the United States should enhance knowledge in these areas.

Education and premorbid intelligence. The potent effects of education in determining performance on many neuropsychological tests are usually well appreciated in substance use research. Even against a backdrop of extended substance use histories, educational differences significantly influence neuropsychological performance (Guerra et al. 1987). Unfortunately, individuals' premorbid levels of functioning are often unknown. This has continued to be particularly disruptive to understanding the neurocognitive effects of alcohol and other drugs. For example, the clinical impression is that abusers of phencyclidine and inhalants often have low premorbid levels of functioning, yet prospective data to test this hypothesis are lacking.

Actuarial estimates of premorbid IQ for Americans are possible with techniques such as Barona and colleagues' (1984) formula based on demographic characteristics. Such formulas are also available for the United Kingdom (Crawford et al. 1989). These estimates are thought to be more useful for subject matching in research (Knight and Longmore 1994) than for individual clinical applications (Sweet et al. 1990). Statistical control of IQ and education in the study of neuropsychological deficits associated with chronic substance use is problematic because of their interdependent influences (Dikmen et al. 1993). If neuropsychological abilities actively influence IQ and educational attainments throughout development, and if use-related neuropsychological deficits sometimes cause low educational attainments and/or IQ scores, then statistically controlling for these variables will attenuate the true relation between use behavior and neuropsychological test scores. In addition, although conceptual distinctions can be made between "intelligence" and neuropsychological competency, in practice the same tests (e.g., the Wechsler Adult Intelligence Scale—Revised [WAIS-R] and the Shipley Institute of Living Scale) (Wechsler 1981; Zachary 1986) are often used to measure both constructs (Benton 1994). A clearer understanding of the relation of premorbid functional levels to subsequent use-related impairment requires prospective study of subjects whose neurocognitive performance was assessed before they began excessive use.

Other characteristics. Other subject characteristics used as inclusion and exclusion criteria in neuropsychological research affect the generality and specificity of study results. In studies of the neurotoxic effects of alcohol, many researchers now routinely exclude those with a history of traumatic brain injury, concurrent psychiatric diagnoses, organic brain syndromes, and other medical conditions that commonly co-occur with chronic substance use and that in their own right may cause neurocognitive impairment. This practice provides more precise information about the neurotoxic effects of alcohol and other drugs separately from other etiological influences. The downside of this strategy is the lack of systematic information for clinicians regarding the range of neuropsychological impairment encountered in treatment settings, where individuals typically present with some of these other characteristics. Although it is important to separate the multiple etiologies of brain damage observed in chronic substance users, a more comprehensive research strategy would be to include large enough numbers of subjects with one or more co-occurring risk factors to more fully describe and compare brain dysfunction across subtypes. Such studies are costly in terms of the larger sample sizes required. Their advantage is in providing common data on significant subtypes of users assessed with a consistent research protocol, thereby increasing the clinical relevance of results.

Measurement of Alcohol and Other Drug Use

A clear understanding of the relation between use of alcohol and other drugs and neurocognitive impairment depends in part on the accuracy of data that can be obtained about individuals' present and past substance use behavior. Urine, saliva, blood, or breath tests may be used to corroborate self-reports of current or recent drug use. The direct assay of drug levels is desirable, especially when more than one substance is involved. For example, in one study, 79% of subjects had positive urine screens for phencyclidine before weekly meetings compared with only 29% self-reporting use, even though a positive screen was not a criterion for treatment discharge and honesty was encouraged (Gorelick et al. 1989). Interestingly, some studies have found no influence of acute drug state on neuropsychological performance using either self-reporting (Guerra et al. 1987; Richards et al. 1992) or urine screens (Rounsaville et al. 1982), whereas other studies have found increased impairment among subjects with positive urine screens (e.g., Grant et al. 1978).

Historical information on substance use patterns almost always comes exclusively from self-report. The veracity of self-reported substance use data is limited by both subject compliance and memory. Recent advances in the use of standardized alcohol consumption interviews (e.g., Sobell and Sobell 1992) and the use of collateral informants have increased the reliability and validity of assessments of chronic consumption patterns.

Neuroanatomical Measurement Techniques

A full understanding of the effects of alcohol and other drugs on the brain and behavior requires research including multiple levels of analysis. Different drugs may have similar cognitive-behavioral effects but different anatomical substrates or physiological mechanisms and thus have different implications for pharmacological or other treatment. There have been many imaging research studies of persons with alcohol and other substance use disorders. However, as a rule, imaging studies offer nonspecific findings that by themselves are not useful diagnostically. Studies that have included both behavioral and imaging assessments have provided some measure of validation for the behavioral findings. A notable exception is the diagnosis of Korsakoff's syndrome. This disorder, which is diagnosed on behavioral grounds, can be substantiated by the atrophy of diencephalic structures that, as a rule, accompanies the diagnosis.

Many imaging modalities have been used in substance abuse research. Structural brain studies, which have predominantly measured levels of atrophy, have used computed tomography (CT) and in recent years magnetic resonance imaging (MRI). The main focus of these studies has been to assess the degree of ventricular enlargement and/or cortical atrophy in subjects with substance use disorders by using qualitative methods, quantitative methods, or both. Many studies have concentrated on measuring cerebrospinal fluid (CSF). More recently, studies have assessed the actual brain parenchyma, measuring proportions of gray and white matter in different regions, or have addressed issues related to tissue water balance by examining the differential magnetic relaxation properties of tissues, which are dependent on their water content. Some of these latter techniques have been thought to be of potential use in monitoring improvement and compliance with treatment. For example, the water shifts in the brain that occur when an individual starts drinking heavily (after abstinence) will result in increased relaxation times and may be reflected in a change in T2-weighted MRI images, which are designed to highlight the signal from water.

Functional imaging techniques have included 1) positron-emission tomography (PET), used to measure the regional distribution of brain glucose utilization and the distribution and kinetic properties of different neurotransmitter systems; 2) single photon emission computed tomography (SPECT), used to assess blood flow or binding to specific receptor systems; and 3) electroencephalography (EEG) and evoked potentials, used to measure the electrical characteristics of different brain regions. Throughout this chapter, when addressing specific findings related to different psychoactive substances, we highlight some of the relevant imaging studies for those substances.

The substance abuse MRI, PET, and SPECT literature shares the measurement concerns and limitations of the imaging literature in general. MRI, with its excellent spatial resolution, can be used to assess specific brain areas. However, the parameters selected (the scan sequence) must maximize both the spatial and the contrast resolution to allow the definition of the boundary between the structure of interest and its surrounding tissue. For example, depending on the parameters selected, the signal from gray and white matter may be differentially affected and thus may influence the relative volumes measured. In addition, an axis of planar sampling must be selected to maximize the number of slices taken through the structure of interest while minimizing contributions from surrounding structures. Elongated structures such as the hippocampus should be imaged perpendicular to its long axis to minimize partial-volume effects. Precise anatomical landmarks must be used to establish such an axis as well as to identify the position of the first and final slices of a series through the structure. In imaging studies, coverage must include the entire head. By using anatomical landmarks to select the slices, the bias related to differences in levels of atrophy in the groups contrasted will be minimized.

Spatial resolution is a limiting factor in PET studies, with a range of 5–10 mm being the norm. Within this range of spatial resolution, anatomical landmarks are unclear, suggesting the need to coregister the functional scan with the MRI to have improved placement of regions of interest. In addition, given the known alcohol-related cerebral atrophy, to measure the brain parenchymal functional activity, CSF must be removed from the regions of interest. If the contribution of CSF is not removed, then the measured functional brain tissue activity will be artificially lowered. Another consideration is whether the functional scan is obtained at rest or while the subject is performing a task. Although the brain may appear normal at rest, when increased demands are made, such as during the performance of a cognitive task, there may not be sufficient reserve, and abnormalities may become evident. Similar concerns pertain to studies with SPECT.

◈ NEUROPSYCHOLOGICAL IMPAIRMENT ASSOCIATED WITH SPECIFIC DRUGS

Alcohol

There has been a sustained research interest in determining whether chronic alcohol ingestion in humans has specific neurotoxic effects, apart from those mediated through hepatic, nutritional, or metabolic abnormalities (Victor 1994; Walton 1994), and, if so, whether specific areas of the brain are particularly susceptible to these neurotoxic effects (Evert and Oscar-Berman 1995; Nixon 1993). However, considerable controversy regarding nosological distinctions based on the etiology of alcohol-related brain impairment currently remains (Bowden 1990; Victor 1994). The classification presented below represents current knowledge of the major chronic conditions resulting in neurocognitive impairment. A summary is provided in Table 9–1 by etiological category. Given the present focus, we do not discuss disorders associated with acute intoxication, withdrawal syndrome, or fetal alcohol syndrome. Further information on the pathological effects of alcohol use associated with cognitive status and mental functioning may be found in reviews by Knight and Longmore (1994), Lehman et al. (1993), and Victor (1992).

Impairment Mediated by Nutritional or Metabolic Disturbances

Deficiencies in glucose, sodium, calcium, phosphorus, and magnesium are common in chronic heavy drinkers and may contribute to altered mental status (Lehman et al. 1993). The incidence of malnutrition has been difficult to estimate because of confounding factors such as socioeconomic status (Marsano 1994). Despite modest but significant correlations between thiamine levels and performance on several neuro-

---

Table 9–1.   Categories of neuropsychological impairment associated with chronic excessive alcohol consumption

---

Impairment mediated by nutritional disturbances

   Wernicke-Korsakoff syndrome

   Alcoholic cerebellar degeneration

Impairment mediated by hepatic disturbance

Impairment of multiple or uncertain etiology

   Marchiafava-Bignami disease

   Central pontine myelinolysis

   Alcohol dementia

Nonspecific brain atrophy, shrinkage, and neuropsychological deficit

---

psychological tests, Molina et al. (1994) found that duration of alcohol intake and education were stronger predictors of performance than was serum thiamine. They suggested that thiamine deficiency is not the main pathogenetic factor related to cognitive deterioration in chronic heavy drinkers. However, thiamine deficiency has a well-documented causative role in precipitating Wernicke-Korsakoff syndrome, one of the most familiar neurological disorders associated with chronic excessive alcohol use.

Wernicke-Korsakoff syndrome.   In chronic heavy drinkers, thiamine deficiency occurs from inadequate dietary intake, reduced gastrointestinal absorption, decreased hepatic storage, and impaired utilization (Charness 1993). In the brain, characteristic lesions are often found symmetrically surrounding the third and fourth ventricles, and the mamillary bodies are almost always involved. Lesions of the medial dorsal nuclei of the thalamus, not the mamillary bodies, are thought to be most crucial to the characteristic memory disorder associated with this syndrome (Victor 1992). About half of patients are reported to show a mild to moderate degree of diffuse EEG slowing (Victor 1992). During the acute phase, Wernicke's encephalopathy is characterized by ataxia, disordered eye movements, and confusion (Walton 1994); however, many patients with acute Wernicke's syndrome do not have this classic triad of symptoms (Charness 1993; Victor 1994).

Most of those who survive Wernicke's encephalopathy develop Korsakoff's syndrome. Verbal abilities may remain intact, as in chronic heavy drinkers without Korsakoff's syndrome; however, an amnestic syndrome develops, involving both anterograde and retrograde memory deficits (Lezak 1995; Parkin 1991; Ryan and Butters 1986). Immediate memory appears normal, yet the affected person has a profound inability to retain new information for more than a few minutes. Retrograde amnesia exhibits a temporal gradient, with better memory for past events spaced farther in time from onset of the disorder. Defective encoding and retrieval processes have been demonstrated in persons with Korsakoff's syndrome; however, the extent to which storage, encoding, or retrieval deficits account for the amnesia of Korsakoff's syndrome is not clear. Research showing improvement in memory function when recall is cued or mnemonic strategies are provided has implicated both encoding and retrieval deficits (Lezak 1995). Much evidence suggests that memory functions are better preserved on tasks that do not rely on intentional reference to a prior learning experience (i.e., procedural, incidental, semantic, implicit, or unconscious memory) (Knight and Longmore 1994).

Some current clinical neuropsychology texts (Lezak 1995) describe the cardinal features of Korsakoff's syndrome as sudden onset, significant lesions in diencephalon structures, marked passivity and emotional blunting, confabulation, profound memory deficit, and lack of potential for improvement. However, neuropathological data and clinical histories suggest that the onset of Wernicke-Korsakoff syndrome may also be slow and that the disorder may be progressive, involving both chronic and acute episodes that result in cumulative damage (Bowden 1990; Charness 1993). Substantial evidence is presented by Bowden (1990) to suggest that 1) persons with Korsakoff's syndrome are much more heterogeneous than previously suspected with respect to the extent of neuropsychological and functional impairment, 2) the classic amnestic deficit may not always characterize Korsakoff's syndrome, and 3) substantial recovery of function sometimes occurs with abstinence.

Before the availability of MRI, the integrity of the diencephalon structures could not be reliably assessed in vivo. For example, the mamillary bodies are best visualized on coronal section (oriented up and down parallel to the face), which was not possible with CT. With the advent of reliable MRI techniques, it has become clear that mamillary bodies and other diencephalic structures may be affected in nonamnesic chronic heavy drinkers (Blansjaar et al. 1992; Davila et al. 1994) and that frontal and temporal abnormalities are also present in amnesic heavy drinkers (Jernigan et al. 1991b; Kulisevsky et al. 1993). Bowden (1990) concluded that because many chronic heavy drinkers with Korsakoff's syndrome are not identified antemortem, their inclusion in studies of chronic heavy drinkers presumed to be neurologically normal may have contributed to inflated assessments of brain damage and overestimated the direct neurotoxic effect of alcohol. Based on MRI examinations revealing similar brain lesions in men with and without Korsakoff's amnestic syndrome, it has alternatively been suggested that the morphological abnormalities typically associated with Wernicke-Korsakoff syndrome are common to both chronic heavy alcohol use and thiamine deficiency (Blansjaar et al. 1992). The use of neuroradiological and neuropathological as opposed to behavioral criteria in diagnostic decision making may lead to somewhat different classifications of the disorder. These data suggest that the presentation of Korsakoff's syndrome is more complex than was previously thought. Perhaps unrecognized thiamine-mediated Korsakoff lesions account for much of what we think of as neurotoxic alcohol effects, or perhaps chronic excessive alcohol use alone (without malnutrition) can cause Korsakoff's amnestic syndrome and the characteristic lesion of the diencephalon is not a necessary condition.

Jernigan and colleagues (1991a) found that the amount of CSF in the cerebral ventricles and in the cortical sulci was significantly increased in nonamnesic chronic heavy drinking men relative to control subjects. The diencephalon, the caudate nucleus, and portions of the cerebral cortex and limbic systems were significantly smaller in the alcoholic patients. Amnesic chronic heavy drinking men showed a similar pattern of brain volume loss with reliably greater losses in the midline diencephalic structure, the mesial temporal region, and the anterior cortex, perhaps accounting for their more severe memory problems (Jernigan et al. 1991b). Graded decrements in visuoperceptive and problem-solving impairment from chronic heavy drinkers with Korsakoff's syndrome to chronic heavy drinkers without Korsakoff's syndrome and to control subjects have been found, suggesting a dual etiology of thiamine deficiency and neurotoxic alcohol effects on the frontal lobes (Butters and Salmon 1986; Jacobson et al. 1990). However, frontal-lobe functions involving active sequential ordering are well preserved in chronic heavy drinkers with Korsakoff's syndrome when retrieval from long-term memory is not involved (Wiegersma et al. 1991). This raises the question of whether some of the frontal-lobe deficits observed in persons with Korsakoff's syndrome may be secondary to amnesia.

Alcohol-related cerebellar degeneration. Cerebellar degeneration may occur after an extended history of heavy drinking and impaired nutrition, and liver disease co-occurs about half of the time (Victor 1992). Abnormalities of stance and gait are notable, but atrophy or shrinkage of the cerebellum may be present in chronic heavy drinkers in the absence of these symptoms (Sullivan et al. 1995b). Both rapid and slow progression over weeks or months may occur. Abstinence and correction of vitamin B deficiency may partially reverse symptoms (Lehman et al. 1993). Victor (1992) suggested that the observed pathological cerebellar changes do not differ from those observed in Wernicke's syndrome and that cerebellar degeneration may represent the same disease process in the absence of ocular and cognitive symptoms. The contribution of cerebellum structure and function to cognitive processes is controversial, as is the relation of cerebellar damage to cognitive dysfunction in alcoholic patients (Sullivan et al. 1995b).

Impairment Mediated by Hepatic Disturbance

The liver filters and detoxifies blood and performs other metabolic functions vital to the integrity of the central nervous system (CNS). Liver inflammation and disease, such as hepatitis and cirrhosis, may cause blood flow abnormalities in the brain and cognitive impairment in the absence of alcohol abuse (O'Carroll et al. 1991; Tarter et al. 1987), presumably via complex disruptions of these functions. *Hepatic encephalopathy* is a general term encompassing marked disruption in mentation and brain function consequent to liver disease (Tarter et al. 1993). One type, portal systemic encephalopathy, is caused by the shunting of venous blood into the general circulation without first going through the liver (Butterworth 1995). As a result of shunting, toxic substances such as ammonia remain in the blood and are thought to interfere with neurotransmitter communication and contribute to neurocognitive impairments. Hepatic encephalopathies are generally progressive from subclinical and low-grade stages through end stages including hepatic coma (Butterworth 1995).

In chronic heavy drinkers, hepatitis and cirrhosis are characterized by inflammatory processes in the liver occurring in response to alcohol or its metabolites (D. H. Adams 1994). Hepatitis and cirrhosis occur in about 40% and 20% of heavy drinkers, respectively, underscoring individual differences in susceptibility that are not well understood (Pratt et al. 1990). Hepatic encephalopathy often develops in chronic heavy drinkers with liver disease (Charness 1993) and is characterized by cognitive and motor dysfunction. Visuospatial skills, reaction time, abstraction, learning and memory, and psychomotor skills may be impaired; verbal skills may not be affected (Tarter et al. 1993).

Chronic heavy drinkers with cirrhosis may have more brain atrophy (Harper and Kril 1991) and neurocognitive deficits (Tarter et al. 1993) than nonheavy drinkers with cirrhosis. Greater cognitive impairment and brain blood flow and EEG abnormalities also have been found in chronic heavy drinkers with cirrhosis than in those without liver disease (Tarter et al. 1993). The severity of liver disease correlates with neuropsychological performance in chronic heavy drinkers at various stages of cirrhosis (Pomier Layrargues et al. 1991). These findings suggest a dual etiology for brain effects in chronic heavy drinkers with cirrhosis: liver disease and neurotoxic alcohol effects. The patterns of findings regarding memory deficits are complex (Arria et al. 1991), and differences in abstracting deficits between cirrhotic and noncirrhotic chronic heavy drinkers have not always been found (Tarter et al. 1995). More research is needed to define precisely the role of hepatic dysfunction in the cognitive impairment of chronic heavy drinkers varying in problem severity, length of abuse, and psychiatric comorbidity.

Impairment of Multiple or Uncertain Etiology

Marchiafava-Bignami disease. Marchiafava-Bignami disease is characterized by degeneration or demyelination of the corpus callosum. It is a rare complication of chronic heavy alcohol use seen primarily in men ages 45–60. Because the clinical presentation varies, ranging from a slowly progressive dementia to stupor or coma, it is difficult to diagnose antemortem. Head trauma and premorbid deficits may increase the idiosyncratic nature of deficit patterns. MRI or CT can identify lesions (Charness 1993). It is uncertain whether this disorder is caused by a metabolic abnormality, malnutrition associated with chronic alcohol consumption, or the direct neurotoxic effects of alcohol (Charness 1993; Victor 1994).

Central pontine myelinolysis. Central pontine myelinolysis, a rare disorder of cerebral white matter, involves demyelinating processes and characteristic lesions that are bilateral and symmetrical in the pyramidal tracts of the pons (Charness 1993; Charness et al. 1989; Knight and Longmore 1994). Lesions in the striatum, thalamus, cerebellum, and cerebral white matter may also be present (Wright et al. 1979). This disorder may occur with chronic malnutrition and an extended history of excessive drinking or with significant electrolyte imbalance in nonheavy drinkers. Supposedly, its cause may also be iatrogenic if the intravenous correction of low levels of blood sodium proceeds too rapidly. Rapid onset with flaccid quadriplegia and paralysis limits patient responsivity, and death may ensue within weeks (Knight and Longmore 1994). Behavioral symptoms may be obscured by other conditions or may include lethargy, confusion, and coma. More than half of cases have been reported in very-long-term heavy drinkers, often in conjunction with Wernicke-Korsakoff syndrome (Victor 1992).

Alcohol dementia. Alcohol dementia involves widespread, generalized cognitive deficits typically following many years of excessive alcohol use. In addition to impaired abstract reasoning, visuospatial skills, and other nonverbal fluid abilities, deficits in crystallized verbal functions such as vocabulary and information occur. Memory and executive impairment are notable (e.g., Ryan and Butters 1986). It is not clear whether this dementia represents a specific disorder. Victor (1992) suggested that data have neither clearly demonstrated that the condition results from a direct toxic effect of alcohol on the brain nor differentiated this condition from established dementias (e.g., Wernicke-Korsakoff syndrome, Marchiafava-Bignami disease) secondary to chronic heavy alcohol use. Clinical distinctions of acute onset and memory impairment in Wernicke-Korsakoff syndrome versus gradual onset and global dysfunction in alcohol dementia no longer seem valid in light of recent research suggesting great heterogeneity of onset and extent of impairment associated with Korsakoff's syndrome. Postmortem studies have found that diagnoses of alcohol dementia were given to many persons who actually had Wernicke-Korsakoff syndrome (e.g., Harper et al. 1986). Lezak (1995) described this disorder as a unique dementia, but Victor's (1994) review of clinical, neuropsychological, radiological, and pathological evidence found little compelling support for a distinct, well-defined syndrome of "alcohol dementia" apart from the disorders primarily mediated through liver dysfunction, malnutrition, or metabolic disturbance. More research is needed on the degree of specificity in the etiology and presentation of this putative syndrome.

Nonspecific Brain Damage and Neuropsychological Impairment

Even in the absence of significant nutritional, metabolic, or hepatic impairment, chronic heavy alcohol use has been consistently associated with impaired neuropsychological and cognitive functioning. The proportion of chronic heavy drinkers with some form of mild to moderate neuropsychological dysfunction is much larger than the proportion found to have one of the specific brain syndromes discussed above (Parsons 1993). About 50%–70% of chronic heavy drinkers entering treatment show some form of clinically significant neuropsychological impairment (P. R. Martin et al. 1986), and these prevalence rates appear to be representative of chronic heavy drinkers in the general population (Løberg and Miller 1986).

Structural and functional brain damage.   Morphological brain abnormalities are typically found in about 50%–60% of unselected samples of chronic heavy drinkers (Ron 1983). More recent data from MRI studies have consistently replicated these findings. Neurological deficits in heavy drug users are more likely to occur from heavy alcohol use than from other psychoactive drugs. Some young people who are heavy drinkers may develop cerebellar atrophy before age 25 (Aasly et al. 1993). The most commonly reported brain sequelae of chronic heavy alcohol use are increased ventricular and sulcal CSF volumes (Pfefferbaum et al. 1992; Wang et al. 1992). However, some studies have documented only cortical atrophy and not ventricular dilation in chronic heavy drinkers compared with control subjects (Wang et al. 1993). These differences may arise from differences in the severity and duration of use by subjects across studies. Some studies reported losses of gray and white matter volume in the cortex, with no particular cortical region being more affected (Pfefferbaum et al. 1993), whereas others found very specific changes such as reduced anterior hippocampal volumes (Sullivan et al. 1995a). Harding and colleagues' (1997) postmortem histopathological study found that hippocampal volume reductions in amnestic and nonamnestic chronic heavy drinkers occurred exclusively in the white matter, suggesting that functional memory deficits are not linked to neuron loss in the hippocampus. Localization of damage is complicated by injuries secondary to head trauma. Head trauma is most likely to affect orbitofrontal and anterior temporal regions because of their position relative to skull bones (Alexander 1982).

Chronic heavy drinkers consistently have reductions in glucose utilization in PET studies (e.g., Volkow et al. 1992, 1994; Wik et al. 1988). Localized frontal PET findings have been related to performance on specific neuropsychological tests (K. M. Adams et al. 1993, 1995). Nicolas et al. (1993) used SPECT and found that deficits in blood flow were more prominent in the frontal areas than in other brain regions of chronic heavy drinkers. However, other researchers who used PET did not find these changes (e.g., Eckardt et al. 1990) and proposed that to ascertain metabolic differences, individuals need to perform a cognitive task during imaging. Other physiological parameters, such as event-related EEG responses, have been reported to be affected by heavy alcohol intake. P3A and P3B event-related potentials may be delayed in abstinent men who were previously chronic heavy drinkers (Biggins et al. 1995), and a reduced P300 amplitude has been inversely correlated with ventricular size and width of cortical sulci (Kaseda et al. 1994).

Theories of behavioral neurocognitive impairment. Despite the unclear cerebral substrate of the behavioral neuropsychological deficits experienced by chronic heavy drinkers, much work has focused on explaining impairment in terms of damage to specific brain regions. Several reviews (e.g., Bowden 1990; Evert and Oscar-Berman 1995; Nixon 1993) have described theories of selective brain vulnerability in chronic heavy drinkers. These include disruption of right-hemisphere functions, damage to frontal and diencephalic brain regions, diffuse cortical damage, and premature aging of the brain. The evidence for each of these hypotheses has been equivocal, highlighting the heterogeneity of deficits observed and the difficulty in adequately specifying and controlling the multitude of factors known or suspected to affect brain structure and function in chronic heavy drinkers.

At present, the diffuse model most adequately captures the range of observed impairment in heavy drinkers, although the frontal and diencephalic systems seem particularly susceptible to damage (Nixon 1993; Oscar-Berman and Hutner 1993). The most apparent weakness of the diffuse model may be its inability to be disproved because it accommodates all varieties and patterns of deficits (Nixon 1993). It is also possible that the tendency of researchers to report group averages has obscured the identification of subtypes of persons with more focal deficits. Tivis and colleagues (1995) sought to determine whether the mild generalized dysfunction often found at the group level in alcohol use disorder samples may be an artifact of averaging together the performance of different subtypes of chronic heavy drinkers. After those with neurological or major medical problems were excluded, hierarchical cluster analysis revealed that 94% of the cases in two independent samples fell within one cluster reflecting mild verbal and nonverbal performance decrements and memory and perceptual skill impairment. Steingass and colleagues (1994) also failed to identify distinctive subgroups of impaired persons in a group of long-term heavy drinkers (average of 16 years) who had been abstinent for an average of 2.5 years. Further study is needed to determine whether the inclusion of large enough numbers of heavy drinkers selected to represent a priori subtypes (e.g., concurrent antisocial personality disorder, history of traumatic head injury) will yield distinct clusters of dysfunction.

The most consistent evidence of behavioral impairment in chronic heavy drinkers has been found in tasks requiring fluid cognitive abilities: visuospatial and visuomotor skills, abstract reasoning, new learning, attention, and certain forms of memory (Bates 1993; Knight and Longmore 1994; Parsons 1993). Overlearned or crystallized verbal skills, such as vocabulary and general information, are less affected. Fluid abilities are often measured with nonverbal tests, peak early in the life span, and are most vulnerable to all types of environmental insult, as well as normal aging effects.

In addition to conceptualizing vulnerable abilities along the fluid-crystallized dimension (Barron and Russell 1992), the distinction between controlled and automatic information processing (e.g., Hasher and Zachs 1979; Schneider et al. 1984; Tracy and Bates, in press) also provides a useful heuristic. The effects of chronic alcohol use on cognition appear to be strongest on controlled, analytic, and effortful information processes involving selective or divided attention, as opposed to overlearned, automatic information processes that make fewer demands on attentional resources (e.g., Smith and Oscar-Berman 1992). The effect of alcohol on controlled, effortful, and attention-demanding information-processing operations may underlie performance decrements across a variety of demanding neuropsychological tasks (Goldman 1995; Ingle and Weingartner 1995; Tracy et al. 1995).

Neurocognitive findings in the chronic alcohol and normal aging literatures share common characteristics. For example, selective right-hemisphere deficits and a decline in executive function (frontal damage) have also been suggested as major neuropsychological changes associated with aging (Libon et al. 1994). The effects of aging, chronic substance use, exposure to occupational and environmental toxins, and traumatic head injury may all be found on "right-hemisphere" tasks, "frontal" tasks, and even "left-hemisphere" or verbally mediated tasks, if they tend to make demands on working memory, effortful information processing, or executive functions (Anger 1990; Ellis and Oscar-Berman 1989; Lezak 1995). Although different brain insults may tend to cause impaired performance on the same tests, use of the double dissociation paradigm (Barron and Russell 1992) and careful analyses of the types of errors made (Cermak et al. 1989) have provided support for different types of information-processing deficits in chronic heavy drinkers compared with nonheavy drinking elderly and other clinical groups. Burger et al. (1987) found that differences in performance on the Luria-Nebraska Neuropsychological Battery (Golden et al. 1985) between age groups were not the same as those found between chronic heavy and nonheavy drinking groups. Although aging and heavy alcohol use were both associated with decreased performance on the motor, visual, and expressive language tests, only age was associated with poorer performance on the memory, intellectual processes, arithmetic, tactile, and perceptive language tests.

Interest in the frontal-lobe deficits associated with chronic alcohol use has increased in recent years. This may be partly due to renewed interest in the importance of "executive functions" in the control of current behavior and the support of future-oriented behavior (Benton 1994). The prefrontal cortex is functionally specialized for strategic planning, use of environmental feedback, working memory, goal selection, and response inhibition (Luria 1973). Executive control functions appear relevant to understanding the development of substance use behaviors, risk of relapse, and other treatment-relevant phenomena. Executive deficits present functionally as poor planning ability, sequencing difficulties, impaired working memory, inflexible thought processes, and difficulty orienting behavior toward future goals (Benton 1994; Goldberg 1986).

Both the executive functioning construct and its neural substrates are complex and heterogeneous. Different prefrontal areas support different component executive processes, and the potential exists for damage in other areas of the brain to affect executive abilities also (Boller et al. 1995; Goldberg and Bilder 1987). Word generation in fluency tasks, for example, involves the left dorsolateral prefrontal cortex, Broca's area, the posterior portion of the midfrontal gyrus, the supplementary motor area, and Wernicke's area (Candon et al. 1997). The frontal-subcortical circuits also have afferent and efferent connections to posterior temporal, parietal, and occipital association areas (Cummings 1995). Although impairment on tests of executive functioning is prevalent in chronic heavy alcohol and other drug users (Morgenstern and Bates, in press), it is not known whether the neural substrates of dysfunction in persons with use disorders tend to be common or unique. Several theoretical models of the etiology of alcohol and other drug use disorders have assigned a critical role to the operation of nonautomatic executive cognitive processes (e.g., Giancola and Moss 1998; Tiffany 1990). In general, such models propose that impairment to working memory, cognitive and behavioral flexibility, response inhibition, and other effortful cognitive processes increases the likelihood that vulnerable individuals will not be able to interrupt or avoid the recurrence of overlearned, inflexible, and automatic alcohol and other drug use behaviors. More research is needed to determine the extent to which specific effortful cognitive processes are needed to prevent the development and/or persistence of seemingly compulsive substance use behaviors.

Focal brain areas may also be vulnerable to effects of chronic alcohol intake, either directly or via episodes of malnutrition. K. M. Adams and colleagues (1993) found that the local cerebral metabolic rate for glucose in the medial frontal region of the cerebral cortex correlated significantly with performance on the Wisconsin Card Sorting Test (Heaton 1985), but not on the Category Test (Reitan and Wolfson 1993), when CT/MRI ratings of anatomical atrophy were statistically controlled. Interestingly, information-processing approaches to understanding the nature of neuropsychological deficits associated with substance use disorders have provided results that may be consonant with neuro-radiological research. Perrine (1993), for example, found that two different information-processing operations (attribute identification and rule learning) primarily determined performance on the Wisconsin Card Sorting Test compared with the Category Test. The integrated study of the effects of alcohol on brain structure, brain function, and the information-processing operations that support neurocognitive competency is needed to determine the correspondence of new knowledge at different levels of analysis and to develop a comprehensive model of alcohol-related effects (Bates 1993; Evert and Oscar-Berman 1995; Nixon 1995). Multilevel research should also provide a more articulated understanding of the effects of chronic alcohol intake effects at the various levels needed for prevention, intervention, and remediation of dysfunction.

Gender Differences

Overall, research on gender differences in alcohol-associated neuropsychological impairment has shown that male and female chronic heavy drinkers have similar patterns and extent of deficit (Acker 1986; Fabian et al. 1981; Glenn and Parsons 1992; Nixon et al. 1995; Steingass et al. 1994). Women develop liver disease and brain damage with lower daily alcohol intake and shorter drinking histories than do men (Lancaster 1994). Thus, women may be at risk earlier for hepatically mediated neurocognitive dysfunction than are men. Gender-related differences in risk of both hepatic and brain damage from alcohol may be related to lower rates of first-pass metabolism by women (Frezza et al. 1990). First-pass metabolism is reported to account for 20%–80% of an ingested dose of alcohol (Julkunen et al. 1985), contributing to the higher rates of absorption, BALs, and areas under the curve for women after oral ingestion (Frezza et al. 1990). Mann and collaborators (1992)—although controlling for liver dysfunction, thiamine deficiency, age, and daily alcohol consumption—did not control for gender-related differences. Despite shorter drinking histories in women, a similar degree of brain shrinkage in both sexes was found. It would be tempting to conclude, as they do, that women may have heightened brain vulnerability to the damaging effects of alcohol. However, given the lack of control over differences in rates of alcohol absorption and in body mass between men and women, further research is needed.

Impairment in Social Drinkers

Little consistent support for the hypothesis of direct neurotoxic effects of alcohol in social drinkers has been forthcoming (Bates 1993; Parsons 1986). Some limited evidence indicates that very recent excessive drinking (Bergman 1985) and frequent high-quantity consumption (Bates and Tracy 1990; Salame 1991) may be related to lower neurocognitive performance and learning levels in nonclinical samples. Heavy social drinkers (> 200 g/week) showed reduced P3 amplitude in an auditory recall task compared with very light drinkers (< 20 g/week) (Nichols and Martin 1996). Taken together, the results in this area suggest that in nonclinical samples, alcohol-related damage does not accrue in a continuous fashion with small to high alcohol doses, but rather that some quantity/frequency threshold of alcohol use must be reached before neurocognitive damage is possible (Parsons and Nixon 1998). Little is known about individual differences in vulnerability in this regard.

Also, standard neuropsychological tests may not be very sensitive to subtle deficits in nonclinical samples of social drinkers. This implies that tests may have different sensitivities dependent on sample characteristics such as age and extent of use, which may affect the detected cognitive sequelae of alcohol use. In addition, cognitive-behavioral systems appear to be flexible and capable of reorganization, whereby intact cognitive skills may compensate for impaired ones without a loss in performance (Luria et al. 1969). From this perspective, standard performance scores may mask alcohol-linked deficits in neurocognitive functioning. Functional cognitive systems (e.g., memory, visual-spatial ability, abstracting ability), operationally defined as latent constructs in a structured equation model, were significantly less associated with one another in heavy social drinkers (Tracy and Bates 1994) and persons with alcoholic use disorders (Ham and Parsons 1997) than in control subjects who abstained or used little alcohol. A more direct test of the compensatory hypothesis will require the prospective longitudinal study of intraindividual changes in the functional organization of cognitive skills in response to excessive alcohol use.

Recovery of Function

Neuropsychological impairment is not static following cessation of excessive drinking. Some data suggest that the most severe impairments may partially resolve in the initial 1–4 weeks following cessation of drinking (Goldman 1987; Page and Linden 1974); however, recovery processes may extend over the course of a year or more (Parsons and Leber 1982). Different neurocognitive abilities show varying amounts and rates of spontaneous, time-dependent recovery (Goldman 1987; Muuronen et al. 1989). Verbal deficits recover within the first few weeks, whereas memory and visuospatial skills show less recovery within the first month (Parsons and Leber 1982). New learning, complex or novel problem solving, and speeded information-processing tasks require the longest recovery times and may show persistent deficits (Goldman 1987, 1995). Imaging studies have confirmed that use-related brain damage appears to be fully or partially reversible, and many researchers now use the term *brain shrinkage* as opposed to *brain damage* to describe the anatomical abnormalities found in many recently abstinent chronic heavy drinkers. Multiple lines of evidence (e.g., Parsons et al. 1990) are consistent with Grant and colleagues' (1986) suggestion that many chronic heavy drinkers experience a slowly reversing, intermediate-duration organic mental disorder. Partial reversal of sulcal atrophy and ventricular dilation has been found (Grant 1987; Grant et al. 1986; Wilkinson 1987). Using imaging quantification of longitudinal brain change, volumetric white matter increases and CSF reductions over a follow-up abstinence interval have been demonstrated (Shear et al. 1994). Pfefferbaum and colleagues (1995) found improvements in cortical gray matter, sulcal, and lateral ventricular volumes after an average of 12–32 days of abstinence. Men who did not resume drinking showed improvement in third ventricular volume later in time (between 2 and 12 months); those who did resume heavy drinking showed arrested ventricular improvement and white matter volume loss. Despite recovery seen behaviorally and on imaging, chronic heavy drinkers may continue to show low P300 amplitudes after 3–10 years of abstinence. Taken together with the results of studies from premorbid, high-risk subjects, the lack of recovery in P300 amplitude after extended abstinence suggests that this abnormality may predate the development of alcoholism (Begleiter et al. 1995).

Persons with alcoholism may show rapid recovery of function over 1–2 weeks, slow recovery over months and years, or little to no recovery of function (P. L. Carlin and Wilkenson 1983; Goldman 1995). Little is known about the moderators of individual differences in recovery, with the exception of age and drinking behaviors. Younger alcoholic patients (Goldman 1983; Parsons and Leber 1982) and those who stop or greatly reduce drinking (Muuronen et al. 1989) are more likely to experience faster and more complete improvements in cognitive functioning than are others, although performance may still not reach normal control levels. Improvements in affective regulation and liver function (K. Schafer et al. 1991) as well as other biological changes (Goldman 1987) affect some of the cognitive recovery of abstinent alcoholic patients.

Other Drugs: General Methodological Considerations

Study of the neurocognitive effects of psychoactive substances is complicated because individuals seldom confine their use to only one drug, except for alcohol (e.g., Brown et al. 1993). Thus, drug effects are often superimposed on those of alcohol and one or more other drugs of concurrent or historical use. This has caused much heterogeneity in drug use classifications in this area of research. Groups of chronic excessive users of a particular drug have been defined in varied ways, including the subject's "drug of preference" and various combinations of concurrent and lifetime diagnoses of other substance use disorders. We discuss individual drug effects and multiple drug effects separately. However, most of the individual drug data also apply to the effects of multiple-substance use on neurocognition.

Available information about drug purity—which varies with time and geographic location—is usually limited. Effects of neurotoxic drugs may be mediated by dose and route of administration. There is a lack of data on the comparability of brain and behavioral effects of drug intake across various routes of administration. The extant information is from samples showing substantial heterogeneity in comorbid psychopathology. Psychiatric, medical, and neurological problems have only sometimes been used as exclusion criteria, and small sample sizes have precluded subtype analyses. Across studies, control groups were heterogeneous in substance use, sometimes comprising subjects with alcohol or other drug use disorders, or control subjects without substance use disorders. Many studies have matched drug use and control groups on age, gender, ethnicity, and years of education. Average age is usually in the late 20s to 30s. Chronic effects in older long-term users are unknown. Many studies have included both sexes; however, women have been underrepresented, and the data usually have been averaged across sexes.

Cocaine

Cocaine abusers have sometimes shown lower premorbid (Barrone estimate) and current IQ estimates than chronic heavy drinkers and control subjects (Beatty et al. 1995). O'Malley and Gawin (1990) found poorer Verbal and Performance IQs in combined freebase and intranasal users than in control subjects matched on age, gender, and race but not when subjects were also matched on socioeconomic status (O'Malley et al. 1992).

Visuospatial construction (Ardila et al. 1991; J. Berry et al. 1993), vigilance in signal detection tasks (Bauer 1994; Manschreck et al. 1990), and memory (Ardila et al. 1991; J. Berry et al. 1993; Herning et al. 1990; O'Malley et al. 1990, 1992) are consistently lower in heavy cocaine users than control subjects in subjects tested between 1 and 20 weeks since last use. Abstracting deficits have been found (Beatty et al. 1995; O'Malley et al. 1992), but they do not seem paramount. Word fluency (Ardila et al. 1991; O'Malley et al. 1992) does not appear to be affected, whereas decrements in Trail Making speed were found in some samples (J. Berry et al. 1993) but not in others (O'Malley et al. 1992).

Little is known about the likelihood of clinically significant impairment in individuals with cocaine use disorders. In a small study of freebase and intranasal cocaine users who were primarily middle-class male Caucasians (average of 24 days after detoxification), O'Malley and colleagues (1992) reported that 50% in the cocaine-dependent group showed impairment on a neuropsychological screening battery compared with 15% in a control group. A comprehensive comparison of chronic heavy cocaine users (primarily freebase) to chronic heavy drinkers and healthy control subjects found similar mild, diffuse dysfunction in the cocaine and alcohol groups relative to control subjects (Beatty et al. 1995). The authors suggested that chronic cocaine use may give rise to diffuse, mild brain dysfunction or to impairment of the frontal limbic system.

Cocaine is a sympathomimetic drug with potent vasoactive properties. It also has significant anesthetic actions. Chronic cocaine use has been associated with cortical and subcortical perfusion defects as seen with SPECT (Holman et al. 1993; Woods 1992). Moreover, perfusion deficits in frontal, periventricular, and temporoparietal areas—which are associated with attention, new learning, visual and verbal memory, word production, and visuomotor integration—remained in subjects who were drug free for at least 6 months (Strickland et al. 1993). Perfusion abnormalities also have been found in chronic crack cocaine users (Weber et al. 1993). A sample of African American men who had been cocaine abstinent for a mean of 66.4 (SD = 26.2) months showed no structural brain abnormalities on MRI compared with control subjects; however, proton MR spectroscopy provided evidence of abnormality in the nonneuronal cells of subcortical brain regions (Chang et al. 1997). Researchers using PET months after detoxification reported reduced glucose utilization in the frontal areas of cocaine users (Volkow et al. 1994) and related these reductions to decreased availability of dopamine D_2 receptors (Volkow et al. 1993).

Cocaine is a potent dopamine reuptake blocker, and with chronic use it can cause dopamine depletion. Neurotransmitter systems in the brain are functionally interconnected. Thus, the marked effects of cocaine on the dopamine system likely affect other neurotransmitter systems such as serotonin. These significant effects on neurotransmitter systems may give rise to psychiatric symptoms ranging from depression to psychosis, which further complicates neuropsychological research on the chronic effects of cocaine use. Current psychiatric symptoms may correlate with daily cocaine doses, lifetime consumption, and length of abstinence (Manschreck et al. 1990), but these factors are not consistently associated with the neurocognitive performance of individuals with cocaine use disorders (Ardila et al. 1991; Beatty et al. 1995; Manschreck et al. 1990). Some relations between use histories and performance have been reported for specific tasks (e.g., O'Malley et al. 1992).

The few behavioral studies of neurocognitive recovery in abstinent cocaine users have been short term and often involved comorbid conditions. Bauer (1994) reported that cocaine-dependent subjects (of whom 36% also had an alcohol use disorder) showed slowing of reaction time (RT) relative to chronic heavy drinkers and control subjects in a vigilance task. The slowing persisted throughout a 15-week test interval following their last use of cocaine. Herning and colleagues (1990) also found slowed RT in a memory task that persisted across 3–4 weeks of testing in a cocaine-dependent group with a high prevalence of antisocial personality disorder. In a study that included statistical controls for high rates of clinical depression, improvements in neuropsychological functioning from 72 hours to 2 weeks from last use were also observed, with memory and psychomotor speed showing the least recovery (J. Berry et al. 1993). Brown and colleagues (1993) noted a similar degree of impairment in a sample of individuals with alcohol problems and also in a sample of persons with both alcohol and cocaine problems at the start of treatment. The two groups also showed similar improvements over 6 months on several WAIS-R subscales, although sample attrition was substantial on subsequent testing.

Inhalants

Most controlled studies of inhalant users have evaluated primary toluene users. Toluene is a widely abused organic solvent found in products such as cement glue, paint thinner, adhesives, and cleaning fluids. It is not entirely clear to what extent other toxic constituents of inhaled products, such as chlorinated hydrocarbons and propane, are also responsible for neurological and neuropsychological damage. As in the cocaine literature, sample sizes have tended to be small, men have been tested primarily, and the data from small numbers of female inhalant users have been averaged with males' data.

People who chronically inhale toluene appear to be at substantial risk for neurocognitive impairment (Allison and Jerrom 1984; Fornazzari et al. 1983; Tsushima and Towne 1977) as well as peripheral neuropathy, cerebellar degeneration, cortical atrophy, temporal-lobe epilepsy, and paranoid psychosis (Byrne et al. 1991; Ehyai and Freemon 1983; Fornazzari et al. 1983; Hormes et al. 1986; Rosenberg et al. 1988). Brain atrophy, especially in the cerebellum, is associated with a behavioral syndrome that includes impairment of motor control, intellect, and memory (Fornazzari et al. 1983).

CT and MRI studies of toluene abusers have confirmed significant multifocal CNS damage. The most common effects are cerebral cortical, cerebellar, and brain-stem atrophy (Lazar et al. 1983; Rosenberg et al. 1988; Xiong et al. 1993). In addition, studies have consistently reported abnormalities in brain-stem evoked potentials, even when no gross brain-stem structural damage was present (Lazar et al. 1983; Rosenberg et al. 1988). A loss of differentiation on MRI between gray and white matter among toluene abusers has also been found (Rosenberg et al. 1988; Xiong et al. 1993). It appears that toluene gets partitioned into the lipid membranes of cells in cerebral tissue, causing a loss of signal (hypointensity) on the MRI in those tissues, and thus is responsible for the hypointensity seen in the basal ganglia of inhalant users (Unger et al. 1994). Given that gray matter may lose signal (appear more like white matter), this mechanism is also probably responsible for the loss of gray-white differentiation.

A large behavioral study compared 68 primary inhalant users with 41 adolescents who were primary users of multiple other drugs. Analyses controlling for age and other drug use showed that primary inhalant users performed significantly poorer on a broad range of neurocognitive measures, including verbal skills, Full-Scale IQ, achievement tests, trail making speed, psychomotor abilities, and visuoperceptive skills (Korman et al. 1981). Other studies also report widespread diffuse deficits in chronic inhalers (Allison and Jerrom 1984; G. J. Berry 1976).

The prevalence of impairment in inhalant users is not known. Fornazzari and colleagues (1983) reported that of 24 solvent abusers (mean age 23) tested the day after last use, 65% showed significant neurological and neuropsychological impairments. In the impaired group, behavioral symptoms correlated with CT scan measurements of cerebellum, ventricles, and cortical sulci, all of which were abnormal compared with control subjects matched on age. The authors noted, however, that subjects were educationally, culturally, and emotionally deprived (Fornazzari et al. 1983). Although the clinical impression is often that chronic inhalant users have low premorbid levels of functioning, longitudinal studies have not been done, and empirical evidence is indirect. Chronic inhalant use by adolescents may also indirectly affect neurocognitive performance by resulting in a failure to use potential skills to acquire education-based knowledge (Mahmood 1983).

The relation between impairment and time of last use and duration of use is not entirely clear. It is unknown whether CNS damage occurs only after several years of regular inhalant use or whether it can occur after relatively limited exposure. Few relations between duration of use and neurological scores were reported for subjects who used inhalants for a mean of about 6 years (Fornazzari et al. 1983). Tsushima and Towne (1977), however, observed a trend toward increasing neurocognitive deficits with increasing length of use in 20 young, low-income solvent inhalers. More recent work found extreme effects in a long-term (mean about 13 years) clinical sample of heavy users in their mid-20s. Of 22 persons who inhaled solvents on a daily basis and who were randomly selected from those being treated at a psychiatric hospital, 18 had developed acute paranoid psychosis, and 2 had documented decreases in IQ of 25 points or more over a period of several years (Byrne et al. 1991).

The long-term neuropsychological consequences of solvent exposure have also been studied in industrial workers chronically exposed to solvents at work. Cherry et al. (1992) found that occupational exposure to solvents was more frequent in patients admitted to a hospital with organic brain damage than with other psychiatric diagnoses. Increased probability of previous solvent exposure was found primarily in those admitted with organic dementia or with cerebral atrophy and an alcohol-related diagnosis. It appeared likely that an interaction between solvent exposure and heavy alcohol consumption contributed to brain damage.

Little is known about the permanence of brain damage and functional impairment associated with inhalant use. Fornazzari et al. (1983) observed recovery of liver functions, but not cognitive functions, over a 2-week period following cessation of use. However, they reported that subjects who remained in the study were those who were either unimpaired or most impaired at the first test. A well-controlled case report (Wiedmann et al. 1987) described a former long-term, high-quantity inhalant user at 3-month intervals over 18 months. Substantial, but not total, recovery of function was observed.

Opiates

The chronic effects of opiate use on neurocognitive functioning have been difficult to specify. Opiate users almost always use alcohol and other drugs, so it is usually not possible to separate multiple drug use effects from those specifically produced by opiates. Within and across studies, subjects may have still been experiencing acute opiate effects (from drugs obtained personally or via participation in a methadone maintenance program) or may have been recently detoxified (e.g., Guerra et al. 1987; Rounsaville et al. 1981). Co-occurring risk factors for neuro-cognitive impairment are also prevalent in opiate-using samples (Grant et al. 1978; Rounsaville et al. 1981). Chronic opiate users have a high prevalence of medical complications unrelated to the substance itself. Intravenous drug users frequently share needles and have a high prevalence of infectious diseases ranging from hepatitis to HIV infection. Complications leading to kidney failure, and heart valve infections leading to microembolisms in the brain and other organs, are common. These medical conditions can have considerable consequences for brain function and integrity. Finally, different conclusions regarding neurocognitive impairment associated with opiate use may be drawn from the same data, depending on whether authors reported the percentage rates of users showing clinically significant impairment (Rounsaville et al. 1981) or highlighted comparisons of users' average performance levels with those of control groups who also showed deficits (Rounsaville et al. 1982).

A 12-year follow-up study of 490 former opiate users who had participated in drug treatment programs throughout the United States reported demographic-based IQ estimates that were similar to those from the WAIS-R standardization sample (Chastain et al. 1986). These data replicated other findings of generally normal IQs in groups of users of opiates and other drugs (Guerra et al. 1987; Rounsaville et al. 1981) and clients maintained on 50- or 80-mg daily doses of methadone (Lombardo et al. 1976). Age-, gender-, education-, and ethnicity-matched samples of primary cocaine versus opiate users showed higher estimated IQ, vocabulary, and abstraction scores (Shipley Institute of Living Scale) in the cocaine group (Montoya et al. 1994).

Several studies of moderately large samples of chronic opiate users, many of whom used other drugs and had histories of childhood hyperactivity and other risk factors, found clinically significant neuropsychological impairment (based on the Halstead-Reitan [Reitan and Wolfson 1993] or similar batteries) in 37%–79% of users (Grant et al. 1978; Rounsaville et al. 1981). Impairment was diffuse, and little evidence was obtained to link deficits to opiate use per se. Rounsaville and colleagues' (1982) subsequent comparison of their opiate-use sample (two-thirds of which also regularly used one to six other drugs) failed to show substantial differences in overall impairment relative to neurologically diagnosed (epileptic) and Comprehensive Employment Training Act (CETA)-applicant control groups. One study (Amir and Bahri 1994) was able to compare the performance of age- and education-matched groups of Arabian heroin-only users, polydrug users, chronic heavy alcohol users, and control subjects screened for head injury, electroconvulsive therapy, and major physical or mental illness. The heavy alcohol and drug use groups made significantly more errors on Benton's Revised Visual Retention Test (BRVRT; Benton 1974) than control subjects. This result is consistent with the outcome of earlier work (Penk et al. 1981) that compared the BRVRT performance of heroin-only, polydrug use, and control groups of United States military veterans. That study found heroin-only and polydrug use groups were two standard deviations below expected performance levels and suggests that visual memory may be vulnerable to chronic opiate–use as well as multiple drug–use effects.

Following detoxification, primary opiate polydrug users (women and men) in their 20s did not show neurocognitive impairment compared with community control subjects who were similar in demographic, educational, and cultural characteristics (Guerra et al. 1987); hospitalized veterans matched on age, sex, and education (Fields and Fullerton 1975); or standard normalization samples (Rodriquez 1993a, 1993b). Thus, although attention, verbal fluency, and memory may be impaired before detoxification (Guerra et al. 1987), deficits do not appear to persist in youthful users with limited use histories. On the other hand, a small sample of long-term (average 32 year) daily opiate polydrug users ages 40–61 showed substantial deficit (Strang and Gurling 1989). In this study, subjects were either using pharmaceutical heroin legally (in England) or had recently stopped. Six of seven subjects showed abnormal CT scans, and five also showed neuropsychological impairment. However, no clear correlations between morphological abnormalities and neuropsychological deficits were found, nor was a consistent pattern of deficits found across tests of visuospatial or perceptual abilities, verbal or visual recognition memory, or abstraction.

Despite apparent use-related differences in damage between young and older samples of primary opiate polydrug users, direct support for the effect of duration of use on impairment is limited. In small group comparisons of control, short-term (1–2 year), and long-term (4–5 year) opiate polydrug users, Cipolli and Galliani (1987) found some suggestion of greater intellectual impairment (via the Rorschach test) in the long-term group. However, most researchers have found little or no correlation between duration or recency of opiate use and neurocognitive impairment (Guerra et al. 1987; Rounsaville et al. 1982). As noted for other drugs of abuse, when intensive use starts at an early age and interferes with educational or occupational attainments, the resultant lifestyle may also give rise to deficits in cognitive development that are separate from direct toxic brain effects (Chastain et al. 1986).

Phencyclidine

Phencyclidine (PCP) is classified medically as a dissociative anesthetic. Its acute effects are generally dose-related, ranging from euphoria and excitement to anxiety, disorganized thoughts, hallucinations, and other psychotic symptomatology. More research has focused on the psychiatric and aggression-associated effects of PCP than on chronic neuropsychological sequelae. PCP appears to affect the actions of multiple CNS neurotransmitter systems (Pearlson 1981) and depresses cell firing in the locus coeruleus and other brain regions. PCP is an N-methyl-D-aspartate (NMDA) channel blocker (Zutkin and Javitt 1990; Zutkin and Zutkin 1992). NMDA receptor function abnormalities have been suggested to underlie psychotic-like symptoms induced by PCP (Tracy et al. 1995; Zutkin and Javitt 1990). PCP blockage of NMDA receptors in the hippocampus has also been proposed to underlie both acute and chronic effects of PCP on memory functions (Cosgrove and Newell 1991).

Chronic users of PCP and multiple drugs have tended to show neurocognitive impairment similar to or somewhat more pervasive than age- and education-matched polydrug users who did not take PCP (A. S. Carlin et al. 1979; Cosgrove and Newell 1991). Cosgrove and Newell found the most substantial impairment on measures of short-term and long-term memory. Most PCP users also showed impaired executive functions as assessed by the Category Test and Trail Making Test Part B (Reitan and Wolfson 1993). Impaired abstraction has been found in chronic PCP users whether or not head trauma and a history of CNS disturbance were used as exclusion criteria (Cosgrove and Newell 1991; Lewis and Hordan 1986).

Significant improvements on global indices of neuropsychological functioning were found in chronic PCP users who either stopped or reduced PCP use over 4 weeks (Cosgrove and Newell 1991). Much of the improvement was in the area of verbal memory. An earlier study of a small sample of chronic PCP polydrug users who had been abstinent an average of about 2 years found neuropsychological deficits suggestive of mild organic mental disorder in half the sample (A. S. Carlin et al. 1979). Subjects with preexisting learning disabilities and head trauma were not excluded, so it is not clear whether these data represented premorbid deficits or the absence of recovery from drug effects.

Marijuana

Unlike alcohol, the chronic excessive use of marijuana has not been associated consistently with neurocognitive impairment across a range of samples varying in age, gender, socioeconomic status, and culture (Fehr and Kalant 1983; Tracy et al. 1995; Weinrieb and O'Brian 1993; Wert and Raulin 1986). Wert and Raulin's (1986) review of nine cross-cultural studies of neurocognitive impairment in cannabis users suggested that the evidence for impairment was weak. In the five studies that did find evidence of impairment, there was an absence of control groups, lack of information on premorbid functional levels, inadequate control of acute intoxication effects and other drug use, lack of clinically significant differences, and potential uncontrolled effects of psychopathology. These shortcomings are not unique to the study of marijuana, but characterize much early neurocognitive drug research. None of the six studies conducted with United States samples through 1981 demonstrated significant differences between chronic users and control subjects. For example, occasional or regular use of marijuana was not associated with deficit in youthful, high-functioning users who were of high socioeconomic status (SES) (Grant et al. 1973; Rochford et al. 1977). Furthermore, 10 subjects who were long-term (> 7 years), high-quantity (2–4 oz mixed with tobacco per day) users who used marijuana as part of religious sect rituals showed no acute or chronic impairments in abstraction, memory, or other cognitive abilities compared to norms. Mean IQ scores were in the superior to very superior range (J. Schaeffer et al. 1981). Such findings argue against generalized neurotoxic effects of marijuana in healthy individuals in the absence of other risk factors.

Some studies from other cultures report more evidence of decrement and decline in neurocognitive skills (e.g., pencil tapping, recent memory) after regular, extended periods of charas smoking and bhang drinking, although it is not clear how differences in culture and method of cannabis intake affected results (e.g., Mendhiratta et al. 1988; Varma et al. 1988). More recently, Block and colleagues (Block and Ghoneim 1993; Block et al. 1992) matched subjects, before initiation of marijuana use, on scores from the fourth grade in the Iowa Tests of Basic Skills (Hieronymus et al. 1982). Their comparison of light (1–4 times/week), intermediate (5–6 times/week), and heavy (7 or more times/week) users with nonusers matched on sex, SES, age, and work status showed that heavy users scored lower than all others on math, verbal expression, and long-term retrieval of high imagery words but not on text learning, paired associate learning, word associations, or psychomotor tests. Tests controlling for group differences in lifetime and recent use of other drugs did not change the significance of results. The authors suggested that the primary group differences between heavy marijuana users and others on tests of acquired knowledge versus new learning may suggest an indirect effect of marijuana on individuals' cumulative learning history over years rather than direct neurotoxic effects.

A carefully controlled study of normal, healthy individuals who had smoked marijuana daily for at least 3 years found no differences in auditory and visual P300 latencies or amplitudes compared with nonusing control subjects (Patrick et al. 1995). In addition, no evoked potential differences were identified in a subsample who had used marijuana daily for more than 15 years. A small sample of chronic marijuana smokers performed an auditory selective attention task more poorly than control subjects and showed enhanced early processing negativity on recorded brain event–related potentials (Solowij et al. 1991). A subsequent comparison of those data with the performance of another group of subjects who had stopped cannabis use found less evidence of attentional deficit among the former users (Solowij 1995).

Research is still needed to remedy limitations of previous studies. Virtually all research has been retrospective, and, even with the inclusion of control groups, it is not clear whether group differences existed prior to cannabis use (Weinrieb and O'Brian 1993; Wert and Raulin 1986). Prospective studies are needed to separate cannabis effects from premorbid characteristics, to identify subjects who may be vulnerable to impairment, and to identify risk factors. High-risk groups such as elderly subjects with a long history of chronic use, children with learning disabilities, and adolescents in treatment have received little attention. A small treatment sample of adolescent marijuana users performed significantly less well on two of seven memory measures compared with drug-free community control subjects, whereas the performance of a control treatment sample without substance use disorders was intermediate (Schwartz et al. 1989). Because of the possibility of individual differences in vulnerability, it may be important to look at impairment classifications of individual subjects, not solely group means (Fehr and Kalant 1983). At present, there is little compelling evidence for neurocognitive damage independently caused by chronic marijuana use.

As a final note, it has been reported that the tetrahydrocannabinol content and potency of marijuana have increased substantially in the past decade (ElSohly and Abel 1988). This might suggest that reliance on earlier data may underestimate the chronic neurotoxic insult of the higher-potency marijuana now available in the United States (Schwartz et al. 1989). This concern is likely unfounded, however, because the apparently higher potency of domestic marijuana in the United States in recent years appears to be an artifact of differences in the origin of the marijuana samples analyzed at the start of the Mississippi Project in 1974 (Morgan 1995).

Polydrug Use

Knowledge of the effects of multiple substance use on the brain and behavior has become especially important given trends toward increased polydrug use. Multiple drug use is prevalent in youthful (C. S. Martin et al. 1993) and adult (C. S. Martin et al. 1996) problem drinkers, and, as noted above, problem drug users seldom confine their use to only one drug type and almost always use alcohol. The simultaneous use of several different psychoactive drugs can produce negative effects on neurocognitive functioning that may be additive or synergistic. Different neurological and neuropsychological consequences may accrue when two or more drugs are used simultaneously rather than in temporally distinct episodes. For example, two drugs may compete for the same enzymes for metabolism, resulting in more sustained levels when taken concomitantly. Systematic research has not addressed these critical issues. Ideally, information should be available on the nature and extent of deficit that is likely to be found in persons who use certain common drug combinations, such as alcohol, marijuana, and cocaine. However, most samples have contained insufficient numbers of persons using specific drug combinations to generate precise information on neurocognitive damage.

Variability in samples and other methodological differences between studies have made it difficult to replicate early data that suggested about half of chronic polydrug users may experience some type of neuropsychological impairment (Grant and Judd 1976; Grant et al. 1979). This is not entirely surprising, because the drugs subjects used varied both within and across studies and included cocaine, inhalants, PCP, opiates, marijuana, hallucinogens, and the non–medically prescribed use of sedative-hypnotics, tranquilizers, and amphetamines. Sample sizes have been mostly small, and the subjects had histories of use that ranged from months to years. Control of premorbid and concurrent risk factors for neurocognitive impairment has been variable. The average age in samples of polydrug users usually fell within the range of early adolescence to the 30s. Such heterogeneity of subject and drug factors permits only the most tentative conclusions to be drawn from this literature.

One study compared 26 adolescents who met DSM-III-R criteria (American Psychiatric Association 1987) for psychoactive substance dependence (mostly polydrug inhalants [solvents and gasoline], marijuana, "basuco" [a preparation of freebase cocaine used in Colombia], and alcohol) with 38 age-, education-, and SES-matched control subjects. No significant differences in verbal skills, perceptual recognition, memory, or motor abilities were found, although control subjects tended to score higher (Bernal et al. 1994). Potentially vulnerable attentional and abstracting abilities were not evaluated. The authors suggested that in young persons with limited exposure histories, polysubstance use may act more to interfere with continued cognitive development than to cause cognitive decline.

Fals-Stewart and Lucente (1994) tested 246 (27% female, mean age 27) inpatients who had more than one Axis I diagnosis of psychoactive substance abuse (alcohol, cocaine, and opioids were most prevalent). One month after admission, 22.4% of subjects were classified as impaired on a test battery including the Category Test, Trail Making Test, WAIS Vocabulary test, Tactual Performance Test (Reitan and Wolfson 1993), Block Design test, and Digit Symbol test (Wechsler 1981). A smaller-scale study of similarly aged men abstinent for 3 weeks to 1 year found that the mean performance of polysubstance abusers on a similar battery fell within the normal to mildly impaired ranges, with much variability and some individuals impaired on each test (J. Schafer et al. 1994a). A more articulated knowledge of the specific neurocognitive impairment patterns that are likely to occur in specific subtypes of polydrug users requires further research that includes larger numbers of persons with common but distinct polyuse patterns.

◈ RISK FACTORS FOR IMPAIRMENT IN PERSONS WITH SUBSTANCE USE DISORDERS

Table 9–2 lists the major risk factors that have been suggested to increase vulnerability to neurocognitive impairment in persons with alcohol and other substance use disorders. With the exception of advancing

Table 9–2.   Putative risk factors for neurocognitive impairment in persons with alcohol and other substance use disorders

Age

Gender

Low education and academic achievement

Childhood behavior problems and attention-deficit disorder

Chronicity, extent, and pattern of substance use

Multiple substance use

Other psychiatric disorders

Personality disorder

Familial alcoholism history

Head trauma

Medical problems associated with central nervous system damage

age, the empirical evidence has been variable regarding the importance of each of these risk factors in determining the likelihood, nature, and extent of damage to the brain and functional abilities of chronic heavy substance users. This has been due, in part, to the substantial methodological difficulties involved in studying the unique effects of risk factors that naturally co-occur in samples of persons with substance use disorders, especially when information is not available concerning the temporal ordering of their presentation. Clinically, the co-occurrence of more than one of these factors in persons presenting for treatment signals an increase in the likelihood of neurocognitive impairment and the need for careful neuropsychological assessment. Knowledge of individual characteristics that mediate neurocognitive risk is helpful in distinguishing persons whose deficits predate their current substance use disorder from those whose impairment may be responsive to improved medical conditions and the cessation of use. This information may be useful for determining how much recovery of function might be expected with abstinence or reduced use, setting realistic expectations for recovery, and identifying treatment needs.

Age

Normative declines in cognitive functioning occur with increasing age, especially in fluid abilities that are not verbally mediated (La Rue 1992). Bornstein's (1986) data showed that conventional cutoff scores, derived from discrimination studies of normal and brain-damaged groups, substantially overestimated impairment in a normal sample as age increased. This was especially evident for individuals older than 60 years with limited education. Nevertheless, greater neurocognitive impairment often has been associated with increased age in subjects with polydrug use disorders (Fals-Stewart and Lucente 1994; Grant et al. 1978) and in chronic heavy alcohol users (Ryan and Butters 1986), even when age-corrected scores were analyzed (Tarbox et al. 1986). The rather consistent finding that deficit severity was related to age in alcoholic samples led to "premature aging" hypotheses, which suggested that alcohol accelerates the effects of aging on the brain or that the brains of older individuals are more vulnerable to the neurotoxic effects of alcohol. Although it is likely that aging and alcoholism affect neurocognitive impairment through different processes (e.g., Kramer et al. 1989), the probability of impairment in persons with substance use disorders increases with advancing age.

Gender

Among chronic heavy alcohol users, neurocognitive impairment is usually equivalent in men and women, although women have shorter drinking histories and smaller quantities of alcohol consumed. The extant research does not address whether this is due to increased vulnerability of women or insufficient knowledge of some other gender-related difference that can account for the perceived increased brain vulnerability in women. Until more is known about gender differences, such as alcohol absorption at the gastric mucosa and other factors discussed above, the issue will remain unresolved.

Low Education and Academic Achievement

Less formal education is associated not only with lower levels of performance on tests of crystallized verbal abilities such as vocabulary and information but also with lower performance on tests of fluid cognitive abilities such as abstracting and on executive function tests (Lezak 1995). Factors such as poor educational records and leaving school early are associated with more severe impairment in persons with alcohol and polysubstance use disorders (e.g., Rounsaville et al. 1981).

Childhood Behavior Problems and Attention-Deficit Disorder

Childhood behavior problems include hyperactivity, impulsivity, learning disabilities, aggressiveness, and attention-deficit disorder. In research, symptoms are often measured with retrospective checklists such as the Childhood Behavioral Disorders Checklist (Tarter et al. 1977), which assesses the presence of symptoms and behaviors before age 13 years. Childhood behavior problems are often more prevalent in alcohol use disorder groups (Glenn and Parsons 1989; Nixon et al. 1995) and other groups with substance use disorders (Beatty et al. 1995; Meek et al. 1989; Rounsaville et al. 1981) than in control groups, and they are suspected to increase risk for the development of substance use disorders. Prospective study also suggests that the early unsanctioned use of alcohol predicts higher levels of—and more rapid growth of—behavior problems from childhood to adolescence (Johnson et al. 1995). Alcohol use may reciprocally contribute to the expression of childhood behavior problems, or both substance use and childhood behavior problems may arise from some more general temperamental predisposition such as sensation seeking or a core antisocial trait (Johnson et al. 1995). These data again point to the poorly understood etiological roots of common personality, cognitive, and behavioral aspects of substance use disorders and certain psychopathology. More childhood behavior problems predicted more severe neuropsychological deficit in several use-disorder samples (Glenn et al. 1993; Workman-Daniels and Hesselbrock 1987), but there have also been negative results (e.g., Beatty et al. 1995). Adult residual attention-deficit disorder may be more prevalent among chronic heavy drinkers than control subjects, but it does not appear to be related to cognitive efficacy (Nixon et al. 1995).

Chronicity, Extent, and Pattern of Substance Use

The relation between duration of alcohol abuse and degree of neuropsychological impairment is not very clear. Imaging studies have provided some evidence for increased damage with increasing duration of alcohol use. For example, frontal, parietal, and temporal glucose utilization was negatively correlated with years of alcohol use (Volkow et al. 1994). Length of addiction correlated significantly with CSF volumes visualized by MRI, after taking age into account (Chick et al. 1989). In relapsing men, lifetime alcohol consumption predicted white matter volume losses and enlargement of the third ventricle when drinking was resumed (Pfefferbaum et al. 1995).

Parsons's (1993) review concluded that no consistent effects of drinking chronicity, quantity, or frequency of use on severity of neuropsychological impairment had been found. Although specific findings have not been replicated across different samples, the significant associations found have been consistently in the direction of greater impairment with greater use. The unreliability of drinking history information in some studies may have contributed to equivocal results. Saarnio's study (1994) of 179 Finnish male alcoholic inpatients randomly assigned to groups tested during either the first, second, or fourth week of abstinence found that duration of problem drinking was associated with neuropsychological functioning only early during abstinence when withdrawal symptomatology was prevalent. Saarnio suggested that individual differences in spontaneous recovery may have masked drinking-duration effects.

With respect to the patterning of alcohol consumption, Hunt (1993) suggested that binge drinkers who go through many withdrawals may be at heightened risk for brain damage because withdrawal from chronic alcohol consumption results in unregulated NMDA and calcium receptors and increased glucocorticoid exposure. Behaviorally, however, Tarbox and colleagues (1986) and Sanchez-Craig (1980) found that bout or episodic drinkers performed better than daily drinkers on short-term memory, internal scanning, and visuospatial-visuomotor skills. One hindrance to research has been the lack of a consistent taxonomy of drinking patterns. Systematic and empirically tested methods of categorizing binge, episodic, sporadic, and steady drinkers (e.g., Epstein et al. 1995) are needed to provide uniform definitions of drinking patterns.

Multiple Substance Use

Comorbid substance use disorders are prevalent in samples of persons seeking treatment for alcohol and other drug use problems (Dinwiddie et al. 1987; Pogge et al. 1992; Rounsaville et al. 1981). To the extent that different drugs induce brain dysfunction to different neural systems or facilitate impairment of the same systems, neurocognitive deficit may be augmented in multiple substance users.

Other Psychiatric Disorders

The prevalence of psychoactive substance use disorders is higher among patients with schizophrenia and affective psychoses than in the general population (Regier et al. 1990). The lifetime prevalence of substance abuse disorders in schizophrenic patients may be as high as 65% (Mueser et al. 1990). As discussed throughout this book, many psychiatric disorders are associated with well-documented neurocognitive abnormalities. The prevalence of co-occurring psychopathology in populations with substance use disorders varies depending on sample characteristics. For example, prevalence among individuals with use disorders who are receiving treatment in psychiatric hospitals would be higher than in an outpatient community treatment setting. Co-occurring affective disorders, especially depression and anxiety, are most common and may independently contribute to poor neurocognitive performance levels. Comorbidity risk is not limited to adult users of psychoactive substances. Pogge et al. (1992) found substantial amounts of Axis I psychopathology in male and female adolescent inpatients with alcohol and other substance use diagnoses. Psychopathology may also be prevalent in heroin-dependent individuals receiving methadone maintenance treatment (Hendriks et al. 1990). Conversely, an earlier review (Craig 1986) found major psychiatric symptomatology was the exception in drug-dependent subjects. Historical changes in methods of diagnosing psychiatric disorders and substance abuse and dependence—or changes in the populations themselves—may have contributed to this apparent discrepancy.

Systematic research on the common and specific neuropsychological deficits in patients dually diagnosed with a substance use disorder and another specific psychiatric disorder is lacking. However, more interest in this area is emerging as the substantial prevalence rates of substance use disorders in persons with other psychiatric diagnoses become known (Mueser et al. 1990). Tracy et al. (1995) reviewed the common and different cognitive effects of substance use disorders and schizophrenia, and they proposed several frameworks for conceptualizing their etiological overlap and common cognitive effects. The frameworks yield testable, alternative models of dually mediated risk such as shared vulnerability and the potentiation or exacerbation by substance use of psychiatrically mediated impairment. These models are of heuristic value to neurocognitive research aimed at understanding the independent and combined effects of substance use disorders and psychopathology.

Personality Disorder

In contrast to the divergent findings above, Craig's (1986) earlier review of about 200 empirical reports from 1925 to 1985 found an increased prevalence of personality disorders in drug-dependent individuals. Subjects diagnosed with abuse of or dependence on alcohol (Fishbein et al. 1989), inhalants (Dinwiddie et al. 1987), cocaine (Bauer 1994), primarily heroin, or multiple drugs (Guerra et al. 1987) show higher rates of comorbid antisocial personality disorder than those without such diagnoses. A multisite study of alcohol treatment samples found that more than half met criteria for at least one personality disorder; antisocial personality disorder was the most prevalent in men (25.7%), whereas women had higher rates of borderline (36.4%) and self-defeating (22.7%) personality disorders (Morgenstern et al. 1997).

Early deficits in executive functions have been found in physically aggressive boys (Seguin et al. 1995), especially in those at risk for a persistent pattern of antisocial behavior (Moffit et al. 1994). Verbal deficits have sometimes been found. The sensation-seeking behaviors of antisocial individuals (Cloninger 1987) and the persistence of executive deficits in physically aggressive individuals (Giancola 1995) may place them at heightened risk for substance use as well as for compound alcohol-related deficits mediated by other factors such as medical disorders and head trauma.

Subjects with substance use (primarily alcohol) disorders and antisocial personality disorder showed more prefrontal deficit (Category Test, Trail Making Test Part B, Block Design test) than those without antisocial personality disorder (Malloy et al. 1990). Similarly, more severe verbal memory deficits have also been found in chronic heavy drinkers with antisocial personality disorder (Malloy et al. 1989, 1990). These studies also found that chronic heavy drinkers with comorbid antisocial personality disorder reported poorer health, earlier onset and heavier alcohol use, and greater abuse of other drugs than those without antisocial personality disorder. In combination with antisocial personality disorder and head trauma, these risk factors all contributed to more severe neurocognitive deficits.

Familial Alcoholism History

Conclusions have diverged regarding the premorbid cognitive status of individuals with a positive family history of alcoholism (Bates 1993; Pihl

et al. 1990; Searles 1988; Sher 1991). Our examination of a large community sample of youths with a positive family history and those with a negative
family history found no reliable family history group differences in male or
female subjects across a range of neuropsychological abilities (Bates and
Pandina 1992; see also Alterman and Hall 1989; Schuckit et al. 1987; Workman-Daniels and Hesselbrock 1987) for negative findings. Well-controlled,
programmatic research by Schandler and colleagues (1995), however, has
provided consistent evidence of inferior learning speed and pattern in
visuospatial information processing from about age 3 years to adulthood in
offspring with a positive family history of alcoholism.

Much evidence for cognitive deficits related to a positive family history
for alcoholism has been obtained from samples containing individuals
who have additional risk factors for neurocognitive deficit such as
psychopathology or personality disorder on the part of offspring or their
parents (e.g., Gabrielli and Mednick 1983; Tarter et al. 1984). When differences are found between offspring with positive and negative family
histories, the most consistent impairments have been in tasks requiring
verbal, abstracting, or visuospatial abilities (Hesselbrock et al. 1991; Pihl
et al. 1990; Sher 1991). Physical abuse, head injury, and parental neglect
may accompany parental alcoholism (Tarter et al. 1984) and antisocial
personality disorder (Malloy et al. 1990) and enhance the likelihood of
deficit in persons with a positive family history of alcoholism.

Some evidence suggests that certain brain abnormalities found in
samples of young subjects with a positive family history, such as decreased P300 amplitude, may normalize during development and thus
not be evident during adulthood in affected populations (Hill et al. 1995;
Steinhauer and Hill 1993). Hill and colleagues suggested that such markers may index a neurobiological developmental delay. The consequences
of such developmental delays on neurocognitive competency and resiliency during adulthood are unknown.

Research in affected populations has also met with mixed results. Detoxified chronic heavy drinkers with a positive family history sometimes
have shown greater neurocognitive deficit than subjects with a negative
family history (K. W. Schaeffer et al. 1988; Turner and Parsons 1988),
but not always (e.g., Alterman et al. 1987; Drake et al. 1995). Differences
in alcohol use intensity and duration, and in other factors that may affect
the cognitive sequelae of use between chronic heavy drinkers with a positive and a negative family history have seldom been controlled. Chronic
heavy drinkers with a positive family history who return to drinking after
a period of abstinence may show greater neurocognitive deterioration

than other persons who resume drinking (Drake et al. 1995). Heightened prevalences of medical and psychiatric disorders in chronic heavy drinkers with a positive family history compared with those with a negative family history may also increase the risk of neurocognitive impairment (Penick et al. 1987).

Positive family history status appears to increase risk for other substance abuse disorders. For example, Byrne and colleagues (1991) found that one-half of patients being treated for solvent inhalation at a psychiatric hospital had a positive family history for alcoholism but not for other psychopathology. As with chronic heavy drinkers, persons with heroin and polydrug use disorders with a positive family history sometimes (e.g., Rodriquez 1993a), but not always (Rodriquez 1993b), show greater deficits relative to those with a negative family history.

Head Trauma

Alcohol use is a well-documented contributing factor to head trauma (Jones 1989), and alcohol dependence is overrepresented among head trauma victims (O'Shanick et al. 1984). Alcohol and head trauma may often compromise the same neuropsychological functions because both affect orbitofrontal and anterior temporal brain regions. One study of a large sample of patients with head injuries found that neuropsychological outcome was independently related to both severity of head injury and severity of alcohol problem (Dikmen et al. 1993). This study identified the clustering of characteristics such as limited education, low levels of verbal and nonverbal abilities, problem drinking, and head injuries, which may represent a subtype. These data again demonstrated the common covariation of multiple risk factors that heighten the expression of, or vulnerability to, neurocognitive deficit.

Medical Problems Associated With Central Nervous System Damage

Neuropathological and other data suggest that thiamine deficiency and liver dysfunction may play important roles in nonspecific alcoholic brain atrophy as well as in the specific syndromes described above (e.g., Harper and Kril 1991). Recent research (Lavoie and Butterworth 1995) points to complex interactions between liver disease, which may facilitate thiamine depletion in alcoholic patients, and reduced activity of thiamine-dependent enzymes in the absence of Wernicke's encephalopathy, which also may contribute to brain damage and cognitive impairment in alcoholic patients. Although the etiology of impairment often is not clear, the presence of clinical or subclinical levels of hepatic impairment, nutritional or metabolic abnormalities, or other medical conditions may independently affect brain function and heighten risk for impairment in individuals with substance use disorders. Subclinical levels of liver dysfunction may give rise to subtle neurocognitive deficits in patients showing no obvious neurological symptoms of brain damage (Butterworth 1995), suggesting the need for neuropsychological assessment in this at-risk group.

◈ Neuropsychological and Cognitive Assessment Approaches

Data on the prevalence of functional and structural neuropsychological abnormalities in chronic heavy drinkers and other individuals with substance use disorders strongly argue for the need to assess impairment in this domain. More than half of chronic heavy alcohol and other drug users show mild to severe impairment in one or more areas of neuropsychological functioning (e.g., Grant et al. 1979; Meek et al. 1989; Parsons 1993), although group averages in many studies do not fall within the impaired range. The heterogeneity of deficit found among individuals calls for assessment approaches designed to capture impairment in multiple domains of functioning. Formal neuropsychological testing is indicated, because many chronic users have intact verbal abilities. Deficits in fluid abilities such as abstraction thus may not be apparent in casual conversations or structured interviews. Recent trends in managed mental health care systems have resulted in reduced treatment times, making the early detection of deficit more critical for clinical decision making (Meek et al. 1989; Weinstein and Shaffer 1993). Limited resources for assessment present the challenge of devising assessment strategies that are cost- and time-efficient, yet broadly focused, sensitive, and clinically applicable to populations with substance use disorders.

Table 9–3 provides examples of different approaches to assessing neuropsychological and cognitive deficits in patients with substance use disorders. A comprehensive description of these, as well as other often-used neuropsychological tests, is provided by Lezak (1995). Nixon (1995) and Weinstein and Shaffer (1993) also outline, within functional domains, many of the alternative tests used in substance use research.

Table 9–3. Assessment methods for detecting neuropsychological impairment and brain damage in persons with alcohol and other substance use disorders

Traditional neuropsychological and achievement batteries

    Halstead-Reitan Battery (HRB; Reitan and Wolfson 1993)

    Wechsler Adult Intelligence Scale—Revised (WAIS-R; Wechsler 1981)

    Shipley Institute of Living Scale (Zachary 1986)

Eclectic and specialized neuropsychological batteries

    National Institute of Mental Health Core Neuropsychological Battery (Butters et al. 1990)

    Meta-Analytic Derived Battery (Chouinard and Braun 1993)

    Decision Tree Battery (Horton 1993)

    Mini-Mental State Exam (MMSE; Folstein et al. 1975)

    Neurobehavioral Cognitive Status Examination (NCSE; Meek et al. 1989)

    Screening Battery (Drebing et al. 1994)

Process-oriented neurocognitive assessments

    WAIS-R Neuropsychological Instrument (Kaplan et al. 1991)

    Product Recall Test (Sussman et al. 1986)

    Piagetian Plant Task (Kuhn and Brannock 1977)

    Rivermead Behavioral Memory Test (Wilson et al. 1985)

Traditional Neuropsychological Batteries

Traditional battery approaches such as the Halstead-Reitan Battery and the WAIS-R have been most used in research and have the advantage of rich historical databases. Extensive age-, sex-, and education-stratified normative data are available (e.g., Heaton et al. 1991). Disadvantages typically include lengthy administration times and limited assessments of memory and executive functions.

Eclectic and Specialized Neuropsychological Batteries

Eclectic neuropsychological batteries are often made up of tests selected from traditional batteries. Eclectic batteries should ideally be composed of tests that tap cognitive abilities known to be particularly vulnerable to alcohol and other drug-associated impairment. Such composite neuropsychological batteries assessing multiple domains of functioning are assumed to be more sensitive to diffuse impairment (Butters et al. 1990; Drebing et al. 1994) and to predict brain dysfunction better than any single measure (Rojas and Bennett 1995).

Recent research with older adults and asymptomatic HIV-positive patients—who, like patients with substance use disorders, show diffuse impairment of fluid functions—provides useful assessment batteries. Early neurocognitive declines in older adults include impaired psychomotor speed, verbal and visual memory, visuospatial and visuoperceptual abilities, and cognitive flexibility–set shifting (Drebing et al. 1994). The diffuse brain dysfunction of asymptomatic HIV-positive patients is suspected to involve similar functional domains, as well as abstraction and attention deficits (Butters et al. 1990). Although the causes of deficits may be different in elderly persons, those with early HIV infection, and those with use disorders, at a functional-behavioral level, assessment advances in these fields are relevant to those with substance use disorders.

Comprehensive eclectic batteries. Butters and colleagues' battery (1990) comprises recommendations of the National Institute of Mental Health (NIMH) Work Group on Neuropsychological Assessment Approaches most sensitive to the early diffuse brain dysfunction of asymptomatic HIV-positive patients. This battery, which takes approximately 7–9 hours to administer, includes multiple tests within eight domains of functioning: attention, memory, speed of processing, language, visuospatial skills, construction abilities, motor abilities, and abstraction.

Chouinard and Braun (1993) conducted a meta-analysis of the relative sensitivity of neuropsychological screening tests used to detect diffuse brain dysfunction within functional domains similar to those of the NIMH work group. The major difference was their addition of assessments in the executive functioning domain. The most sensitive and brief tests in each domain were identified. The results of their meta-analyses may be used by clinicians to construct a time-efficient, sensitive, and functionally broad battery. However, interrelationships of test sensitivity were not evaluated for tests in different domains, leaving the question unanswered whether tests from each of the domains need to be included for screening purposes.

Brief and screening batteries. A particularly time-efficient assessment strategy, designed to meet screening, severity classification, and treatment selection needs, is represented by Horton's (1994) decision tree model. For example, screening decisions are made by first administering the Trail Making Test Part B; depending on performance on this test, a subsequent test of lesser (Mini-Mental State Exam [MMSE; Folstein et al. 1975]) or greater (Shipley Institute of Living Scale) difficulty is given. The decision tree approach offers a systematic way to increase flexibility in matching assessments to an individual's functional level.

The sensitivity of the MMSE in detecting diffuse impairment was compared with that of a brief eclectic screening battery (WAIS-R Digit Symbol, Trail Making Test Parts A and B, Rey Auditory-Verbal Learning Test [Rey 1964], Rey-Osterrieth Complex Figure copy and delayed recall [Corwin and Bylsma 1993]) in a high-functioning, older population (Drebing et al. 1994). The alternative battery proved more sensitive than the MMSE, with two individual tests achieving correct classification rates near those of the full battery: the Digit Symbol Substitution Test and the Trail Making Test Part B. These data suggested that multiple-measure batteries may not always greatly improve sensitivity to diffuse deficit. However, sensitivity to focal impairment of abilities not assessed by these two measures was enhanced by administration of the full battery.

Meek and colleagues (1989) compared the Neurobehavioral Cognitive Status Examination (NCSE; Schwamm et al. 1987), the screening test for the Luria-Nebraska Neuropsychological Battery, and the Trail Making Test in a veterans' substance abuse program. The data suggested that the NCSE could be administered by nonprofessionals to assess orientation, attention, memory, language fluency and comprehension, naming, visuospatial construction, calculation, abstraction, and judgment. Most tasks begin with a screening item, and for individuals unable to perform the screen, easier metric items quantify the degree of impairment. Performance in each area is classified as normal or mildly, moderately, or severely impaired.

Tests to screen for specific types of deficits in subgroups with substance use disorders are also available. For example, one brief assessment technique detects executive functioning deficits in geriatric populations (Royall et al. 1992). This clinically based bedside screen focuses on behavioral sequelae such as loss of spontaneity and environmental intrusions. It was able to discriminate four groups of elderly subjects ranging from residents of independent living apartments to residents of an Alzheimer's special care unit; scores also correlated well with traditional tests of executive functions such as the Trail Making Test, Wisconsin Card Sorting Test, and Test of Sustained Attention (Lezak 1995). Further research is needed to determine the applicability and relative utility of various brief screening tests with specific subtypes of substance use disorders.

In summary, eclectic neurocognitive batteries offer the advantage of deficit assessment across multiple functional domains, specifically tailored to the types of dysfunction most prevalent in patients with substance use disorders. Batteries composed of well-studied, preexisting tests also enjoy the advantage of rich normative and comparative databases. However, there is a persisting research need for validation studies at the level of the battery rather than composite tests.

Process-Oriented Neurocognitive Assessments

A cognitive science approach to the assessment of functional deficits in persons with substance use disorders involves process-oriented assessments. This approach seeks to establish the relation between brain structure, process, and behavioral performance on specific cognitive tasks (Polster 1993). Performance on most traditional neuropsychological tasks is multidetermined, and a single poor performance score may alternately reflect impairment in attention, working memory, abstracting abilities, or response selection. Cognitive process assessments can help determine which of these component processing operations is undermining performance in complex neuropsychological tests.

Process-oriented assessment approaches have included the modification of established neuropsychological batteries (WAIS-R Neuropsychological Instrument; Kaplan et al. 1991), the development of new standardized batteries (Rivermead Behavioral Memory Test; Wilson et al. 1985), and the use of individual tests (Product Recall Task) (Sussman et al. 1986). Kaplan and colleagues' (1991) modification of the WAIS-R clarifies information-processing errors that underlie poor performance on WAIS-R subtests. Their approach provides a standardized method of evaluating qualitative aspects of performance strategies (Lezak 1995). Nixon and Parsons (1991) have proposed a process-oriented method of assessing cognitive impairment that focuses on differences in access, availability, and efficiency of information processing. They used the Plant Task (Kuhn and Brannock 1977), based on Piagetian constructs of formal operations, to show that male and female chronic heavy drinkers were less able than control subjects to ignore irrelevant information when using feedback from the environment, yet they were not deficient in information availability. Performance on the Plant Task has also predicted completion of alcohol treatment (Erwin and Hunter 1984). The utility of process-oriented tasks in applied settings will be enhanced by research to determine their overlap with established neuropsychological measures and by the development of normative, comparative databases.

Additional Considerations in Selecting Tests

An important concern in selecting assessments is that alternative tests of performance within the same functional domain often do not provide interchangeable information. For example, although the Wisconsin Card Sorting Test and the Category Test are both widely used to assess abstraction, concept formation, and executive functioning, the common variance shared between the two tests is only between 12% and 30% (e.g., Perrine 1993). Similarly, our examination of tests commonly used to measure frontal or executive functions (e.g., Trail Making Test Part B, Stroop Test [Golden 1978], Category Test, Wisconsin Card Sorting Test perseveration errors, Word Fluency [Benton 1973]) showed only slight to moderate diagnostic equivalence in a sample with substance use disorders (Bates et al. 1996). Given that time-efficient screens for impairment typically include only one or two tests per functional domain, future research should be responsive to clinicians' need for more knowledge about the diagnostic equivalence of well-known tests.

The relative sensitivity of neurocognitive assessment batteries is also a function of test-retest reliability, test difficulty, test intercorrelations, and the number of summary scores derived (Chouinard and Braun 1993). As Siu (1991) noted for dementia, no standardized, practical criteria exist for most neurocognitive problems. Some studies have used diagnoses assigned by clinicians or physicians, whereas others used neuroimaging or neuropathological findings. As discussed above, the use of behavioral versus anatomical criteria may lead, for example, to different persons being given the diagnosis of Korsakoff's syndrome (cf. Blansjaar et al. 1992; Bowden 1990). Critical research needs are to determine appropriate criterion measures of impairment, to assess the sensitivity and specificity of screening batteries to impairment in populations with substance use disorders, and to evaluate their ability to predict functional competence in areas relevant to treatment success (Gillen et al. 1991).

◈ IMPLICATIONS FOR TREATMENT

Neurocognitive Deficit, Treatment Process, and Treatment Outcome

The idea that cognitive impairment may interfere with individuals' ability to profit from treatment for substance use disorders has considerable intuitive and conceptual appeal. Cognitive factors support patients' ability to attend, to learn and remember new information, to integrate new knowledge and skills with prior learning experiences, and to plan and implement behavioral strategies as alternatives to substance use. The diffuse cortical and frontal damage found in many patients with alcohol and other substance use disorders may substantially interfere with the attentional and controlled information-processing operations required by many treatments (Goldman 1990; Weinstein and Shaffer 1993).

Empirical study has supported the idea that neurocognitive impairment may interfere with treatment process and outcome in alcoholic patients (Parsons et al. 1987). Overall, however, the ability of neuropsychological impairment to predict outcome has been quite modest across studies, and sometimes no relation has been found between extent of impairment and outcome (e.g., Bergman 1987). It appears likely that information regarding neurocognitive deficit in individuals with substance use disorders will be most clinically useful when evaluated within the broader constellation of intrapersonal capabilities and environmental supports of the individual. Recent study has begun to provide more articulated information in this area. The following section discusses clinical perspectives and current research findings that examine the association of neurocognitive deficits to treatment issues within models involving other relevant patient characteristics.

Implications for Clinical Decision Making and Management

From an applied perspective, neurocognitive assessment is generally believed to provide information useful for clinical decision making with patients with alcohol and other substance use disorders (Horton 1993; Meek et al. 1989). Neurocognitive assessment is initially useful to determine patients' level of cognitive competence at the start of treatment. One study found that it is possible to obtain psychometrically and clinically stable estimates of neuropsychological functioning within the first week of addictions treatment entry, or the week following medical detoxification, if required (Bates 1997). In addition to providing information useful in matching patients to the cognitive demands of various interventions, assessment of neurocognitive deficit may influence the attitudes and expectations of clinicians and of patients themselves (Weinstein and Shaffer 1993). Impressions of patients considered to be resistant and in denial appeared to change when treatment providers and staff members were given information regarding memory deficits and other cognitive problems that might otherwise have been interpreted as lack of patient cooperation (Meek et al. 1989). Neurocognitive impairment in the early weeks of treatment may explain some of the inattention, distractibility, unreliability, and lack of motivation described by therapists of individuals with use disorders (Grant and Judd 1976).

Clinical interpretation of neurocognitive performance should take into account length of abstinence, features of withdrawal, anxiety, depression, motivation, practice effects, trauma, and medical status, as well as standard socioeconomic and sociodemographic factors (Glass 1991). Variability in neurocognitive impairment among users suggests that treatments may need to be tailored to various cognitive levels (Meek et al. 1989). For patients with opiate and polydrug use disorders and neuropsychological impairment, highly structured, problem-oriented, and reality-based interventions including simple and straightforward communications may be most appropriate (Grant and Judd 1976; Grant et al. 1978). Polysubstance users with antisocial personality disorder may not fare well in intensive residential treatments, because these make many demands on sustained attention, concentration, and memory. Fals-Stewart and Lucente (1994) suggested a graded approach to treatment with such clients, including initial placement in a supervised living setting and, once cognitive function returns, movement to more intensive treatment.

Cognitive deficits will not always or fully remediate, depending on the cause of deficit and the degree of brain damage. Reassessment of neuropsychological functioning over time provides information regarding the extent and rate of recovery so that treatment may be adapted to maximize benefits (Meek et al. 1989; Weinstein and Shaffer 1993). Treatment strategies need to address chronic limitations in learning and behavioral flexibility (Grant et al. 1978) and to acknowledge the possibility of long-lasting cognitive deficits that may affect both the performance of complex tasks and the ability to learn (Schwartz et al. 1989). Repetition of material to compensate for attentional, concentration, and memory deficits, and the use of concrete examples to compensate for impaired abstraction, are techniques that may facilitate learning.

In addition to the cognitive recovery that occurs spontaneously over time with abstinence, neurocognitive efficacy may also be enhanced by providing "experience" with certain neuropsychological tasks (Goldman 1990) or specific cognitive retraining (Wetzig and Hardin 1990). Neurocognitive process approaches provide information at a level that can be useful in the design of remediation strategies (Nixon 1995). For example, Wetzig and Hardin (1990) used an information-processing approach to design a remedial training program in strategy planning and use of environmental feedback. They found that for neurocognitively impaired chronic heavy drinkers, this training resulted in improved performance that generalized beyond the original training task.

A number of cognitive remediation strategies and other techniques that have been developed for different populations may prove useful for maximizing treatment efficacy with individuals who have use disorders. Interventions that have been successful in persons with head injuries may be applied to those with substance use disorders and neurocognitive damage. Weinstein and Shaffer (1993) discuss and extend Morse and Montgomery's (1992) summaries of clinical strategies to remediate specific neurocognitive problems (e.g., attention, executive deficits, and memory), in relation to individual and group therapy for populations with use disorders. For example, clinicians can specifically modify treatment for patients with a memory storage problem by using preorganization, cuing, and other strategies developed to improve attention and encoding; using compensatory strategies such as writing in a notebook; and focusing on procedural memory abilities in learning specific tasks. Such strategies have broad applicability because they may be flexibly applied to various kinds of patients over time, and they allow cognitive remediation to become an integral component of treatment within varied settings such as therapeutic communities, methadone maintenance programs, outpatient treatment centers, and family intervention programs (Weinstein and Shaffer 1993).

Finally, there is a lack of available data to link relevant intrapersonal characteristics to the efficacy of different treatments for specific types of persons (Mattson et al. 1994). Research has just begun to provide more information about treatment efficacy for neurocognitively impaired individuals with substance use disorders and common co-occurring conditions such as antisocial personality disorder. Fals-Stewart and Lucente

(1994) found that polysubstance abusers in residential treatment with antisocial personality tendencies and cognitive impairment stayed in the treatment program a shorter amount of time, were rated by clinical staff as participating in treatment less positively, and were removed more frequently from treatment for rule violations than others. Neurocognitive impairment and antisocial personality tendencies independently affected and interactively combined to affect treatment tenure. Chronic inhalant abusers also may be particularly resistant to treatment because of high rates of antisocial personality disorder (Dinwiddie et al. 1987), acute or persistent paranoid psychosis, or temporal-lobe epilepsy (Byrne et al. 1991). Concurrent confusional states may remit within several weeks or may persist. The combined socioeconomic, intellectual, and psychological vulnerabilities that characterize many inhalant abusers make this disorder particularly challenging to treat (Dinwiddie et al. 1987).

The effects of brain damage on mood, judgment, self-esteem, learning, motivation, social stability, and related factors may moderate or mediate the relation of neurocognitive impairment to outcome (Glass 1991; Roehrich and Goldman 1993). Neuropsychological impairment may indirectly affect relapse through its direct effects on competency in other life areas such as skill acquisition, interpersonal functioning, and the control of negative affect (Goldman 1990; J. Schafer et al. 1994a). These latter factors would then be the more proximal determinants of relapse. J. Schafer and colleagues' (1994a) study of polysubstance abusing men and their nonabusing wives found that husbands with lower neurocognitive performance (verbal, abstracting, and executive abilities) engaged in more frequent negative communications and fewer positive communications and reported increased levels of violence during conflicts. Given that negative interpersonal interactions are a risk factor for relapse among chronic heavy drinkers, the authors suggested that a similar dynamic may be involved with polysubstance abusers. The need for remediation of interpersonal problems in cognitively impaired persons with alcohol use disorders may underlie Cooney and colleagues' (1991) unanticipated finding that neuropsychologically impaired persons placed in interactional group therapy showed better outcomes than did those in behavioral skills training therapy.

◈ CONCLUSION

Chronic heavy users of alcohol often experience neuropsychological impairment, structural brain damage, and functional brain abnormalities.

Much of this damage appears to be driven by nutritional, metabolic, and hepatic dysfunction. Further research is needed to determine the role of direct neurotoxic alcohol effects in humans. Diffuse impairment across one or more domains of cognitive functioning is common; abstraction, executive functioning, memory, new learning, and complex visuospatial skills appear to be most vulnerable. Chronic heavy drinkers whose neuropsychological dysfunction is secondary to alcohol abuse may achieve substantial recovery of brain structure and function when they stop drinking, especially if they are young and do not have an extensive history of abuse. The data point to the importance of selecting the right types of neuropsychological assessments to identify and track multidimensional deficit patterns over time. Specialized neuropsychological batteries appear to be best suited to accomplish these goals. Clinically, knowledge of individuals' neuropsychological status is considered necessary to inform treatment selection and determine the need for cognitive remediation.

Drugs such as cocaine, opioids, PCP, marijuana, and inhalants have been far less studied than alcohol. Moreover, the potential neurotoxic effects of specific drugs are difficult to delineate because of individuals' tendency to use multiple psychoactive substances. Although many drug abusers have neurocognitive impairment, evidence for a direct or indirect causal relationship between drug use (perhaps with the exception of inhalants) and deficit is much less compelling than for alcohol. The literature to date has not adequately separated the influence of deficits that predate drug abuse or arise from co-occurring conditions from neuropsychological impairment consequent to drug use. For these reasons, we thought it would be premature and misleading to present a simple table of the kinds of neurocognitive impairments caused by the use of different drugs. The reader may be frustrated by what is unknown about the nature and extent of neuropsychological and cognitive impairments mediated by drug abuse, their prevalences, and recovery courses. For the multitude of reasons discussed herein, research in this area is very difficult. Yet, with the use of prospective longitudinal designs and structural and functional brain imaging techniques, multilevel research methodologies can now begin to answer these questions. We hope these methodologies are pursued with vigor, because understanding of the origins and mechanisms of brain damage associated with psychoactive substance abuse has important implications for prevention as well as for the development of behavioral and pharmacological interventions.

◈ REFERENCES

Aasly J, Storsaeter O, Nilsen G, et al: Minor structural brain changes in young drug abusers: a magnetic resonance study. Acta Neurol Scand 87:210–214, 1993

Acker C: Neuropsychological deficits in alcoholics: the relative contributions of gender and drinking history. British Journal of Addiction 81:395–403, 1986

Adams DH: Leucocyte adhesion molecules and alcoholic liver disease. Alcohol Alcohol 29:249–260, 1994

Adams KM, Gilman S, Koeppe RA, et al: Neuropsychological deficits are correlated with frontal hypometabolism in positron emission tomography studies of older alcoholic patients. Alcohol Clin Exp Res 17:205–210, 1993

Adams KM, Gilman S, Koeppe R, et al: Correlation of neuropsychological function with cerebral metabolic rate in subdivisions of the frontal lobes of older alcoholic patients measured with [18 F] fluorodeoxyglucose and positron emission tomography. Neuropsychology 9:275–280, 1995

Adams RL, Boake C, Crain C: Bias in a neuropsychological test classification related to education, age, and ethnicity. J Consult Clin Psychol 50:143–145, 1982

Alexander M: Traumatic brain injury, in Psychiatric Aspects of Neurologic Disease. Edited by Benson DF, Blumer D. New York, Grune & Stratton, 1982, pp 219–249

Allison WM, Jerrom DWA: Glue sniffing: a pilot study of the cognitive effects of long-term use. International Journal of the Addictions 19:453–458, 1984

Alterman AI, Hall JG: Effects of social drinking and familial alcoholism risk on cognitive functioning: null findings. Alcohol Clin Exp Res 13:799–803, 1989

Alterman AI, Gerstley LJ, Goldstein G, et al: Comparisons of the cognitive functioning of familial and nonfamilial alcoholics. J Stud Alcohol 48:425–429, 1987

American Psychiatric Association: Diagnostic and Statistical Manual of Mental Disorders, 3rd Edition, Revised. Washington, DC, American Psychiatric Association, 1987

Amir T, Bahri T: Effect of substance abuse on visuographic function. Percept Mot Skills 78:235–241, 1994

Anger WK: Worksite behavioral research: results, sensitive methods, test batteries and the transition from laboratory data to human health. Neurotoxicology 11:629–720, 1990

Ardila A, Rosselli M, Strumwasser S: Neuropsychological deficits in chronic cocaine abusers. Int J Neurosci 57:73–79, 1991

Arria AM, Tarter RE, Kabene MA, et al: The role of cirrhosis in memory functioning of alcoholics. Alcohol Clin Exp Res 15:932–937, 1991

Barona A, Reynolds CR, Chastian R: A demographically based index of premorbid intelligence for the WAIS-R. J Consult Clin Psychol 52:885–887, 1984

Barron JH, Russell EW: Fluidity theory and neuropsychological impairment in alcoholism. Archives of Clinical Neuropsychology 7:175–188, 1992

Bates ME: Psychology, in Recent Developments in Alcoholism, Vol 11. Edited by Galanter M. New York, Plenum, 1993, pp 45–72

Bates ME: Stability of neuropsychological assessments early in alcoholism treatment [published erratum appears in J Stud Alcohol 59:236, 1998]. J Stud Alcohol 58:617–621, 1997.

Bates ME, Pandina RJ: Familial alcoholism and premorbid cognitive deficit: a failure to replicate subtype differences. J Stud Alcohol 53:320–327, 1992

Bates ME, Tracy JI: Cognitive functioning in young "social drinkers": is there impairment to detect? J Abnorm Psychol 99:242–249, 1990

Bates ME, Labouvie EW, Rotgers F: Diagnostic concordance of six executive function tests (abstract). The Clinical Neuropsychologist 10:343, 1996

Bauer LO: Vigilance in recovering cocaine-dependent and alcohol-dependent patients: a prospective study. Addict Behav 19:599–607, 1994

Beatty WW, Katzung VM, Moreland VJ, et al: Neuropsychological performance of recently abstinent alcoholics and cocaine abusers. Drug Alcohol Depend 37:247–253, 1995

Begleiter H, Reich T, Hesselbrock V, et al: The collaborative study on the genetics of alcoholism. Alcohol Health Res World 19:228–248, 1995

Benton AL: Test de praxie constructive tri-dimensionnelle: forme alternative pour la clinique et la recherche. Revue de Psychologie Appliquee 23:1–5, 1973

Benton AL: Revised Visual Retention Test. New York, Psychological Corporation, 1974

Benton AL: Neuropsychological assessment. Annu Rev Psychol 45:1–23, 1994

Bergman H: Cognitive deficits and morphological cerebral changes in a random sample of social drinkers, in Recent Developments in Alcoholism, Vol 3. Edited by Galanter M. New York, Plenum, 1985, pp 265–275

Bergman H: Brain dysfunction related to alcoholism: some results from the KARTAD Project, in Neuropsychology of Alcoholism: Implications for Diagnosis and Treatment. Edited by Parsons OA, Butters N, Nathan PE. New York, Guilford, 1987, pp 21–44

Bernal B, Ardila A, Bateman JR: Cognitive impairments in adolescent drug-abusers. Int J Neurosci 75:203–212, 1994

Berry GJ: Neuropsychological Assessment of Solvent Inhalers: Final Report to the National Institute on Drug Abuse. Washington, DC, U.S. Government Printing Office, 1976

Berry J, van Gorp WG, Herzberg DS, et al: Neuropsychological deficits in abstinent cocaine abusers: preliminary findings after two weeks of abstinence. Drug Alcohol Depend 32:231–237, 1993

Biggins CA, MacKay S, Poole N, et al: Delayed P3A in abstinent elderly male chronic alcoholics. Alcohol Clin Exp Res 19:1032–1042, 1995

Blansjaar BA, Vielvoye GJ, van Dijk JG, et al: Similar brain lesions in alcoholics and Korsakoff patients: MRI, psychometric and clinical findings. Clin Neurol Neurosurg 94:197–203, 1992

Block RI, Ghoneim MM: Effects of chronic marijuana use on human cognition. Psychopharmacology 110:219–228, 1993

Block RI, Farinpour R, Braverman K: Acute effects of marijuana on cognition: relationships to chronic effects and smoking techniques. Pharmacol Biochem Behav 43:907–917, 1992

Boller F, Traykov L, Dao-Casellana M, et al: Cognitive functioning in "diffuse" pathology: role of prefrontal and limbic structures. Ann N Y Acad Sci 769:23–29, 1995

Bornstein RA: Classification rates obtained with "standard" cut-off scores on selected neuropsychological tests. J Clin Exp Neuropsychol 8:413–420, 1986

Bowden SC: Separating cognitive impairment in neurologically asymptomatic alcoholism from Wernicke-Korsakoff syndrome: is the neuropsychological distinction justified? Psychol Bull 107:355–366, 1990

Brown TG, Seraganian P, Tremblay J: Alcohol and cocaine abusers 6 months after traditional treatment: do they fare as well as problem drinkers? J Subst Abuse Treat 10:545–552, 1993

Burger MC, Botwinick J, Storandt M: Aging, alcoholism, and performance on the Luria-Nebraska Neuropsychological Battery. J Gerontol 42:69–72, 1987

Butters N, Salmon D: Etiology and neuropathology of alcoholic Korsakoff's syndrome: new findings and speculations, in Neuropsychiatric Correlates of Alcoholism. Edited by Grant I. (Monograph Series) Washington, DC, American Psychiatric Press, 1986, pp 61–108

Butters N, Grant I, Haxby J, et al: Assessment of AIDS-related cognitive changes: recommendations of the NIMH Workgroup on neuropsychological assessment approaches. J Clin Exp Neuropsychol 12:963–978, 1990

Butterworth RF: The role of liver disease in alcohol-induced cognitive defects. Alcohol Health Res World 19:122–129, 1995

Byrne A, Kirby B, Zibin T, et al: Psychiatric and neurological effects of chronic solvent abuse. Can J Psychiatry 36:735–738, 1991

Candon B, Montaldi D, Wilson JTL, et al: The relation between MRI neuroactivation changes and response rate on a word-fluency task. Applied Neuropsychology 4:201–207, 1997

Carlin AS, Grant I, Adams KM, et al: Is phencyclidine (PCP) abuse associated with organic mental impairment? Am J Drug Alcohol Abuse 6:273–281, 1979

Carlin PL, Wilkenson DA: Assessment of neurological dysfunction and recovery in alcoholics: CT scanning and other techniques. Substance and Alcohol Actions/Misuse 4:191–197, 1983

Cermak LS, Verfaellie M, Letourneau L, et al: Verbal and nonverbal right hemisphere processing by chronic alcoholics. Alcohol Clin Exp Res 13:611–616, 1989

Chang L, Mehringer CM, Ernst T, et al: Neurochemical alterations in asymptomatic abstinent cocaine users: a proton magnetic resonance spectroscopy study. Biol Psychiatry 42:1105–1114, 1997

Charness ME: Brain lesions in alcoholics. Alcohol Clin Exp Res 17:2–11, 1993

Charness ME, Simon RP, Greenberg DA: Ethanol and the nervous system. N Engl J Med 321:442–454, 1989

Chastain RL, Lehman WEK, Joe GW: Estimated intelligence and long-term outcomes of opioid addicts. Am J Drug Alcohol Abuse 12:331–340, 1986

Cherry NM, Labreche FP, McDonald JC: Organic brain damage and occupational solvent exposure. British Journal of Industrial Medicine 49:776–781, 1992

Chick JD, Smith MA, Engleman HM, et al: Magnetic resonance imaging of the brain in alcoholics: cerebral atrophy, lifetime alcohol consumption, and cognitive deficits. Alcohol Clin Exp Res 13:512–518, 1989

Chouinard M-J, Braun CMJ: A meta-analysis of the relative sensitivity of neuropsychological screening tests. J Clin Exp Neuropsychol 15:591–607, 1993

Cipolli C, Galliani I: Addiction time and intellectual impairment in heroin users. Psychol Rep 60:1099–1105, 1987

Cloninger CR: Neurogenetic adaptive mechanisms in alcoholism. Science 236:410–416, 1987

Convit A, de Leon M, Hoptman MJ, et al: Age-related changes in brain, I: magnetic resonance imaging measures of temporal lobe volumes in normal subjects. Psychiatr Q 66:343–355, 1995

Cooney NL, Kadden RM, Litt MD, et al: Matching alcoholics to coping skills or interactional therapies: two-year follow-up results. J Consult Clin Psychol 59:598–601, 1991

Corwin J, Bylsma FW: Translations of excerpts from Andre Rey's Psychological Examination of Traumatic Encephalopathy and P.A. Osterrieth's The Complex Figure Copy Test. The Clinical Neuropsychologist 7:3–15, 1993

Cosgrove J, Newell TG: Recovery of neuropsychological functions during reduction in use of phencyclidine. J Clin Psychol 47:159–169, 1991

Craig RJ: The personality structure of heroin addicts, in Neurobiology of Behavioral Control in Drug Abuse (NIDA Res Monogr No 74). Washington, DC, U.S. Government Printing Office, 1986, pp 25–36

Crawford JR, Stewart LE, Cochrane RHB, et al: Estimating premorbid IQ from demographic variables: regression equations derived from a UK sample. Br J Clin Psychol 28:275–278, 1989

Cummings JL: Anatomic and behavioral aspects of frontal-subcortical circuits. Ann N Y Acad Sci 769:1–13, 1995

Davila MD, Shear PK, Lane B, et al: Mammillary body and cerebellar shrinkage in chronic alcoholics: an MRI and neuropsychological study. Neuropsychology 8:433–444, 1994

De Santi S, de Leon MJ, Convit A, et al: Age-related changes in brain, II: positron emission tomography of frontal and temporal lobe glucose metabolism in normal subjects. Psychiatr Q 66:356–368, 1995

Dikmen SS, Donovan DM, Loberg T, et al: Alcohol use and its effects on neuropsychological outcome in head injury. Neuropsychology 7:296–305, 1993

Dinwiddie SH, Zorumski CF, Rubin EH: Psychiatric correlates of chronic solvent abuse. J Clin Psychiatry 48:334–337, 1987

Di Sciafani V, Ezekiel F, Meyerhoff DJ, et al: Brain atrophy and cognitive function in older abstinent alcoholic men. Alcohol Clin Exp Res 19:1121–1126, 1995

Drake AI, Butters N, Shear PK, et al: Cognitive recovery with abstinence and its relationship to family history for alcoholism. J Stud Alcohol 56:104–109, 1995

Drebing CE, Van Gorp WG, Stuck AE, et al: Early detection of cognitive decline in higher cognitively functioning older adults: sensitivity and specificity of a neuropsychological screening battery. Neuropsychology 8:31–37, 1994

Eckardt MJ, Rohrbaugh JW, Rio DE, et al: Positron emission tomography as a technique for studying the chronic effects of alcohol on the human brain. Ann Med 22:341–345, 1990

Ehyai A, Freemon FR: Progressive optic neuropathy and sensorineural hearing loss due to chronic glue sniffing. J Neurol Neurosurg Psychiatry 46:349–351, 1983

Ellis RJ, Oscar-Berman M: Alcoholism, aging and functional cerebral asymmetries. Psychol Bull 106:128–147, 1989

ElSohly MA, Abel CT: Quarterly Report: Potency Monitoring Project (Report No. 24, Oct-Dec 1987). University City, MS, Research Institute of Pharmaceutical Sciences, 1988

Epstein EE, Kahler CW, McCrady BS, et al: An empirical classification of drinking patterns among alcoholics: binge, episodic, sporadic, and steady. Addict Behav 20:23–41, 1995

Erwin JE, Hunter JJ: Cognitive predictors of program completion in the treatment of alcoholism, in Advanced Concepts in Alcoholism: Advances in the Biosciences, Vol 47. Edited by Tittmar HG. New York, Pergamon, 1984, pp 149–162

Eslinger PJ, Grattan LM: Frontal lobe and frontal-striatal substrates for different forms of human cognitive flexibility. Neuropsychologia 31:17–28, 1993

Evert DL, Oscar-Berman M: Alcohol-related cognitive impairments: an overview of how alcoholism may affect the workings of the brain. Alcohol Health Res World 19:89–96, 1995

Fabian MS, Jenkins RI, Parsons OA: Gender, alcoholism and neuropsychological functioning. J Consult Clin Psychol 49:139–140, 1981

Fals-Stewart W, Lucente S: Effect of neurocognitive status and personality functioning on length of stay in residential substance abuse treatment: an integrative study. Psychology of Addictive Behaviors 8:179–190, 1994

Fehr KO, Kalant H: Long-term effects of cannabis on cerebral function: a review of the clinical and experimental literature, in Cannabis and Health Hazards: Proceedings of an ARF/WHO Scientific Meeting on Adverse Health and Behavioral Consequences of Cannabis Use. Edited by Fehr KO, Kalant H. Toronto, Addiction Research Foundation, 1983, pp 501–576

Fields FRJ, Fullerton JR: Influence of heroin addiction on neuropsychological functioning. J Consult Clin Psychol 43:114, 1975

Fishbein DH, Herning RI, Pickworth WB, et al: EEG and brainstem auditory evoked response potentials in adult male drug abusers with self-reported histories of aggressive behavior. Biol Psychiatry 26:595–611, 1989

Folstein MF, Folstein SE, McHugh PR: Mini-Mental State: a practical method for grading the cognitive state of patients for the clinician. J Psychiatr Res 12: 189–198, 1975

Fornazzari L, Wilkinson DA, Kapur BM, et al: Cerebellar, cortical and functional impairment in toluene abusers. Acta Neurol Scand 67:319–329, 1983

Frezza M, Di Padova C, Pozzato G, et al: High blood ethanol levels in women: the role of decreased gastric alcohol dehydrogenase activity and first pass metabolism. N Engl J Med 322:95–99, 1990

Gabrielli WF, Mednick SA: Intellectual performance in children of alcoholics. J Nerv Ment Dis 171:444–447, 1983

Giancola PR: Evidence for dorsolateral and orbital prefrontal cortical involvement in the expression of aggressive behavior. Aggressive Behavior 21:431–450, 1995

Giancola PR, Moss HB: Executive cognitive functioning in alcohol use disorders, in Recent Developments in Alcoholism. Edited by Galanter M. New York, Plenum, 1998

Gillen RW, Kranzler HR, Kadden RM, et al: Utility of a brief cognitive screening instrument in substance abuse patients: initial investigation. J Subst Abuse Treat 8:247–251, 1991

Glass IB: Alcoholic brain damage: what does it mean to patients? British Journal of Addiction 86:819–821, 1991

Glenn SW, Parsons OA: Alcohol abuse and familial alcoholism: psychosocial correlates in men and women. J Stud Alcohol 50:116–127, 1989

Glenn SW, Parsons OA: Efficiency measures in male and female alcoholics. J Stud Alcohol 53:546–552, 1992

Glenn SW, Errico AL, Parsons OA, et al: The role of antisocial, affective, and childhood behavioral characteristics in alcoholics' neuropsychological performance. Alcohol Clin Exp Res 17:162–169, 1993

Goldberg E: Varieties of perseveration: a comparison of two taxonomies. J Clin Exp Neuropsychol 8:710–726, 1986

Goldberg E, Bilder RM Jr: The frontal lobes and hierarchical organization of cognitive control, in The Frontal Lobes Revisited. Edited by Perecman E. New York, IRBN Press, 1987, pp 159–187

Golden CJ: Stroop Color and Word Test: A Manual for Clinical and Experimental Uses. Chicago, IL, Stoelting, 1978

Golden CJ, Purisch AD, Hammeke TA: Luria-Nebraska Neuropsychological Battery: Forms I and II. Los Angeles, CA, Western Psychological Services, 1985

Goldman MS: Cognitive impairment in chronic alcoholics: some cause for optimism. Am Psychol 38:1045–1054, 1983

Goldman MS: The role of time and practice in the recovery of function in alcoholics, in Neuropsychology of Alcoholism: Implications for Diagnosis and Treatment. Edited by Parsons OA, Butters N, Nathan PE. New York, Guilford, 1987, pp 291–321

Goldman MS: Experience-dependent neuropsychological recovery and the treatment of chronic alcoholism. Neuropsychol Rev 1:75–101, 1990

Goldman MS: Recovery of cognitive functioning in alcoholics: the relationship to treatment. Alcohol Health Res World 19:148–154, 1995

Gorelick DA, Wilkins JN, Wong C: Outpatient treatment of PCP abusers. Am J Drug Alcohol Abuse 15:367–374, 1989

Grant I: Alcohol and the brain: neuropsychological correlates. J Consult Clin Psychol 55:310–324, 1987

Grant I, Judd LL: Neuropsychological and EEG disturbances in polydrug users. Am J Psychiatry 133:1039–1042, 1976

Grant I, Rochford J, Fleming T, et al: A neuropsychological assessment of the effects of moderate marijuana use. J Nerv Ment Dis 156:278–280, 1973

Grant I, Adams KM, Carlin AS, et al: The neuropsychological effects of polydrug abuse: the results of the national collaborative study, in Polydrug Abuse: The Results of a National Collaborative Study. Edited by Adams KM, Carlin AS, Wesson DR. San Francisco, CA, Academic Press, 1978, pp 223–261

Grant I, Reed R, Adams K, et al: Neuropsychological function in young alcoholics and polydrug abusers. Journal of Clinical Neuropsychology 1:39–47, 1979

Grant I, Adams KM, Reed R: Intermediate-duration (subacute) organic mental disorder of alcoholism, in Neuropsychiatric Correlates of Alcoholism (Monograph Series). Edited by Grant I. Washington, DC, American Psychiatric Press, 1986, pp 37–60

Guerra D, Sole A, Cami J, et al: Neuropsychological performance in opiate addicts after rapid detoxification. Drug Alcohol Depend 20:261–270, 1987

Ham HP, Parsons OA: Organization of psychological functions in alcoholics and nonalcoholics: a test of the compensatory hypothesis. J Stud Alcohol 58:67–74, 1997

Harding AJ, Wong A, Svoboda M, et al: Chronic alcohol consumption does not cause hippocampal neuron loss in humans. Hippocampus 7:78–87, 1997

Harper C, Kril J: If you drink your brain will shrink: neuropathological considerations. Alcohol Alcohol Suppl 1:375–380, 1991

Harper CG, Giles M, Finlay-Jones R: Clinical signs in the Wernicke-Korsakoff complex: a retrospective analysis of 131 cases diagnosed at necropsy. J Neurol Neurosurg Psychiatry 49:341–345, 1986

Hasher L, Zachs R: Automatic and effortful processes in memory. J Exp Psychol Gen 108:356–388, 1979

Heaton RK: Wisconsin Card Sorting Test. Odessa, FL, Psychological Assessment Resources, 1985

Heaton RK, Grant I, Matthews CG: Comprehensive Norms for an Expanded Halstead-Reitan Battery: Demographic Corrections, Research Findings, and Clinical Applications. Odessa, FL, Psychological Assessment Resources, 1991

Helms JE: Why is there no study of cultural equivalence in standardized cognitive ability testing? Am Psychol 47:1083–1101, 1992

Hendriks VM, Steer RA, Platt JJ, et al: Psychopathology in Dutch and American heroin addicts. International Journal of the Addictions 25:1051–1063, 1990

Herning RI, Glover BJ, Koeppl B, et al: Cognitive Deficits in Abstaining Cocaine Abusers (NIDA Res Monogr No 101). Washington, DC, U.S. Government Printing Office, 1990, pp 167–178

Hesselbrock V, Bauer LO, Hesselbrock MN, et al: Neuropsychological factors in individuals at high risk for alcoholism, in Recent Developments in Alcoholism, Vol 9. Edited by Galanter M. New York, Plenum, 1991, pp 21–40

Hieronymus AN, Lindquist EF, Hoover HD: Manual for School Administrators, Iowa Tests of Basic Skills. Chicago, IL, Riverside Publishing, 1982

Hill SY, Steinhauer S, Locke J: Event-related potentials in alcoholic men, their high-risk male relatives, and low-risk male controls. Alcohol Clin Exp Res 19:567–576, 1995

Holman BL, Mendelson J, Garada B, et al: Regional cerebral blood flow improves with treatment in chronic cocaine polydrug users. J Nucl Med 34:723–727, 1993

Hormes JT, Filley CM, Rosenberg NL: Neurologic sequelae of chronic solvent vapor abuse. Neurology 36:698–702, 1986

Horton AM Jr: Future directions in the development of addiction assessment instruments, in National Institute on Drug Abuse: Diagnostic Sourcebook on Drug Abuse Research and Treatment. Edited by Rounsaville BJ, Tims FM, Horton AM Jr, et al. Washington, DC, U.S. Government Printing Office, 1993, pp 87–92

Horton AM Jr: Identification of neuropsychological deficit: levels of assessment. Percept Mot Skills 79:1251–1255, 1994

Hunt WA: Are binge drinkers more at risk of developing brain damage? Alcohol 10:559–561, 1993

Ingle KG, Weingartner HJ: Cognitive deficits in alcoholism: approaches to theoretical modeling. Alcohol Health Res World 19:155–158, 1995

Jacobson RR, Acker CF, Lishman WA: Patterns of neuropsychological deficit in alcoholic Korsakoff's syndrome. Psychol Med 20:321–334, 1990

Jernigan TL, Butters N, DiTraglia G, et al: Reduced cerebral grey matter observed in alcoholics using magnetic resonance imaging. Alcohol Clin Exp Res 15:418–427, 1991a

Jernigan TL, Schafer K, Butters N, et al: Magnetic resonance imaging of alcoholic Korsakoff patients. Neuropsychopharmacology 4:175–186, 1991b

Johnson EO, Arria AM, Borges G, et al: The growth of conduct problem behaviors from middle childhood to early adolescence: sex differences and the suspected influence of early alcohol use. J Stud Alcohol 56:661–671, 1995

Jones GA: Alcohol abuse and traumatic brain injury. Alcohol Health Res World 13:105–109, 1989

Julkunen RJK, Di Padova C, Lieber CS: First pass metabolism of ethanol: a gastrointestinal barrier against systemic toxicity metabolism of ethanol. Life Sci 37:567–573, 1985

Kaplan E, Fein D, Morris R, et al: WAIS-R as a Neuropsychological Instrument. San Antonio, TX, Psychological Corporation, 1991

Kaseda Y, Miyazato Y, Ogura C, et al: Correlation between event-related potentials and MR measurements in chronic alcoholic patients. Japanese Journal of Psychiatry and Neurology 48:23–32, 1994

Knight RG, Longmore BE: Clinical Neuropsychology of Alcoholism. Hillsdale, NJ, Lawrence Erlbaum, 1994

Korman M, Matthews RW, Lovitt R: Neuropsychological effects of abuse of inhalants. Percept Mot Skills 53:547–553, 1981

Kramer JH, Blusewicz MJ, Preston KA: The premature aging hypothesis: old before its time? J Consult Clin Psychol 57:257–262, 1989

Kuhn D, Brannock J: Development of the isolation of variables scheme in experimental and "natural experiment" contexts. Dev Psychol 13:9–14, 1977

Kulisevsky J, Pujol J, Junque C, et al: MRI pallidal hyperintensity and brain atrophy in cirrhotic patients: two different MRI patterns of clinical deterioration? Neurology 43:2570–2573, 1993

Lancaster FE: Gender differences in the brain: implications for the study of human alcoholism. Alcohol Clin Exp Res 18:740–746, 1994

La Rue A: Adult development and aging, in Handbook of Neuropsychological Assessment: A Biopsychosocial Perspective. Edited by Puente AE, McCaffrey RJ. New York, Plenum, 1992, pp 81–120

Lavoie J, Butterworth RF: Reduced activities of thiamine-dependent enzymes in brains of alcoholics in the absence of Wernicke's encephalopathy. Alcohol Clin Exp Res 19:1073–1077, 1995

Lazar RB, Ho SU, Melen O, et al: Multifocal central nervous system damage caused by toluene abuse. Neurology 33:1337–1340, 1983

Lehman LB, Pilich A, Andrews N: Neurological disorders resulting from alcoholism. Alcohol Health Res World 17:305–309, 1993

Lewis JE, Hordan RB: Neuropsychological assessment of phencyclidine abusers, in Phencyclidine: An Update (Research Monograph Series No 64). Rockville, MD, National Institute on Drug Abuse, 1986, pp 190–208

Lezak MD: Neuropsychological Assessment, 3rd Edition. New York, Oxford University Press, 1995

Libon DJ, Glosser G, Malamut BL, et al: Age, executive functions, and visuospatial functioning in healthy older adults. Neuropsychology 8:38–43, 1994

Lin K-M, Poland RE, Silver B: Overview: the interface between psychobiology and ethnicity, in Psychopharmacology and Psychobiology of Ethnicity. Edited by Lin K-M, Poland RE, Nakasaki G. Washington, DC, American Psychiatric Press, 1993, pp 11–35

Lishman WA: Alcohol and the brain. Br J Psychiatry 156:635–644, 1990

Loberg T, Miller WR: Personality, cognitive, and neuropsychological correlates of harmful alcohol consumption: a cross-national comparison of clinical samples. Ann N Y Acad Sci 472:75–97, 1986

Lombardo WK, Lombardo B, Goldstein A: Cognitive functioning under moderate and low dosage methadone maintenance. International Journal of the Addictions 11:389–401, 1976

Luria AR: The Working Brain: An Introduction to Neuropsychology. New York, Basic Books, 1973

Luria AR, Naydin VL, Tsvetkova LS, et al: Restoration of higher cortical function following local brain damage, in Handbook of Clinical Neurology, Vol 3: Disorders of Nervous Activity. Edited by Vinken PJ, Bruyn GW. New York, Wiley, 1969, pp 368–433

Mahmood Z: Cognitive functioning of solvent abusers. Scott Med J 28:276–280, 1983

Malloy PF, Noel N, Rogers S, et al: Risk factors for neuropsychological impairment in alcoholics: antisocial personality, age, years of drinking, and gender. J Stud Alcohol 50:422–426, 1989

Malloy P, Noel N, Longabaugh R, et al: Determinants of neuropsychological impairment in antisocial substance abusers. Addict Behav 15:431–438, 1990

Mann K, Batra A, Gunthner A, et al: Do women develop alcoholic brain damage more readily than men? Alcohol Clin Exp Res 16:1052–1056, 1992

Manschreck TC, Schneyer ML, Weisstein CC: Freebase cocaine and memory. Compr Psychiatry 31:369–375, 1990

Marsano L: Alcohol and malnutrition. Addictions Nursing 6:62–71, 1994

Martin CS, Arria A, Mezzich AC, et al: Patterns of polydrug use in adolescent alcohol abusers. Am J Drug Alcohol Abuse 19:511–521, 1993

Martin CS, Clifford P, Maisto S, et al: Polydrug use in an inpatient treatment sample of problem drinkers. Alcohol Clin Exp Res 20:413–417, 1996

Martin PR, Adinoff B, Weingartner H: Alcoholic organic brain disease: nosology and pathophysiologic mechanism. Prog Neuropsychopharmacol Biol Psychiatry 10:147–164, 1986

Mattson ME, Allen JP, Longabaugh R, et al: A chronological review of empirical studies matching alcoholic clients to treatment. J Stud Alcohol Suppl 12: 16–29, 1994

Meek PS, Clark HW, Solana VL: Neurocognitive impairment: the unrecognized component of dual diagnosis in substance abuse treatment. J Psychoactive Drugs 21:153–160, 1989

Mendhiratta SS, Varma VK, Dang R, et al: Cannabis and cognitive functions: a re-evaluation study. British Journal of Addiction 83:749–753, 1988

Moffit TE, Lynam DR, Silva PA: Neuropsychological tests predicting persistent male delinquency. Criminology 32:277–300, 1994

Molina JA, Bermejo F, del Ser T, et al: Alcoholic cognitive deterioration and nutritional deficiencies. Acta Neurol Scand 89:384–390, 1994

Montoya ID, Hess JM, Covi L, et al: A comparative study of psychopathology and cognitive functions between cocaine- and opiate-dependent patients. Am J Addict 3:36–42, 1994

Morgan JP: Cannabis update 1995. Paper presented at the Plenary Session of the Ninth International Conference on Drug Policy Reform, Santa Monica, CA, October 20, 1995

Morgenstern J, Bates ME: Effects of executive function impairment on change processes and substance use outcomes in 12-Step treatment. J Stud Alcohol (in press)

Morgenstern J, Langenbucher J, Labouvie E, et al: The comorbidity of alcoholism and personality disorders in a clinical population: prevalence rates and relation to alcohol typology variables. J Abnorm Psychol 106:74–84, 1997

Morse P, Montgomery D: Neuropsychological evaluation of traumatic brain injury, in Clinical Syndromes in Neuropsychology: The Practitioner's Handbook. Edited by White RF. Amsterdam, Elsevier, 1992, pp 85–176

Mueser KT, Yarnold PR, Levinson DF, et al: Prevalence of substance abuse in schizophrenia: demographic and clinical correlates. Schizophr Bull 16:31–56, 1990

Muuronen A, Bergman H, Hindmarsh T, et al: Influence of improved drinking habits on brain atrophy and cognitive performance in alcoholic patients: a 5-year follow-up study. Alcohol Clin Exp Res 13:137–141, 1989

Nichols JM, Martin F: The effect of heavy social drinking on recall and event-related potentials. J Stud Alcohol 57:125–135, 1996

Nicolas JM, Catafau AM, Estruch R, et al: Regional cerebral blood flow-SPECT in chronic alcoholism: relation to neuropsychological testing. J Nucl Med 34: 1452–1459, 1993

Nixon SJ: Application of theoretical models to the study of alcohol-induced brain damage, in Alcohol-Induced Brain Damage (Monograph No 22, NIH Publ No 93-3549). Edited by Hunt WA, Nixon SJ. Bethesda, MD, National Institute of Alcohol Abuse and Alcoholism Research, 1993, pp 213-228

Nixon SJ: Assessing cognitive impairment. Alcohol Health Res World 19:97–103, 1995

Nixon SJ, Parsons OA: Alcohol-related efficiency deficits using an ecologically valid test. Alcohol Clin Exp Res 15:601–606, 1991

Nixon SJ, Tivis R, Parsons OA: Behavioral dysfunction and cognitive efficiency in male and female alcoholics. Alcohol Clin Exp Res 19:577–581, 1995

O'Carroll RE, Hayes PC, Ebmeier KP: Regional cerebral blood flow and cognitive function in patients with chronic liver disease. Lancet 337:1250–1253, 1991

O'Malley S, Gawin FH: Abstinence Symptomatology and Neuropsychological Impairment in Chronic Cocaine Abusers. (NIDA Res Monogr No 101). Washington, DC, U.S. Government Printing Office, 1990, pp 179–190

O'Malley S, Adamse M, Heaton RK, et al: Neuropsychological impairment in chronic cocaine abusers. Am J Drug Alcohol Abuse 18:131–144, 1992

Oscar-Berman M, Hutner N: Frontal lobe changes after chronic alcohol ingestion, in Alcohol-Induced Brain Damage (Research Monograph No 22, NIH Publication No 93-3549). Edited by Hunt WA, Nixon SJ. Rockville, MD, National Institute on Alcohol Abuse and Alcoholism, 1993, pp 121–156

O'Shanick G, Scott R, Peterson L: Psychiatric referral after head trauma. Psychiatric Medicine 2:131–137, 1984

Page RD, Linden JD: "Reversible" organic brain syndrome in alcoholics. Quarterly Journal of Studies on Alcohol 35:98–107, 1974

Parkin AJ: The relationship between anterograde and retrograde amnesia in alcoholic Wernicke-Korsakoff syndrome. Psychol Med 21:11–14, 1991

Parsons OA: Cognitive functioning in sober social drinkers: a review and critique. J Stud Alcohol 47:101–114, 1986

Parsons OA: Impaired neuropsychological functioning in sober alcoholics, in Alcohol-Induced Brain Damage (Research Monograph No 22, NIH Publ No 93-3549). Edited by Hunt WA, Nixon SJ. Rockville, MD, National Institute on Alcohol Abuse and Alcoholism, 1993, pp 173–194

Parsons OA, Leber WR: Alcohol, cognitive dysfunction and brain damage, in Biomedical Processes and Consequences of Alcohol Use (Alcohol and Health Monograph No 2). Rockville, MD, National Institute on Alcohol Abuse and Alcoholism, 1982, pp 213–253

Parsons OA, Nixon SJ: Cognitive functioning in sober social drinkers: a review of the research since 1986. J Stud Alcohol 59:180–190, 1998

Parsons OA, Butters N, Nathan PE: Neuropsychology of Alcoholism: Implications for Diagnosis and Treatment. New York, Guilford, 1987

Parsons OA, Sinha R, Williams HL: Relationships between neuropsychological test performance and event-related potentials in alcoholic and nonalcoholic samples. Alcohol Clin Exp Res 14:746–755, 1990

Patrick G, Straumanis JJ, Struve FA, et al: Auditory and visual P300 event related potentials are not altered in medically and psychiatrically normal chronic marijuana users. Life Sci 56:2135–2140, 1995

Pearlson GD: Psychiatric and medical syndromes associated with phencyclidine (PCP) abuse. The Johns Hopkins Medical Journal 148:25–33, 1981

Penick EC, Powell BJ, Bingham SF, et al: A comparative study of familial alcoholism. J Stud Alcohol 48:136–146, 1987

Penk WE, Brown AS, Roberts WR, et al: Visual memory of black and white male heroin and nonheroin drug users. J Abnorm Psychol 90:486–489, 1981

Perrine K: Differential aspects of conceptual processing in the Category Test and Wisconsin Card Sorting Test. J Clin Exp Neuropsychol 15:461–473, 1993

Pfefferbaum A, Lim KO, Zipursky RB, et al: Brain gray and white matter volume loss accelerates with aging in chronic alcoholics: a quantitative MRI study. Alcoholism: Clinical and Experimental Research 16:1078–1089, 1992

Pfefferbaum A, Lim KO, Zipursky RB, et al: Increase in brain cerebrospinal fluid volume is greater in older than in younger alcoholic patients: a replication study and CT/MRI comparison. Psychiatry Res 50:257–274, 1993

Pfefferbaum A, Sullivan EV, Mathalon DH, et al: Longitudinal changes in magnetic resonance imaging brain volumes in abstinent and relapsed alcoholics. Alcoholism: Clinical and Experimental Research 19:1177–1191, 1995

Pihl RO, Peterson J, Finn P: Inherited predisposition to alcoholism: characteristics of sons of male alcoholics. J Abnorm Psychol 99:291–301, 1990

Pogge DL, Stokes J, Harvey PD: Psychometric vs. attentional correlates of early onset alcohol and substance abuse. J Abnorm Child Psychol 20:151–162, 1992

Polster M: Drug-induced amnesia: implications for cognitive neuropsychological investigations of memory. Psychol Bull 114:477–493, 1993

Pomier Layrargues G, Nguyen NH, Faucher C, et al: Subclinical hepatic encephalopathy in cirrhotic patients: prevalence and relationship to liver function. Can J Gastroenterol 5:121–125, 1991

Pratt OE, Rooprai HK, Shaw GK, et al: The genesis of alcoholic brain tissue injury. Alcohol Alcohol 25:217–230, 1990

Regier DA, Farmer ME, Rae DS, et al: Comorbidity of mental disorders with alcohol and other drug abuse. JAMA 264:2511–2518, 1990

Reitan RM, Wolfson D: The Halstead-Reitan Neuropsychological Test Battery: Theory and Clinical Interpretation. Tucson, AZ, Neuropsychology Press, 1993

Rey A: L'examen clinique en psychologie. Paris, France, Presses Universitaires de France, 1964

Richards M, Sano M, Goldstein S, et al: The stability of neuropsychological test performance in a group of parenteral drug users. J Subst Abuse Treat 9:371–377, 1992

Rochford J, Grant I, LaVigne G: Medical students and drugs: further neuropsychological and use pattern considerations. Int J Addict 12:1057–1065, 1977

Rodriquez M: Cognitive functioning, family history of alcoholism, and antisocial behavior in female polydrug abusers. Psychol Rep 73:19–26, 1993a

Rodriquez M: Cognitive functioning in male polydrug abusers with and without family history of alcoholism. Percept Mot Skills 77:483–488, 1993b

Roehrich L, Goldman MS: Experience dependent neuropsychological recovery and the treatment of alcoholism. J Consult Clin Psychol 61:812–821, 1993

Rojas DC, Bennett TL: Single versus composite score discriminative validity with the Halstead-Reitan Battery and the Stroop Test in mild brain injury. Archives of Clinical Neuropsychology 10:101–110, 1995

Ron MA: The alcoholic brain: CT scan and psychological findings. Psychol Med 3 (suppl):31–33, 1983

Rosenberg NL, Spitz MC, Filley CM, et al: Central nervous system effects of chronic toluene abuse—clinical, brainstem evoked response and magnetic resonance imaging studies. Neurotoxicol Teratol 10:489–495, 1988

Rounsaville BJ, Novelly RA, Kleber HD: Neuropsychological impairment in opiate addicts: risk factors. Ann N Y Acad Sci 362:79–90, 1981

Rounsaville BJ, Jones C, Novelly RA, et al: Neuropsychological functioning in opiate addicts. J Nerv Ment Dis 170:209–216, 1982

Royall DR, Mahurin RK, Gray KF: Bedside assessment of executive cognitive impairment: the executive interview. J Am Geriatr Soc 40:1221–1226, 1992

Ryan C, Butters N: Neuropsychology of alcoholism, in The Neuropsychology Handbook. Edited by Wedding D, Horton AM Jr, Webster JS. New York, Springer, 1986, pp 376–409

Saarnio P: Measuring the effect of the duration of problem drinking on cognitive functions in alcoholics. Arukoru Kenkyuto Yakubutsu Ison 29:108–113, 1994

Salame P: The effects of alcohol on learning as a function of drinking habits. Ergonomics 34:1231–1241, 1991

Sanchez-Craig M: Drinking pattern as a determinant of alcoholics' performance on the Trail Making Test. J Stud Alcohol 41:1082–1090, 1980

Schaeffer J, Andrysiak T, Ungerleider JT: Cognition and long-term use of ganja (cannabis). Science 213:465–466, 1981

Schaeffer KW, Parsons OA, Errico AL: Abstracting deficits and childhood conduct disorder as a function of familial alcoholism. Alcohol Clin Exp Res 12:617–618, 1988

Schafer J, Birchler GR, Fals-Stewart W: Cognitive, affective and marital functioning of recovering male polysubstance abusers. Neuropsychology 8:100–109, 1994a

Schafer J, Blanchard L, Fals-Stewart W: Drug use and risky sexual behavior. Psychology of Addictive Behaviors 8:3–7, 1994b

Schafer K, Butters N, Smith T, et al: Cognitive performance of alcoholics: a longitudinal evaluation of the role of drinking history, depression, liver function, nutrition, and family history. Alcohol Clin Exp Res 15:653–660, 1991

Schandler SL, Thomas CS, Cohen MJ: Spatial learning deficits in preschool children of alcoholics. Alcohol Clin Exp Res 19:1067–1072, 1995

Schneider W, Dumais ST, Shiffrin RM: Automatic and control processing and attention, in Varieties of Attention. Edited by Parasuraman R, Davies DR. New York, Academic Press, 1984, pp 1–25

Schuckit MA, Butters N, Lyn L, et al: Neuropsychologic deficits and the risk for alcoholism. Neuropsychopharmacology 1:45–53, 1987

Schwamm LH, VanDyke C, Kiernan RJ, et al: The Neurobehavioral Cognitive Status Examination. Ann Intern Med 107:486–491, 1987

Schwartz RH, Gruenewald PJ, Klitzner M, et al: Short-term memory impairment in cannabis-dependent adolescents. American Journal of Diseases of Children 143:1214–1219, 1989

Searles JS: The role of genetics in the pathogenesis of alcoholism. J Abnorm Psychol 97:153–167, 1988

Seguin JR, Pihl RO, Harden PW, et al: Cognitive and neuropsychological characteristics of physically aggressive boys. J Abnorm Psychol 104:614–624, 1995

Shear PK, Jernigan TL, Butters N: Volumetric magnetic resonance imaging quantification of longitudinal brain changes in abstinent alcoholics. Alcohol Clin Exp Res 18:172–176, 1994

Sher KJ: Children of Alcoholics: A Critical Appraisal of Theory and Research. Chicago, IL, University of Chicago Press, 1991

Siu AL: Screening for dementia and investigating its causes. Ann Intern Med 115:122–132, 1991

Smith ME, Oscar-Berman M: Resource-limited information processing in alcoholism. J Stud Alcohol 53:514–518, 1992

Sobell LC, Sobell MB: Timeline follow-back: a technique for assessing self-reported alcohol consumption, in Measuring Alcohol Consumption: Psychosocial and Biochemical Methods. Edited by Litten RZ, Allen JP. Totowa, NJ, Humana Press, 1992, pp 41–69

Solowij N: Do cognitive impairments recover following cessation of cannabis use? Life Sci 56:2119–2126, 1995

Solowij N, Michie PT, Fox AM: Effects of long-term cannabis use on selective attention: an event-related potential study. Pharmacol Biochem Behav 40: 683–688, 1991

Steingass HP, Sartory G, Canavan AGM: Chronic alcoholism and cognitive function: general decline or patterned impairment. Personality and Individual Differences 17:97–109, 1994

Steinhauer SR, Hill SY: Auditory event-related potentials in children at high risk for alcoholism. J Stud Alcohol 54:408–421, 1993

Strang J, Gurling H: Computerized tomography and neuropsychological assessment in long-term high-dose heroin addicts. British Journal of Addiction 84: 1011–1019, 1989

Strickland TL, Mena I, Villanueva-Meyer J, et al: Cerebral perfusion and neuropsychological consequences of chronic cocaine use. J Neuropsychiatry Clin Neurosci 5:419–427, 1993

Sullivan EV, Marsh L, Mathalon DH, et al: Anterior hippocampal volume deficits in nonamnestic, aging chronic alcoholics. Alcohol Clin Exp Res 19:110–122, 1995a

Sullivan EV, Rosenbloom MJ, Deshmukh A, et al: Alcohol and the cerebellum: effects on balance, motor coordination, and cognition. Alcohol Health Res World 19:138–141, 1995b

Sussman S, Rychtarik RG, Mueser K, et al: Ecological relevance of memory tests and the prediction of relapse in alcoholics. J Stud Alcohol 47:305–310, 1986

Sweet JJ, Moberg PJ, Tovian SM: Evaluation of Wechsler Adult Intelligence Scale—Revised premorbid IQ formulas in clinical populations. Psychol Assess 2:41–44, 1990

Tarbox AR, Connors GJ, McLaughlin EJ: Effects of drinking pattern on neuropsychological performance among alcohol misusers. J Stud Alcohol 47:176–179, 1986

Tarter RE, McBride H, Buonpane N, et al: Differentiation of alcoholics. Arch Gen Psychiatry 34:761–768, 1977

Tarter RE, Hegedus A, Winsten N, et al: Neuropsychological, personality and familial characteristics of physically abused juvenile delinquents. Journal of the American Academy of Child Psychiatry 23:668–674, 1984

Tarter RE, Hegedus AM, Van Thiel DH, et al: Neurobehavioral correlates of cholestatic and hepatocellular disease: differentiation according to disease specific characteristics and severity of the identified cerebral dysfunction. International Journal of Neurology 32:901–910, 1987

Tarter RE, Arria A, Van Thiel DH: Liver-brain interactions in alcoholism, in Alcohol Induced Brain Damage (Research Monograph No 22, NIH Publication No 93–3549). Edited by Hunt WA, Nixon SJ. Rockville, MD, National Institute of Alcohol Abuse and Alcoholism, 1993, pp 415–430

Tarter RE, Switala J, Lu S, et al: Abstracting capacity in cirrhotic alcoholics: negative findings. J Stud Alcohol 56:99–103, 1995

Tiffany ST: A cognitive model of drug urges and drug-use behavior: role of automatic and nonautomatic processes. Psychol Rev 97:147–168, 1990

Tivis R, Beatty WW, Nixon SJ, et al: Patterns of cognitive impairment among alcoholics: are there subtypes? Alcohol Clin Exp Res 19:496–500, 1995

Tracy JI, Bates ME: Models of functional organization as a method for detecting cognitive deficits: data from a sample of social drinkers. J Stud Alcohol 55: 726–738, 1994

Tracy JI, Bates ME: The selective effects of alcohol on automatic and controlled memory processes. Neuropsychology (in press)

Tracy JI, Josiassen RC, Bellack AS: Neuropsychology of dual diagnosis: understanding the combined effects of schizophrenia and substance use disorders. Clin Psychol Rev 15:67–97, 1995

Tsushima WT, Towne WS: Effects of paint sniffing on neuropsychological test performance. J Abnorm Psychol 86:402–407, 1977

Turner J, Parsons OA: Verbal and nonverbal abstracting-problem solving abilities and familial alcoholism in female alcoholics. J Stud Alcohol 49:281–287, 1988

Unger E, Alexander A, Fritz T, et al: Toluene abuse: physical basis for hypointensity of the basal ganglia on T-2 weighted MR images. Radiology 193:473–476, 1994

Varma VK, Malhotra AK, Dang R, et al: Cannabis and cognitive functions: a prospective study. Drug Alcohol Depend 21:147–152, 1988

Victor M: The effects of alcohol on the nervous system, in Medical and Nutritional Complications of Alcoholism: Mechanisms and Management. Edited by Lieber CS. New York, Plenum, 1992, pp 413–457

Victor M: Alcoholic dementia. Can J Neurol Sci 21:88–99, 1994

Volkow ND, Hitzemann R, Wang GJ, et al: Decreased brain metabolism in neurologically intact healthy alcoholics. Am J Psychiatry 149:1016–1022, 1992

Volkow ND, Fowler JS, Wang GJ, et al: Decreased dopamine D_2 receptor availability is associated with reduced frontal metabolism in cocaine abusers. Synapse 14:169–177, 1993

Volkow ND, Wang GJ, Hitzemann R, et al: Recovery of brain glucose metabolism in detoxified alcoholics. Am J Psychiatry 151:178–183, 1994

Walton JN: Brain's Diseases of the Nervous System, 10th Edition. Oxford, England, Oxford University Press, 1994

Wang GJ, Volkow ND, Hitzemann R, et al: Brain imaging of an alcoholic with MRI, SPECT, and PET. American Journal of Physiologic Imaging 7:194–198, 1992

Wang GJ, Volkow ND, Roque CT, et al: Functional importance of ventricular enlargement and cortical atrophy in healthy subjects and alcoholics as assessed with PET, MR imaging, and neuropsychologic testing. Radiology 186:59–65, 1993

Weber DA, Franceschi D, Ivanovic M, et al: SPECT and planar brain imaging in crack abuse: iodine-123-iodoamphetamine uptake and localization. J Nucl Med 34:899–907, 1993

Wechsler D: Wechsler Adult Intelligence Scale—Revised. San Antonio, TX, Psychological Corporation, 1981

Weinrieb RM, O'Brian CP: Persistent cognitive deficits attributed to substance abuse, in Neurologic Complications of Drug and Alcohol Abuse, Vol 11. Edited by Brust JCM. Philadelphia, PA, WB Saunders, 1993, pp 663–691

Weinstein CS, Shaffer HJ: Neurocognitive aspects of substance abuse treatment: a psychotherapist's primer. Psychotherapy 30:317–333, 1993

Wert RC, Raulin ML: The chronic cerebral effects of cannabis use, II: psychological findings and conclusions. International Journal of the Addictions 21: 629–642, 1986

Wetzig DL, Hardin SI: Neurocognitive deficits of alcoholism: an intervention. J Clin Psychol 46:219–229, 1990

Wiedmann KD, Power KG, Wilson JTL, et al: Recovery from chronic solvent abuse. J Neurol Neurosurg Psychiatry 50:1712–1713, 1987

Wiegersma S, de Jong E, van Dieren M: Subjective ordering and working memory in alcoholic Korsakoff patients. J Clin Exp Neuropsychol 13:847–853, 1991

Wik G, Borg S, Sjogren I, et al: PET determination of regional cerebral glucose metabolism in alcohol-dependent men and healthy controls using ^{11}C-glucose. Acta Psychiatr Scand 78:234–241, 1988

Wilkinson DA: CT scan and neuropsychological assessments of alcoholism, in Neuropsychology of Alcoholism: Implications for Diagnosis and Treatment. Edited by Parsons OA, Butters N, Nathan PE. New York, Guilford, 1987, pp 76–102

Wilson B, Cockburn J, Baddeley, AD: The Rivermead Behavioral Memory Test. Bary St Edmunds Suffolk, UK, Thames Valley Test Company, 1985

Woods S: Regional cerebral blood flow imaging with SPECT in psychiatric diseases: focus on schizophrenia, anxiety disorders, and substance abuse. J Clin Psychiatry 53:20–25, 1992

Workman-Daniels KL, Hesselbrock VM: Childhood problem behavior and neuropsychological functioning in persons at risk for alcoholism. J Stud Alcohol 48:187–193, 1987

Wright DG, Laureno R, Victor M: Pontine and extrapontine myelinolysis. Brain 102:361–385, 1979

Xiong L, Matthes JD, Li J, et al: MR imaging of "spray heads": toluene abuse via aerosol paint inhalation. AJNR Am J Neuroradiol 14:1195–1199, 1993

Yoshida A: Genetic polymorphism of alcohol-metabolizing enzymes related to alcohol sensitivity and alcoholic disease, in Psychopharmacology and Psychobiology of Ethnicity. Edited by Lin K-M, Poland RE, Nakasaki G. Washington, DC, American Psychiatric Press, 1993, pp 169–183

Zachary RA: Shipley Institute of Living Scale: Revised Manual. Los Angeles, CA, Western Psychological Services, 1986

Zutkin SR, Javitt DC: Mechanisms of phencyclidine (PCP)-n-methyl-d-aspartate (NMDA) receptor interaction: implications for drug abuse research, in National Institute on Drug Abuse: Problems of Drug Dependence 1989 (NIDA Res Monogr 95). Washington, DC, U.S. Government Printing Office, 1990, pp 247–254

Zutkin SR, Zutkin RS: Phencyclidine, in Substance Abuse: A Comprehensive Textbook, 2nd Edition. Edited by Lowinson JH, Ruiz P, Millman RB. Baltimore, MD, Williams & Wilkins, 1992, pp 290–302

10

NEUROPSYCHOLOGICAL MANAGEMENT, TREATMENT, AND REHABILITATION OF PSYCHIATRIC PATIENTS

Judith Jaeger, Ph.D., M.P.A., and
Stefanie Berns, Ph.D. candidate

THE READER WHO has arrived at this point having read the preceding chapters will realize how surprising it is that neuropsychological factors are almost never considered in the clinical management and rehabilitation of psychiatric patients. Such an oversight can be detrimental to the diagnosis, treatment, and rehabilitation of individuals who have these disor-

This work was supported in part by the National Institute of Mental Health (NIMH)–funded Clinical Research Center for the Study of Schizophrenia (Principal Investigator, John Kane, M.D. [P50 MH41960]) and an NIMH grant to Dr. Jaeger (R01 MH55585). The authors are grateful to three anonymous reviewers who provided valuable critical comments and suggestions.

ders. In this chapter, we hope to correct this oversight by describing some specific ways in which neuropsychological factors may be of benefit in the clinical setting. After providing some historical insight into the surprising delay of neuropsychology's entrance into the mainstream in psychiatric treatment settings, we introduce the clinical importance of impaired role functioning in psychiatric disorders. Within this context, the present and future role of neuropsychology in psychiatric rehabilitation is then discussed.

◈ THE EMERGING ROLE OF NEUROPSYCHOLOGY IN PSYCHIATRY

Until recently, neuropsychology has been absent from clinical psychiatric treatment planning and implementation. Historically, the reasons for this absence are not related to inadequacies in the knowledge base, but rather to differences in basic points of view between neuropsychology and psychiatry, between neuropsychology's foundation in the neurosciences and the "functional" methods of explanation that, until recently, had dominated clinical psychiatry since the time of Freud. A brief review of selected points in the history of psychiatry is most useful for understanding why neuropsychologists have only recently been in a position to make substantive contributions to psychiatry, not only for assessment, as has been excellently illustrated in the preceding chapters, but also for clinical management, treatment, and rehabilitation.

A key starting point is Emil Kraepelin's remarkable definition and formulation of the endogenous psychoses (dementia praecox and manic-depressive insanity) at the beginning of the twentieth century. Kraepelin's method and approach were quickly abandoned by psychiatry after his death. The tradition he led, of pursuing a rigorously empirical line of investigation into the signs, symptoms, course, and outcome of psychiatric disturbances with the aim of identifying the neurophysiological genetic etiological factors underlying their presentation, was virtually discarded from daily practice and research in favor of the literary fiction of psychoanalysis. The origin of the appeal to "rule out organicity" familiar to neuropsychologists was based on the false distinction between "organic" and "functional" disease entities that emerged with the dominance of psychoanalysis. "Functional" disease entities were those that were believed to be the result of psychological stressors or "existential crises" from life experience independent of any physiological cause. Since the time of Freud and his followers, psychodynamic descriptions and explanations came to dominate psychiatry and, remarkably, remain influential in some psychiatric settings even today.

With the abandonment of any rigorously empirical clinical nosology, as exemplified by Kraepelin's approach, virtually all idiopathic neuropsychiatric disorders, with the qualified exception of epilepsy, came to be termed *functional* disorders, and their neurological characterization was deemed clinically superfluous. In most cases, only psychiatric disorders with recognized etiopathologies or known external causes such as those from traumatic brain injury, neoplastic disease, vascular event, infectious agents, or intoxication were viewed as "organic" and worthy of further consideration with respect to neurological or neuropsychological characterization or treatment. In the absence of obvious trauma or known pathophysiology, there were additional cases in which "organicity" was also suspected. The identification of these cases was based on patterns of the findings of psychological tests that were routinely administered in the attempt to further characterize psychodynamic processes as well as to provide basic measures of intelligence (e.g., the Bender Gestalt test and the Wechsler Adult Intelligence Scale [WAIS]) (Anastasi 1976; Wechsler 1981). Particular profiles or subtest patterns came to be accepted as suggestive of organicity even though little or no systematic research supported an accurate and reliable use of such tests to identify putative brain dysfunction. The use of such psychological testing methods should not be considered as part of the systemic development of neuropsychology as a clinical and research discipline emerging out of the neurosciences. For example, the most well known of these quasi-neuropsychological tests, the Bender Gestalt test, was never designed as a neuropsychological assessment tool based on research in the neurosciences. It was originally developed as a projective test to study personality, and its use as a screening tool for organicity was incidental to its intent (Lezak 1995). That the Bender-Gestalt test came to be widely used as a screening tool for organicity is most likely the result of factors such as its ease of administration and its acceptable pedigree.

Although the discipline of neuropsychology was developing, drawing on the empirical foundations of the neurosciences, psychiatrists initially looked to neuropsychologists as they had to clinical psychologists: solely for the purposes of "ruling out organicity" in patients with psychiatric disorders. Entering psychiatry while still in its predominantly psychoanalytic era, neuropsychology was placed in the untenable position of being asked to make the wholly illusory distinction between organic and functional disorders.

How did neuropsychology come to be placed in such a position? Signs and symptoms of psychosis virtually identical to those observed in so-called primary psychiatric disorders had been described in patients with known neurological conditions (Slater et al. 1963). The usefulness of neuropsychological assessments in neurology became more and more appreciated during the 1960s and 1970s, in particular for characterizing individuals with focal brain disease and at times even for the accurate localizing of lesions in surgical cases in the absence of tomographic imaging techniques. The demonstrated usefulness of neuropsychological testing in neurological settings suggested the usefulness of these findings as providing a relatively simple and noninvasive method for ruling out unrecognized neurological disease among psychiatric patients. Despite the field's overwhelming reliance on psychodynamic-functional explanations at the time, practicing clinical psychiatrists could not ignore the possibility of unrecognized neurological disease among their patients, nor could they responsibly rule out the possibility of misdiagnosis. Thus came the introduction of neuropsychological assessment into psychiatry.

The role of neuropsychological assessment in psychiatry was severely limited from the onset, however. Only if a patient presented with a neuropsychological assessment profile similar to that of a patient with focal brain injury would it be seriously considered that brain pathology—that is, "organic factors"—might be playing a role in the clinical presentation of the psychiatric disease. For example, only in such a case would a psychotic disorder be viewed as other than functional in origin. In cases in which the findings of neuropsychological assessments indicated deficits that were not localized, psychiatrists viewed these deficits as being either "psychological" in origin (i.e., emanating from the damaged psyche) or secondary to other symptoms of functional psychopathology, which typically fluctuated over time and were therefore not "reliable" as assessment findings. Thus, if a psychiatric patient performed poorly on a test of attention while experiencing a thought disorder, the test results would typically be discounted as unreliable.

Clinicians did not seriously consider the finding of neuropsychological deficits for better understanding the clinical presentation or for improving clinical management because psychiatry's viewpoint at the time prevented systematic empirical consideration of neuropsychology or its potential as a whole. Even the obvious functional disabilities in seriously ill psychiatric patients were understood and managed without reference to the data of neuropsychology. Functional disability was assumed to be either a product of psychopathology—expected to be spontaneously reversed with the management of psychopathology—or the epiphenomenon of "institutionalization" and thus amenable to vocational rehabilitation.

In addition to the very limited inclusion of neuropsychological assessment data into clinical psychiatric practice and treatment planning, two lines of investigation dating from the late 1970s further contributed to the broadened and more serious consideration of neuropsychology in clinical psychiatry and psychiatric rehabilitation. The first were reports that neuropsychological deficits could be reliably observed in patients with psychiatric disorders (Heaton et al. 1978a; see also review by Rogers 1996) and evidence that these deficits may have a neurological basis (Heaton et al. 1979). The clinical relevance of these findings became increasingly difficult to ignore in light of reports that the severity of performance decrements on neuropsychological tests appeared to be directly associated with the level of vocational disability (Heaton et al. 1978b; Newnan et al. 1978).

The second line of investigation contributing to a role for neuropsychology in psychiatric treatment came indirectly from the World Health Organization's International Pilot Study of Schizophrenia (IPSS; Strauss and Carpenter 1978). One of the most important findings for both psychiatric nosology and neuropsychology was the remarkably small association between psychopathological symptoms and functional disability (Carpenter and Strauss 1991; Strauss and Carpenter 1978) among individuals who met consensus criteria for the diagnosis of schizophrenia. This finding has persisted with the slightly more restrictive diagnostic criteria of DSM-IV (American Psychiatric Association 1994) and raises two questions: 1) From a nosologic point of view, does this dissociation suggest the need to question critically the currently accepted diagnostic criteria? It would seem that the symptoms that are considered to be core or fundamental features of a given disease entity should bear some relationship to the presence and severity of the morbid consequences of that disease. 2) From a purely practical point of view, if the psychopathological symptoms of schizophrenia are such poor determinants of disability, then is it sufficient to target these symptoms as we consider standards for clinical management? If not, then the determinants of disability (e.g., functional or vocational) must be identified through further research so that our efforts toward clinical management may be more appropriately directed.

In contrast to psychiatric diagnosis alone, neuropsychological assessment represents an objective and reliable technique for characterizing dimensions of psychological functioning that are impaired in schizophrenia and that might be responsible for difficulties with independent functioning. However, the influence of neuropsychology in psychiatric thinking at the time of the IPSS was sharply delimited, as we described earlier. The dissociation between symptoms and functioning was not further explored at the time, and the possibility that neuropsychological measures might shed light on this seeming paradox was most likely not even considered.

In summary, as a result of events of the past two decades, the role of the clinical neuropsychologist in the psychiatric setting began to evolve from occasional consultant for ruling out organicity to member of a neuropsychiatric treatment team. Increasingly, one sees the use of neuropsychological profiling for understanding not only the diagnostic picture but also the patient's demonstrated strengths and limitations in everyday functioning. Under development in the laboratory are neuropsychologically informed approaches to psychiatric rehabilitation, as well as potentially useful remediation methods adapted from those used with patients with head injuries. Perhaps more futuristic is the notion that neuropsychological science will return to its roots in experimental psychology and psychophysiology and will spearhead efforts to develop measurement approaches that improve the accuracy and reliability of psychiatric diagnosis, consequently improving opportunities for treatment, rehabilitation, and support. To appreciate the potential of these developments for improving psychiatric care and their impact on opportunities for rehabilitation, one must consider the prevalence and effect of functional disability in serious neuropsychiatric disorders, especially in light of "deinstitutionalization" and the proliferation of community-based treatment and rehabilitation programs.

◆ FUNCTIONAL DISABILITY: A CRITICAL DIMENSION OF PSYCHIATRIC DISORDERS

The vast majority of individuals with severe mental illnesses remain compromised by impairments in independent functioning despite optimal medical management. These impairments are often more devastating in their effect on the patient's life than the symptoms of psychopathology. They often persist throughout the person's lifetime and are estimated to exact a financial cost to society three to four times that of the cost of direct patient care (Andrews et al. 1985; Fein 1958; Gunderson and Mosher 1975; Hall et al. 1985).

As mentioned earlier, the relation between chronic symptoms of psychopathology and functional disabilities in independent life functioning is overestimated by most clinicians and is in fact only a modest one (Anthony and Jansen 1984; Meltzer 1992; Strauss and Carpenter 1972, 1978; Strauss et al. 1974). This seeming paradox continues to surprise and frustrate clinicians as well as patients and their families, who so anxiously await a return to ordinary life as acute symptoms stabilize.

A follow-up report from the Washington IPSS sample indicated that psychopathological signs and symptoms are less important for explaining 11-year outcome than nonsymptom prognostic variables such as previous interpersonal relationships, previous hospitalizations, and—notably for our present discussion—extent of cognitive symptoms (Carpenter and Strauss 1991). Several studies have reported only modest cross-sectional associations between negative symptoms and work (Lysaker and Bell 1995) or social skill acquisition (Mueser et al. 1992). These findings are problematic because the determination of selected negative symptoms and their severity was based on independent functioning, the very variable for which the association was being investigated (e.g., vocational functioning is used for the determination of the avolition/apathy rating on the Scale for the Assessment of Negative Symptoms) (Andreasen 1984).

The failure to understand or appreciate the relation between the presence and severity of psychopathological symptoms in psychiatric patients and the capacity to live independently has had tragic consequences. In large measure, this failure resulted in the often reckless deinstitutionalization during the 1970s that followed the advent of neuroleptic drugs. Overestimating the importance of psychopathological symptoms alone led to the untested assumption that the effects of such drugs—which appeared to ameliorate psychopathological symptoms—could also be generalized to an increased capacity for independent living. Furthermore, the development of new approaches to psychiatric rehabilitation and the allocation of resources to empirically tested methods of delivering support services was significantly delayed. (Paradoxically, pressures from public managed behavioral health care and the demand for accountability have done more to propel psychiatry toward an emphasis on rehabilitation and optimizing support services than calls for such a shift coming from traditional clinical research and practice.)

An emphasis on functional disability would contribute greatly to improvements in psychiatric nosology. In considering a nosologic system, it would seem reasonable to postulate that for a particular disease the types and severity of functional disability should be associated with the severity of its core symptoms (as identified in a purely clinical assessment). If they are not, this would suggest that the nosologic system used should reconsider its emphasis on or understanding of those core symptoms. In other words, in a particular group of patients with a diagnosis of schizophrenia, if the course and outcome of symptoms such as hallucinations, delusions, and formal thought disorder are not closely correlated with the types and severity of functional disability, then perhaps these particular symptoms or features should not be considered the essential clinical indicators of the disease entity in such patients. The descriptive study of the functional morbidity of schizophrenia and its mutability (or sometimes lack thereof) in the presence of high-quality individualized rehabilitation and support represents an important opportunity for clarifying the clinical and biological heterogeneity of schizophrenia as it is currently delimited.

There has long been an implicit assumption that functional disability was among the disease dimensions being targeted in the somatic treatment of psychiatric disorders. However, studies of pharmacotherapeutic efficacy do not adequately focus on this dimension, and decisions to market or recommend specific drug treatments are not made on the basis of their ability to increase a patient's capacity for independent productive activity. Rather, the efficacy of new drugs is assessed by the use of narrowly focused clinical observations recorded with the use of rating scales that are administered in the artificially restricted setting of a research interview. Until recently, neither cognitive performance nor capacity to function or engage in productive activity has been "visible" to those studying pharmacotherapeutic treatments. There is an adage in clinical scientific research: "If you don't measure it, it doesn't exist." To date, we know of no psychotropic drug that has been brought to market on the basis of demonstrated efficacy to improve functional capacity in the areas of work or independent living in individuals with idiopathic psychiatric disorders.

In contrast to somatic treatments, psychosocial treatments have come to emphasize functioning and to employ atheoretical, although arguably more successful, supportive approaches for disabled individuals regardless of diagnosis or "clinical picture." There has been a surge of interest in supported employment and the widespread acceptance of the need for ongoing supports to achieve sustained improvements in independent functioning (Becker and Drake 1993, 1994; Bond 1992; Drake et al. 1994; Gervey and Bedell 1994; Gervey et al. 1995; Torrey et al. 1995; Trotter et al. 1988). A parallel interest has evolved in models of supported education (e.g., Cook and Solomon 1993) as well as supported living (e.g., Jones et al. 1994). Such approaches emphasize ongoing, individualized supports reflecting an awareness of the imperviousness of these functional deficits to existing pharmacological, psychotherapeutic, and skills training interventions. In the vocational domain, it is widely accepted that the greatest challenge lies in *sustaining* acquired job roles (Cook and Pickett 1994; Cook and Razzano 1992), recognizing that the underlying impairment continues to take its toll on the patient. The promise of these methods depends on an improved psychiatric nosology that fully incorporates the spectrum of impairments underlying the disabilities and handicaps that are the targets of our rehabilitation and support efforts. Neuropsychological impairments have been striking for their absence in these discussions, in part because their promise for improving psychiatric diagnosis has not yet been realized. However, much remains to be done, and how neuropsychological impairments influence disability and handicap in psychiatric patients has not been properly studied.

In summary, functional disability is a critical domain of psychiatric illness that does not appear to be explained by the presence or severity of clinical psychiatric symptoms (as these are generally characterized and monitored). Over the course of their illness, some patients with significant residual symptoms still manage to function better than other patients with mild residual symptomatology, and many with few or no manifest symptoms remain functionally disabled. This observation should compel those interested in developing a valid psychiatric nosology to revisit the classification of schizophrenia in particular. The fact that symptom management with neuroleptic treatments may not translate into long-term functional recovery has not been widely addressed by researchers studying treatments for schizophrenia. However, interest is growing in advancing clinical efforts in psychiatric rehabilitation. Psychiatric rehabilitation programs seek to support the patient's recovery from disability. This is optimally accomplished through counseling and skills training involving patient-directed goal setting and developing individualized supports for maintaining the patient in a role that can be maximally successful and satisfying. To the degree that neuropsychological deficits figure in among the determinants of functional disability, there resides the promise of neuropsychology, particularly for patients eager to recover a productive role, for improving methods of clinical management and rehabilitation.

◈ ARE NEUROPSYCHOLOGICAL DEFICITS CLINICALLY RELEVANT IN PSYCHIATRIC PATIENTS?

The prevalence and nature of neuropsychological deficits in schizophrenia are described elsewhere (see Calev, Chapter 2, in this volume). However, their presence and severity alone do not betoken their consequence for disability. Does a high rate of perseverative responding on the Wisconsin Card Sorting Test (WCST) translate into difficulties with learning or using new skills or with the ability to sustain employment or to live independently? In this section, we briefly consider the clinical and functional correlates of neuropsychological deficits in psychiatric patients. Evidence indicates that neuropsychological deficits (in contrast to psychopathology) may be responsible for the intractability of impaired life functioning and the limitations of rehabilitation. Consideration of such data might provide a rational basis for the development and use of remediative interventions and/or individually targeted supports in the service of a patient's rehabilitation goals.

Performance on neuropsychological tests has been shown to be correlated with capacity to work (Cook and Razzano 1994; Heaton et al. 1978b; Lysaker et al. 1995; Newnan et al. 1978; Silverstein et al. 1991; Weaver and Brooks 1963), social competence (Penn et al. 1995; Penny et al. 1995), social perception and problem solving (Corrigan et al. 1994a; Penn et al. 1993), and even self-care (Corrigan et al. 1994b). Our own studies have also demonstrated a predictive association between neuropsychological deficits and instrumental role-functioning outcome 3 months later.

The association between performance on neuropsychological tests and clinical symptomatology is less clear, however. Blunted affect, an essential component of all the various conceptualizations of deficit schizophrenia, has been observed to correlate with a variety of motor functions that depend on the integrity of the frontostriatal circuits (Cox and Ludwig 1979; Manschreck 1983; Manschreck and Ames 1984). As indicated above, ratings of negative symptoms have been shown to be correlated with independent functioning but also with neurobehavioral signs of prefrontal impairment (Breier et al. 1991; Merriam et al. 1990) and with learning and memory (Paulsen et al. 1995) in chronically ill patients. A small sample of patients with schizophrenia who had been hospitalized for a short time were seen to have reduced attentional capacity at baseline that was associated with higher residual negative symptoms but not with positive symptoms after 4 weeks of neuroleptic treatment (Goldman et al. 1993). Baseline memory deficits were associated with poor functional status in these patients 1 year later. A general pattern in these studies is that when neuropsychological deficits are associated with symptoms or treatment response, the association is generally present with negative symptoms but not positive symptoms. This appears at first to be inconsistent with the previously discussed findings that neuropsychological deficits are associated with functional disability, whereas symptoms are only modestly so associated. However, as indicated earlier, there may be an unintended confounding in these studies: negative symptom rating scales often incorporate work and independent functioning as signs used to rate avolition and apathy (Andreasen 1981; Kay et al. 1987). Thus, what appears to be a correlation between independent functioning and negative symptoms may actually be a replication of measurement within a single construct that is distinct from the construct of other symptoms of psychopathology. This explains at least one finding in which neuropsychological tests of frontal-lobe functioning were correlated with *both* negative symptoms and social functioning on follow-up (Breier et al. 1991).

What remains to be established is an understanding of the relation between neuropsychological deficits and independent functioning. Are there patterns of neuropsychological deficits that coexist with patterns of course of psychopathology and represent distinct etiopathological entities with distinct patterns of functional outcome?

A multinational study employing Q-factor analysis with 495 subjects with mixed psychiatric diagnoses reported that the association between neuropsychological test performance and social and occupational history and background may follow a functionally specific pattern (Townes et al. 1985). For example, patients with good verbal and memory functions in contrast to poor complex problem solving and motor functioning tended to be older, well-educated, unemployed women. On the other hand, patients with poor verbal and memory functioning and good visuospatial problem solving and motor functioning tended to be younger, less educated men with histories of unskilled employment, learning disability, and drug abuse. Replication and further studies are needed in this area.

To the degree that neuropsychological tests reflect distinct pathophysiological abnormalities that are associated with severity and mutability of impaired role functioning, they may be useful in the development of a more reliable and biologically meaningful psychiatric nosology. An interesting development in this area is the finding of a robust relation between sylvian fissure volumes and employment outcome an average of 46 months after onset in a sample of 140 patients with "functional psychoses of recent onset" who had undergone computed tomography (CT) scanning (van Os et al. 1995). This relation was upheld even when premorbid rate of unemployment (which was also associated with sylvian fissure volumes) was accounted for statistically. A less robust relation with third ventricle volumes was observed and was mediated by cognitive deficits. Further understanding of the underlying determinants of disability is important not only for the advance of psychiatric rehabilitation methodologies and the strategic deployment of supports. Such an understanding may lead to new approaches to psychiatric nosology with the potential for new thinking in the development and testing of best practices for treatment.

Our own studies began in 1990 with several modest attempts to examine the prevalence of neuropsychological deficits in ambulatory patients seeking psychiatric rehabilitation services and to examine the association between neuropsychological deficits and independent functioning. In one study we conducted comprehensive neuropsychological assessments (a 4-hour battery of commonly used neuropsychological tests) in a sample of patients with mixed psychiatric diagnoses. Subjects were 73 consecutively admitted patients to a clinic-based psychiatric rehabilitation program who were seeking comprehensive psychiatric rehabilitation services at least 3 days per week. Three groups—consisting of 22 patients with chart diagnoses of schizophrenia, 16 with schizoaffective disorder, and 25 with affective disorder, obsessive-compulsive disorder, or anxiety disorder—were descriptively characterized relative to a normative population and compared with one another using a series of one-way analyses of variance. All three groups had significant impairments relative to published norms on almost all the tests administered (Figure 10–1). The left portion of Figure 10–1 displays the mean standard score on several neuropsychological measures. The dotted line represents the 50th per-

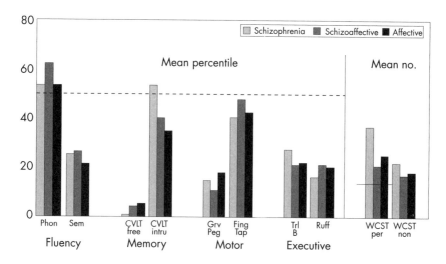

Figure 10–1. Diagnostic comparisons of neuropsychological tests. Phon = phonemic, Sem = semantic, free = free recall, intru = free intrusions, CVLT = California Verbal Learning Test, Grv Peg = Grooved Pegboard, Fing Tap = Finger Tapping Test, Trl B = Trail Making Test Part B, Ruff = Ruff Figural Fluency Test, WCST = Wisconsin Card Sorting Test, per = perseverative errors, non = nonperseverative errors.

centile taken from published norms for each test given. Several of the tests show profound deficits compared with these normative values. On the right side of the figure, the mean number of WCST (Heaton 1985) perseverative and nonperseverative errors are displayed. All three groups, particularly the schizophrenia group, significantly exceed the published cutoff score (as indicated by the solid line).

One-way analyses of variance comparing the three diagnostic group classes revealed few group differences (despite the considerable risk of type I error with the multiple comparisons conducted). The only significant group differences that were seen were on WCST perseverative errors ($P = .03$) and categories ($P = .01$) and on several measures from the California Verbal Learning Test (CVLT; Delis et al. 1986) in which the schizophrenia group was significantly more impaired than the other two groups. Table 10–1 lists the neuropsychological measures classified according to whether they met criteria of statistical significance of diagnostic difference.

These findings are particularly striking for the similarity of the affec-

Table 10–1.   Diagnostic differences on neuropsychological tests

Neuropsychological domain	Nonsignificant differences	Significant differences
Verbal	Phonemic and Semantic Fluency	
Visuospatial	Rey Complex Figure Test: Copy	
Memory	CVLT: Free Recall	CVLT: Free Intrusions
Executive	Ruff Figural Fluency Test WCST: Non-Perseverative Errors Trail Making Test Part B	WCST: Perseverative Errors WCST: Categories
Motor	Finger Tapping Test Grooved Pegboard	

Note.   CVLT = California Verbal Learning Test, WCST = Wisconsin Card Sorting Test.

tive-anxiety disorders group compared with samples of patients with schizophrenia and schizoaffective disorder. Although patients with affective and anxiety disorders do show neuropsychological deficits (Austin et al. 1992; Cassens et al. 1990), most studies comparing similarly selected acute samples confirm the presence of significantly more severe deficits in schizophrenia (Goldberg et al. 1993a). Our failure to find this discrimination can best be interpreted as a function of sampling, confirming our hypothesis that neuropsychological deficit is the common factor found among patients with disability sufficient to seek comprehensive psychiatric rehabilitation services: some patients with affective disorders may not seek rehabilitation services because they do not experience severe long-term disability. When their clinical symptoms resolve, these patients tend to return to the community. It may be that those patients who do not return to productive community roles and instead seek rehabilitative services are also the most neuropsychologically impaired subgroup of the population with affective and anxiety disorders. Thus, neuropsychological deficits may be a reliable predictor of disability status. However, these findings suggest that their specificity in distinguishing among clinical diagnoses is very poor.

In view of these findings and to determine whether they would hold in a schizophrenia-only sample meeting research diagnostic criteria, we conducted the following examination in collaboration with Dr. Robert Bilder and Jeffrey Lieberman at Hillside Hospital: We examined the correlation between the WCST and global ratings from the Social Adjustment Scale (SAS; Schooler et al. 1979), a commonly used measure of independent functioning, among a subset of patients from a study of first-episode schizophrenia.[1]

We summarize here data we previously reported from a subset of the full sample available at the time (Jaeger and Douglas 1992). In 33 first-episode patients from this sample, a battery of neuropsychological tests (including the WCST) was administered within 12 months of the beginning of neuroleptic treatment (baseline); 19 of these patients were also retested within 18 months of administration of the first test. No significant correlations were found between these variables at baseline (not surprisingly, because this was the point of initial stabilization). However, on retesting, perseverative errors were positively and significantly correlated with the SAS global rating for Instrumental Role Functioning ($r = .47, P = .05$, two-tailed), with trends for Social Leisure Functioning ($r = .44, P = .07$) and General Adjustment ($r = .40, P = .10$). Interestingly, WCST perseverative errors at baseline were significantly correlated with several SAS global scores on retesting (Instrumental Role Functioning, $r = .57, P = .01$; General Adjustment, $r = .48, P = .04$; Household Functioning, $r = .40, P = .09$; Social Leisure Functioning, $r = .42$, $P = .08$). This suggests not only that executive deficit as measured by the WCST is associated with level of independent functioning (IF) at follow-up (concurrent validity), but also that this neuropsychological measure may be predictive of future IF (predictive validity).

We further examined correlations between SAS global ratings and composite neuropsychological scores of language, memory, attention, executive, visuospatial, and motor functions derived for each as the average of the z-transformed scores on neuropsychological tests that measure that area. This approach was selected a priori—further exploratory analyses of individual neuropsychological test parameters were not conducted because of power constraints and the ongoing nature of this study. With one-tailed criteria, significant correlations ($P < .05$) were observed at baseline between Attention and Social Leisure ($r = .30$) and

---

[1] *Note:* To guard against type I error, these were the *only* correlations performed for this set of analyses. WCST perseverative errors were selected a priori because of the substantial literature on the importance of this executive functioning measure in schizophrenia and its apparent mediation by dorsolateral prefrontal cortex. Nonperseverative errors were selected for examination to permit evaluation of the specificity of any observed associations to executive deficits.

General Adjustment ($r = .35$), between Executive and Instrumental Role ($r = .31$), Social Leisure ($r = .42$), and General Adjustment ($r = .34$), and between Motor and Social Leisure ($r = .30$).

Our current efforts are to replicate and extend these preliminary findings in a larger sample, over a longer follow-up period, using a statistical model that permits us to examine the role of symptoms of psychopathology in the relation between performance on neuropsychological tests and functional disability. In addition, we have recently begun a large-scale replication in a more chronically ill subset of schizophrenic patients who may be more frequent subjects of our rehabilitation efforts.

Along these lines, we examined the predictive relation between the WCST and SAS global ratings (using our own published anchors for Instrumental Role Functioning) (Jaeger et al. 1992) in a diagnostically mixed sample of patients. Subjects were 31 consenting patients (9 with schizophrenia, 8 with schizoaffective disorder, 6 with affective disorders, and 8 with personality and anxiety disorders) consecutively discharged from a clinic-affiliated psychiatric rehabilitation program during a 15-month period. Immediately after discharge, they were given the WCST, the WAIS-R Information and Vocabulary subtests, the Brief Psychiatric Rating Scale (BPRS; Overall and Gorham 1962), the SAS, and a vocational history and status interview. All subjects were retested on the BPRS, the SAS, and vocational history and status interview 3 and 6 months thereafter.

A stepwise multiple regression revealed that ratings on the SAS Instrumental Role Functioning test administered 3 months after discharge could be predicted by the WCST perseverative error score at baseline ($P < .04$) but not by nonperseverative errors (indicating the specificity of the relationship to perseverations). This finding was unchanged after removal of the independent contributions of diagnosis, follow-up BPRS total score (a measure of level of psychopathology), and WAIS-R Information and Vocabulary subtests (an estimate of verbal IQ). The R-square —as a measure of change—indicated that the WCST explained 17% of the outcome variance.

There were no diagnostic differences (patients with schizophrenia compared with other diagnoses) in SAS ratings, in WCST performance, or in the predictive value of WCST for determining SAS instrumental role functioning. However, WCST at baseline did not predict SAS at the 6-month follow-up point. Diagnosis was the only predictor at this point ($P < .019$). To determine the direction of this diagnosis effect we conducted a 2×2 repeated measure analysis of variance comparing the two diagnostic groups on change in SAS scores from 3 to 6 months after discharge. There was no significant main effect of group or time but a significant group by time interaction such that schizophrenic patients showed a deterioration in SAS score, whereas nonschizophrenic patients improved.

Unfortunately, we had not repeated the WCST at 3 and 6 months after discharge to determine whether a change in WCST was related to this change in role functioning. However, data from a previous administration of the WCST were available for a subset of these patients who had participated in another study employing the WCST on admission to this ambulatory rehabilitation program (ranging from 1 to 26 months before the discharge assessment). Intraclass correlation coefficients (ICCs) to measure test-retest comparability of WCST perseverative errors, percentage of perseverative errors, and perseverative responses at the two time points (admission and discharge) resulted in negligible coefficients, suggesting that WCST performance is heavily state dependent. We failed to find any significant correlations between the magnitude or direction of change in WCST scores and a wide range of demographic and clinical variables in the subset for whom previous WCST data had been obtained. The lack of long-term stability in WCST scores in psychiatric populations has been reported previously (Seidman et al. 1991).

To summarize, evidence indicates that deficits measured with neuropsychological tests may be associated with the severity of functional disability among patients with schizophrenia and in mixed diagnostic groups of psychiatric patients with disability in independent life functioning. Measured cross-sectionally, neuropsychological tests do not discriminate among diagnostic groups, and their ability to predict ongoing functional disability may be limited to a few months. Performance on neuropsychological tests, although partially a reflection of trait features, probably also fluctuates as a function of psychiatric state in certain individuals. In one small study we found that neuropsychological test performance predicted functional outcome in a mixed ambulatory sample 3 months but not 6 months later. Having a diagnosis of schizophrenia predicted poor functional outcome 6 months later. If neuropsychological status is associated with functional disability, this would suggest that incorporating an understanding of a patient's cognitive limitations into the planning of rehabilitation and support interventions might be useful. However, studies employing repeated neuropsychological evaluations are needed that might determine which components of neurobehavioral deficit represent trait characteristics and which reflect state features that fluctuate with the changing clinical presentation of a patient. It would be important to determine the relevance of these distinct types of deficit for the short-term and long-term course of independent functioning. Neurobehavioral measures that distinguish individuals with good and poor long-term outcome are more likely to have relevance for a reliable clinical nosology than those that are associated with short-term course characteristics.

◈ HOW CAN NEUROPSYCHOLOGY BE USED TO BENEFIT THE PSYCHIATRIC PATIENT?

Some historical points are in order. The past decade has seen dramatic successes in traumatology and emergency medicine leading to the survival of record numbers of head trauma victims. At the same time, the clinical challenge for neuropsychologists working in neurological settings has evolved from the old "find the lesion" approach, which was prevalent before the availability of neuroimaging technology, to the challenge of explaining clinical progress and residual disability in terms of neuropsychological deficits. This seems a simple task on the face of it, but any neuropsychologist working with brain trauma who has been faced with such questions knows otherwise. Questions such as "can this patient drive?" have to be answered with almost no available data on the relationship between actual driving ability and type and severity of neurocognitive deficit. And the conservative "better safe than sorry" approach may be sensible in the absence of data, but the consequences of our ignorance may be harsh in a patient residing in a rural or suburban setting where a proscription from driving may profoundly impede recovery and quality of life. Thus emerged a new mandate for neuropsychology: to examine the relation between measured deficits and functional disability with a view toward improving the quality of life in individuals with brain injuries.

Neuropsychologists in psychiatric settings have been slow to embrace this mandate, largely for historic reasons alluded to earlier. Outcome-oriented rehabilitation in psychiatry has been the purview of applied vocational counseling, rehabilitation counseling, counseling psychology, and behavior therapy, disciplines in which training in neuropsychology and neurocognition is virtually absent. (Excluded here are self-proclaimed "therapies" often inappropriately referred to as rehabilitation, such as recreation, music, and art therapy, which in their best form are valuable in providing pleasant diversionary activities for suffering individuals but are clearly not "therapeutic" to any known outcome.) Psychiatric rehabilitation has made great strides in recent years, clarifying its mandate in functional terms, namely, to maximize patients' ability to function as and where they choose with the least possible day-to-day professional intervention (Anthony et al. 1990).

The analogy to physical disabilities is often embraced in this context. Targeted remediation is applied where possible and feasible for deficits that interfere with an individual's own goals, and accommodation through outside supports are provided where remediation falls short. The potential for neuropsychology to make productive contributions along these lines in psychiatry must be pursued through extensive investigation. Neuropsychological assessments may identify potential barriers to achievement of goals, indicate areas in which direct remediation may be useful, and facilitate the development of "cognitive aids" or strategies to assist cognition that may promote independent functioning.

These lines of evidence support a working model that we put forth in 1992 (Jaeger and Douglas 1992) and present in a somewhat revised version in Figure 10–2.

Our assumption is that the closer a treatment is to the causative agent, the more effective it is likely to be. Thus, finding a cure is predicated on the identification of the cause, a goal that continues to elude us in psychiatry. Short of this, management of selected elements of a disease's presentation can be accomplished through perturbation of a physiological system known to be responsible for a particular symptom (e.g., an anxiolytic agent treating the putative physiological mechanism for anxiety). At the other end of the spectrum, providing shelter, meals, or even recreational opportunities may be essential to sustain the health

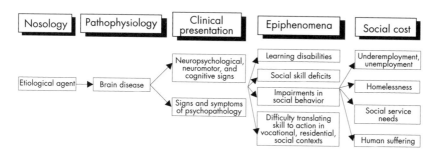

Figure 10–2. A model of psychiatric disease and disability (Jaeger and Douglas 1992).

and comfort of the patient but does little to reduce the severity of illness. At present, drug treatments for symptoms exist only with respect to symptoms of psychopathology, and, for the most part, the basis for the presumed therapeutic effect is largely speculative or altogether unknown. Treatments for neuropsychological deficits are not typically pursued, *yet they may be the primary precursors to skill deficits that are the subject of our rehabilitation treatment.* It will be critical for the advance of this field to validate each of the causative associations hypothesized in this model. Increasing our understanding of the relationships between the neuropsychological deficits and the skill deficits that are responsible for impaired independent role functioning would finally provide a basis for improved rehabilitation and supports.

◈ NEUROPSYCHOLOGICALLY INFORMED APPROACHES TO REHABILITATION

Psychiatric rehabilitation as it is practiced is most fundamentally a patient-driven process. The process serves the group of patients who, regardless of other symptoms or cognitive capacity, retain sufficient will and interest to recover whatever independent productive level of functioning may be possible. Patients characterized by persistent severe avolition or disorganization are typically unable to engage in the rehabilitation process at all. However, it is critical to reevaluate patients continually, as changes in clinical state can naturally occur.

The first challenge in psychiatric rehabilitation is to evaluate the appropriateness of engaging in the often protracted process at a particular point in time with a patient. The past decade has seen a strong movement in favor of overinclusiveness rather than risk excluding an individual who might succeed in achieving some functional recovery with the appropriate supports. This is an understandable and humane response to decades-long practices in which patients were given no choices, and authoritarian psychiatric treatment teams uniformly imposed "therapeutic activities" that were demeaning and unrelated either to the illness, its rational treatment, or the patient's wish to engage in meaningful activity and recover function. This approach led to missed opportunities for individuals capable of productive independent lives, as became apparent following the deinstitutionalization of patients in state psychiatric centers around the country. Although many were seriously harmed by the inappropriateness of their discharge and the absence of adequate community supports, a significant number (as many as one-third) who had been virtually incarcerated with a diagnosis of schizophrenia found productive lives outside the hospital with minimal professional assistance (Harding et al. 1987). (Findings were essentially unchanged when the original patients studied by Harding et al. were rediagnosed retrospectively with DSM-IV criteria.) This illustrates the profound and continuous inadequacy of the current psychiatric diagnostic system for planning or prescribing rehabilitation interventions.

Psychiatry is sorely in need of methodologies capable of reliably characterizing mental functions or syndromes that are correlated to the functional outcome of psychiatric patients. Neuropsychology can provide such objective characterization of selected state and trait features of an individual patient's disorder, and evidence indicates that this characterization is associated with functional disability. Although we are far from the point of a meaningful integration of neuropsychological findings within psychiatric diagnosis, results from neurocognitive and neuromotor assessments can already provide some guidance in the rehabilitation process.

With respect to neurocognitive remediation with psychiatric patients, there have been only a few modest attempts, and preliminary findings have not been optimistic. One reason may be that these attempts are premature, having been conducted before the performance of sufficient studies addressing the question of which neurobehavioral domains (e.g., attention, memory) are critical to disability. In the absence of a clear target for remediation, the development of optimal techniques has been forced to proceed in the dark. In addition, it may be critical to first determine which domains are causatively associated with impaired functioning and which are illness markers only indirectly associated with the severity of overall clinical presentation (e.g., impaired smooth pursuit eye tracking.)

One can view the advent of supported employment, supported education, and supported housing programs as a constructive response to the absence of a systematic fund of knowledge regarding the causes of disability in psychiatric patients. The success of these programs derives from the individualized assessment of support needs, based on observed skills and abilities rather than psychiatric diagnosis.

Despite only limited understanding of the nature of the associations between neurobehavioral deficits and disability (e.g., which specific neurobehavioral factors are associated with dysfunction and by what mechanism, and how these associations fluctuate within the course of the illness), preliminary attempts at cognitive remediation may never-theless be useful. From attempts at cognitive remediation we can learn more about the mutability of particular types of deficits (Bellack et al. 1990; Goldberg 1992; Goldberg et al. 1993b), the potential of improved neuropsychological capacity (should this be achieved) for enhancing par-ticular life skills and ultimately role functioning, and the interaction of these factors with the inherently phasic clinical course of persistent psy-chiatric illnesses (Spaulding et al. 1994). In neuropsychological assess-ment we frequently "test limits" as a technique for understanding the depth of an observed impairment. Until we know more, cognitive remediation can be considered an intensive testing of limits that may or may not generalize to further improvements in cognitive functional ca-pacity but can certainly teach us about the mutability of certain deficits in particular types of patients.

In addition to the (seemingly remote) hope of cognitive remediation, neuropsychological evaluation may provide more immediate benefit in identifying opportunities for targeted support or the use of "cognitive prostheses." Sohlberg and Mateer (1989) divide neuropsychological re-habilitation (in the context of traumatic brain injury) into two compo-nents: restorative methods that attempt to recoup functions lost due to brain damage and compensatory methods that train patients to use alter-native means to accomplish impaired functions. Along these lines, Diller (1987) presented a taxonomy of cognitive remediation models. *Defi-ciency* models assume deficient functioning is a result of lack of use sec-ondary to neurological deficit and its treatment. It assumes that the deficit is not irretrievably lost. Remediation involves exposure or enrich-ment in the deficient area for the purposes of relearning or retraining. In contrast, the *interference* model assumes some permanent loss and pos-its that lack of functional competence arises as a result of the direct in-terference of the neurocognitive deficit with normal functioning. Remediation is thus a teaching method for removal of the interference by suppressing, isolating, and/or bypassing it (i.e., developing alternative cognitive strategies, as when a visuospatially impaired individual uses a sequence of verbal instructions to accommodate for the deficit). Finally, *absence* models assume an intrinsic and, for practical purposes, immuta-ble lack or loss of function that can be compensated for only by pros-thetic aids and support in the environment.

Most psychiatric social skills training paradigms use an interfer-ence-model approach in which alternative strategies are taught to over-come functional impairments. An example is integrated psychological therapy (IPT) (Brenner et al. 1992). IPT assumes that social dysfunction is caused by cognitive deficits through two "vicious cycles" in which elementary cognitive deficits produce more complex cognitive dysfunctions (impaired social perception). These dysfunctions diminish coping skills (poor verbal communication), increase social stressors, and thereby further diminish cognitive and functional capacity. The proposed solution is found in a hierarchical model designed to abort the cycle of deficits initially through basic cognitive remediation exercises and later through training in social perception and interpersonal problem solving. A controlled trial comparing IPT to an intensive social learning–based behavior therapy in an inpatient sample was conducted by Spaulding and colleagues in Lincoln, Nebraska. Reported findings suggest that IPT was not uniquely effective and that both treatments produce similar improvements in measures of executive functioning (Spaulding et al. 1994).

We have previously described some of our early attempts at cognitive remediation in the domain of executive functioning (Jaeger and Douglas 1992, pp. 86–88). Our work with the Executive Board System of Zec and colleagues (1992) contributed to the notion of pursuing a hierarchical approach to remediation in favor of the "mosaic" approach (which implies that a single circumscribed domain of cognitive deficit can be remediated in isolation from all others). The hierarchy we proposed was adopted from the work of Sohlberg and Mateer (1989), developed in the context of head trauma patients. It involves training to an a priori criterion in sustained attention, followed by selective attention, alternating attention, and divided attention. These training exercises assume a deficiency or interference model of attentional functioning and are intended to be restorative. Training is directed at the increase in absolute cognitive capacity through repeated exposure and use of the cortical systems involved, with the implication that neuronal plasticity allows for such an increased capacity.

We have also explored the potential of prospective memory training (Sohlberg and Mateer 1986), which assumes interference and absence models and is intended to be compensatory (as opposed to restorative). Prospective memory refers to the ability to remember to respond or to do something at a designated time point in the future. Examples include remembering to mail a letter on the way out the door, remembering to pick up some bread on the way home tonight, or remembering a doctor's appointment in 2 weeks. Neurocognitively, this is a complex construct that includes executive processes (planning and executing a method for ensuring that the person will remember the critical information at some future time), selective attention and associative learning (when the person sees or notices the mailbox on the way to the bus stop, it will remind him or her to mail the letter), and metamemory (remembering to remember to look at a written agenda at a critical future time). Functionally, prospective memory is critical, and many psychiatric patients struggle in this area. The neurocognitive complexity of prospective memory prevents (given our current state of neuroscientific knowledge) any direct restorative remediation approach outside of the global improvements in mental functions that can accompany an improvement in clinical state. We therefore use an absence model, assuming that the deficit is intractable.

Simply stated, our approach involves the design of individualized cognitive aids and the training and support of the patient around the use of these aids. In the case of prospective memory training, it involves a notebook or card system or, when feasible, could even involve the use of portable electronic devices. In our very preliminary experience with the notebook system, we have found that patients with schizophrenia continue to require support in the use of the notebook even after development and training stages have been satisfactorily completed. In addition, the content and complexity of the notebook is largely determined by the patient's circumstances and must be revised continuously as these change. A patient residing in a group home and attending a psychosocial club most of the day may in fact have little use for such a notebook. However, as such a patient chooses to pursue goals that require more complex time organization, its potential for benefit becomes apparent.

We have no conclusive evidence of the efficacy of this or any other remediative approach at this time. We have previously addressed the difficulties of objectively evaluating such approaches (Jaeger et al. 1992). Controlled testing of cognitive remediation poses many challenges. These challenges must be addressed both by researchers and by clinicians interested in trying approaches such as those described in small groups of patients. A particular challenge is in the selection of the outcome measure, a problem linked with the issue of transfer and generalizability of training. The scientific rationale for the particular remediation approach being used is critical in this decision. For example, the scientific rationale for remediative attention training is to make use of the neurophysiological redundancy of attentional functioning and of the brain's putative plasticity to increase the attentional capacity of the patient. Thus, it is intended to be restorative of attentional capacity, and the outcome measures would include tests of attention as well as measures that might reflect any increase in functional capacity that might follow. On the other hand, the use of a prospective memory prosthesis notebook is intended as a compensatory intervention and would not be expected to result in improvements on neuropsychological tests. Regardless of the remediative method being examined or the particular neuropsychological or functional measures being used for evaluating efficacy, it is advisable to employ multiple baseline assessments over the course of a period of at least 2–3 months in stable patients before initiating any cognitive remediation regimen in a patient. This will allow the clinician and the patient to be assured that the deficits they manifest are stable and unlikely to remit spontaneously and to increase the likelihood that any improvement seen on follow-up is associated with the intervening treatments. (Multiple follow-up assessments over a similar 2- to 3-month period will also help ensure that measured improvements are stable and reliable.)

The use of criterion-based advancement through each phase in a hierarchical remediation regimen requires that exposure to treatment must necessarily vary as a function of the rate of the patient's progress. The considerable individual variability we have seen in the rate of progression through the phases of attention process training (ranging from 6 to 24 months in our experience so far) poses challenges for both research and clinical planning. On the other hand, remediation programs that limit training in a particular phase to some arbitrarily selected duration run the risk of prematurely abandoning exercises that might be useful if patients were given sufficient time to benefit from them. We also caution against haphazard, atheoretical approaches such as simply placing patients in front of computers running cognitive remediation software and waiting to see whether "something happens." Although they are inexpensive, such approaches are unlikely to bear fruit and contribute to cynicism about the potential benefit of any remediation techniques. It would seem critical while developing remediation protocols to adopt and sustain a clear theoretical framework. For example, it would be important to distinguish carefully between restorative approaches, which may yield enduring results but are limited in the domains amenable to their use, and compensatory approaches, which are likely to yield more immediate (as well as more modest) results. Computers may be of use in either approach but must be conscientiously employed within such a framework.

One further caution relates to the tendency throughout psychiatry when developing skills training protocols to implement these protocols without first making the determination that the particular deficit being addressed is in some way critical to functional improvement being sought by the patient. An important contribution from what is now known as the Boston University Model for psychiatric rehabilitation (Anthony et al. 1990) is the notion that the patient's expressed and manifest goals must be primary and a determining factor in pursuing such interventions. Although it is likely that neurocognitive deficits pose critical barriers for most severely disabled psychiatric patients, readiness on the part of the patient to engage actively in the process of overcoming such barriers is essential to neurocognitive remediation. Such readiness assumes that the patient has some interest or goal that might be overcome by these interventions. A patient who is satisfied living in a group home and attending a psychosocial club with no other challenges is unlikely to engage actively in the development of a reminder notebook to compensate for deficits in prospective memory. Neurocognitive remediation does not replace psychiatric rehabilitation. Rather, it represents a potential tool in the context of a comprehensive process of rehabilitation and recovery of functioning.

◈ WHAT WE CAN DO NOW

We have taken a number of steps in our own clinical work that have yielded some benefits as we await more solid data before proceeding. Many clinic psychiatrists, accustomed to focusing on manifest psychopathology, do not, as a matter of course, comprehensively evaluate the details of their patients' daily living practices. Yet the psychotropic drugs prescribed by these physicians have many side effects that impede independent functioning in ways that are already understood. The most apparent is their sedative effect, common to most neuroleptics and benzodiazepines. In our clinical experience with ambulatory patients, we have been struck by the frequency of fatigability and early-morning sleepiness of which *the treating psychiatrist is unaware*. In the course of working with patients who have difficulty during morning activities, we have observed that the therapeutic directive to take the final daily dose "at bedtime" may be too vague. Some patients take their evening dose on turning out the lights, often only hours before daybreak, resulting in peak blood values near the time they would have to rise to arrive at a job on time. Some patients who have difficulty getting to sleep take their medications later than those who have no such difficulty. The potential value of the evening dose for improved sleep may be intended by the psychiatrist but may be lost on the patient if explicit instructions are not provided and feedback obtained. We have noted significant improvements in functioning after years of disability following a review with the psychiatrist of the impact of daytime sleepiness on the patient's functioning. Such feedback from rehabilitation staff is critical to allow the treating psychiatrist, under ever-increasing time pressure, to pay explicit attention to the impact of dosing and timing of psychotropic drugs on the patient's quality of life.

Neuroleptic-induced movement disorders and their management are another problematic area for independent life functioning. The social stigmatization added by movement disorders poses a significant barrier in obtaining employment, housing, and social networks. This is explicit in tardive dyskinesia, but we have seen devastating social rejection even with rather subtle parkinsonian effects such as muted affective expressivity due to facial muscle hypomobility and reductions in gesturing, eye blinking, and affirming head nodding and nonverbal vocalizations. Our concern that functional disability could occur at levels of impairment in this area that are too subtle to be detected with the prevailing rating instruments for assessing drug-induced parkinsonism led us to develop the Gestural and Expressive Stigmata Scale (GESS). Our preliminary data confirming the presence of a significant relationship between GESS ratings and social leisure functioning in a small ambulatory sample has led us to pursue expanded studies in this area, which are now under way. However, clinically, the importance of such effects must be considered in the process of weighing risks and benefits of various pharmacotherapies. Unfortunately, the use of anticholinergic agents to ameliorate such effects may constitute a "catch-22" because these produce known effects on memory functioning.

Until more can be done to improve medication strategies for symptom management, awareness of the effect of side effects on important aspects of independent functioning is critical in the management of the patient's rehabilitation treatment. Acknowledgment of these barriers permits the development of supports. For example, a job coach in a supported work program can inform the employer that a patient's apparent boredom on the job may instead be a reflection of the patient's facial immobility as a result of drug-induced parkinsonism. Counselors in a supported housing program can directly address the need for additional sleep and the timing of bedtime medications in patients who experience daytime sleepiness. Supported employment programs can acknowledge diurnal needs by matching patients' work hours with their periods of peak functional capacity.

Until more is known about the specific manner in which neuropsychological deficits impede functional capacity, increased awareness of the presence of such deficits may itself be beneficial. The possibility for a particular patient that such a deficit may explain a particular difficulty in the rehabilitation process may lead to the development of individualized assistive methods. Examples might include individualized mnemonic systems, environmental supports such as an employer or job coach who provides extra direction for a patient with impairments in sequencing or organizing tasks, or placement of patients in an environment that provides sufficient cuing to help them overcome difficulties in attention and concentration. In addition to suggesting more possibilities for supportive or compensatory rehabilitation methods, awareness of neurobehavioral deficits and their impact on functional capacity has had the critical effect of removing the basis for the pejorative undertone that often arises in the staff's interactions with patients.

◈ Conclusion

Neuropsychologically informed interventions hold great promise for individuals with psychiatric disorders. However, the future of this line of inquiry is likely to be long and hard. Some reasons for this are 1) the difficulty inherent in proving the absence of an effect when various alternative methods are tested, 2) the challenge of determining the critical outcome measure and then quantifying that effect in a set of illnesses that are by nature labile and multidimensional, and 3) continued confusion and controversy concerning critical biological issues (e.g., a "true" psychiatric nosology including discrimination of genetic types and neurodevelopmental versus neurodegenerative characterizations) that may be relevant to the remediation approach employed. The development of treatment techniques should evolve through a rational and coherent process. New approaches and the proposed methods for testing them should be informed by neurobiological considerations as well as clinical ones. Neurocognitive remediation, as with all aspects of psychiatric rehabilitation, is likely to be extremely labor intensive and to require treatments that are long in duration. The tendency by some authors (e.g., Benedict et al. 1994) to dismiss the whole enterprise out of hand after a single unsuccessful attempt seems discriminatory in light of the persistence of such efforts in patients with traumatic head injury (Spring and Ravdin 1992). This is particularly the case when the absence of significant change is observed in only a single domain of measures (multidimensional outcomes are critical in this area) after a single type of remediative technique is used for relatively short periods. On the other hand, caution will also be required to avoid the inevitable grasping at the latest remediation fad. The risk for this is augmented by the desperation of the patients themselves and their families, which often leads to the uncritical adoption of a new technique that is then precipitously abandoned (often without adequate systematic examination) when the expected dramatic recovery is not forthcoming. We cannot overemphasize the need for well-controlled, systematic studies with disprovable hypotheses in this field. What psychiatry does not need is another set of dogmatic beliefs to replace those most recently dispelled. Obscure "neuropsychobabble" does not constitute an advance over the familiar "psychobabble" if our mission is to enhance the quality of life and reduce the devastating costs of mental illness.

◈ REFERENCES

American Psychiatric Association: Diagnostic and Statistical Manual of Mental Disorders, 4th Edition. Washington, DC, American Psychiatric Association, 1994

Anastasi A: Psychological Testing, 4th Edition. New York, Macmillan, 1976

Andreasen NC: Scale for the Assessment of Negative Symptoms (SANS). Iowa City, IA, University of Iowa, 1981

Andreasen NC: Modified Scale for the Assessment of Negative Symptoms. NIMH Treatment Strategies in Schizophrenia Study. Washington, DC, Alcohol, Drug Abuse, and Mental Health Administration, 1984

Andrews G, Hall W, Goldstein G, et al: The economic costs of schizophrenia: implications for public policy. Arch Gen Psychiatry 42:537–543, 1985

Anthony WA, Jansen MA: Predicting the vocational capacity of the chronically mentally ill: research and policy implications. Am Psychol 39:537–544, 1984

Anthony WA, Cohen M, Farkas MD: Psychiatric Rehabilitation. Boston, MA, Center for Psychiatric Rehabilitation, 1990

Austin MP, Ross M, Murray C, et al: Cognitive function in major depression. J Affect Disord 25:21–29, 1992

Becker DR, Drake RE: A Working Life: The Individual Placement and Support (IPS) Program. Dartmouth, NH, Dartmouth Psychiatric Research Center, 1993

Becker DR, Drake RE: Individual placement and support: a community mental health center approach to vocational rehabilitation. Community Ment Health J 30:193–206, 1994

Bellack AS, Mueser KT, Morrison RL, et al: Remediation of cognitive deficits in schizophrenia. Am J Psychiatry 147:1650–1655, 1990

Benedict RHB, Harris AE, Markow T, et al: Effects of attention training on information processing in schizophrenia. Schizophr Bull 20:537–546, 1994

Bond GR: Vocational rehabilitation, in Handbook of Psychiatric Rehabilitation. Edited by Liberman RP. New York, Macmillan, 1992, pp 244–275

Breier A, Schreiber JL, Dyer J, et al: National Institute of Mental Health longitudinal study of chronic schizophrenia: prognosis and predictors of outcome. Arch Gen Psychiatry 48:239–246, 1991

Brenner HD, Hodel B, Roder V, et al: Treatment of cognitive dysfunctions and behavioral deficits in schizophrenia. Schizophr Bull 18:21–26, 1992

Carpenter WT, Strauss JS: The prediction of outcome in schizophrenia, IV: eleven-year follow-up of the Washington IPSS cohort. J Nerv Ment Dis 179: 517–525, 1991

Cassens G, Wolfe L, Zola M: The neuropsychology of depressions. J Neuropsychiatry Clin Neurosci 2:202–213, 1990

Cook JA, Pickett SA: Recent trends in vocational rehabilitation for people with psychiatric disability. American Rehabilitation 20:2–12, 1994

Cook JA, Razzano L: Natural vocational supports for persons with severe mental illness: Thresholds Supported Competitive Employment Program. New Dir Ment Health Serv 56:23–41, 1992

Cook JA, Razzano L: Predictive validity of the McCarron-Dial Testing Battery for employment outcomes among psychiatric rehabilitation clientele. Vocational Evaluation and Work Adjustment Bulletin Summer:39–47, 1994

Cook JA, Solomon M: The community scholar program: an outcome study of supported education for students with severe mental illness. Psychosocial Rehabilitation Journal 17:83–97, 1993

Corrigan PW, Green MF, Toomey R: Cognitive correlates to social cue perception in schizophrenia. Psychiatry Res 53:141–151, 1994a

Corrigan PW, Wallace CJ, Schade ML, et al: Learning medication self-management skills in schizophrenia: relationships with cognitive deficits and psychiatric symptoms (abstract). Behavior Therapy 25:5–15, 1994b

Cox SM, Ludwig AM: Neurological soft signs and psychopathology: findings in schizophrenia. J Nerv Ment Dis 167:161–165, 1979

Delis D, Kramer J, Fridlund A, et al: California Verbal Learning Test. San Antonio, TX, Psychological Corporation, 1986

Diller L: Neuropsychological rehabilitation, in Neuropsychological Rehabilitation. Edited by Meier M, Benton A, Diller L. New York, Guilford, 1987, pp 3–18

Drake RE, Becker DR, Biesanz JC, et al: Rehabilitative day treatment vs. supported employment, I: vocational outcomes. Community Ment Health J 30:519–532, 1994

Fein R: Economics of Mental Illness. New York, Basic Books, 1958

Gervey R, Bedell JR: Supported employment in vocational rehabilitation, in Psychological Assessment and Treatment of Persons With Severe Mental Disorders. Edited by Bedell JR. Washington, DC, Taylor & Francis, 1994, pp 151–175

Gervey R, Parrish A, Bond G: Survey of exemplary supported employment programs for persons with psychiatric disabilities. Journal of Vocational Rehabilitation 5:115–125, 1995

Goldberg TE: Implications of cognitive deficits in schizophrenia (abstract), in American Psychiatric Association Annual Meeting Proceedings. Washington, DC, American Psychiatric Association, 1992, p 298

Goldberg TE, Gold JM, Greenberg R, et al: Contrasts between patients with affective disorders and patients with schizophrenia on a neuropsychological test battery. Am J Psychiatry 150:1355–1362, 1993a

Goldberg TE, Greenberg RD, Griffin SJ, et al: The effect of clozapine on cognition and psychiatric symptoms in patients with schizophrenia [see comments]. Br J Psychiatry 162:43–48, 1993b

Goldman RS, Axelrod BN, Tandon R, et al: Neuropsychological prediction of treatment efficacy and one-year outcome in schizophrenia. Psychopathology 26:122–126, 1993

Gunderson JG, Mosher LR: The cost of schizophrenia. Am J Psychiatry 132: 901–906, 1975

Hall W, Goldstein G, Andrews G, et al: Estimating the economic costs of schizophrenia. Schizophr Bull 11:598–610, 1985

Harding CM, Brooks GW, Ashikaga T, et al: The Vermont longitudinal study of persons with severe mental illness, II: long-term outcome of subjects who respectively met DSM-III criteria for schizophrenia. Am J Psychiatry 144:727–735, 1987

Heaton RK: Wisconsin Card Sorting Test. Odessa, FL, Psychological Assessment Resources, 1985

Heaton RK, Baade LE, Johnson KL: Neuropsychological test results associated with psychiatric disorders in adults. Psychol Bull 85(1):141–162, 1978a

Heaton RK, Chelune GJ, Lehman RAW: Using neuropsychological and personality tests to assess the likelihood of patient employment. J Nerv Ment Dis 166:408–416, 1978b

Heaton RK, Vogt AT, Hoehn MM, et al: Neuropsychological impairment with schizophrenia vs. acute and chronic cerebral lesions. J Clin Psychol 35:46–53, 1979

Jaeger J, Douglas E: Neuropsychiatric rehabilitation for persistent mental illness. Psychiatr Q 63(1):71–94, 1992

Jaeger J, Berns S, Tigner A, et al: Remediation of neuropsychological deficits in psychiatric populations: rationale and methodological considerations. Psychopharmacol Bull 28:367–390, 1992

Jones K, Colson P, Valencia E, et al: A preliminary cost effectiveness analysis of an intervention to reduce homelessness among the mentally ill. Psychiatr Q 65:243–256, 1994

Kay SR, Fiszbein S, Opler LA: The Positive and Negative Syndrome Scale (PANSS) for schizophrenia. Schizophr Bull 13:261–276, 1987

Lezak M: Neuropsychological Assessment, 3rd Edition. New York, Oxford University Press, 1995

Lysaker P, Bell M: Negative symptoms and vocational impairment in schizophrenia: repeated measurements of work performance over six months. Acta Psychiatr Scand 91:205–208, 1995

Lysaker P, Bell M, Beam-Goulet J: Wisconsin Card Sorting Test and work performance in schizophrenia. Psychiatry Res 56:45–51, 1995

Manschreck TC: Psychopathology of motor behavior in schizophrenia. Progress in Experimental Personality Research 12:53–94, 1983

Manschreck TC, Ames D: Neurologic features and psychopathology in schizophrenic disorders. Biol Psychiatry 19:703–719, 1984

Meltzer HY: Dimensions of outcome with clozapine. Br J Psychiatry Suppl 17:46–53, 1992

Merriam AE, Kay SR, Opler LA, et al: Neurological signs and the positive-negative dimension in schizophrenia. Biol Psychiatry 28:181–192, 1990

Mueser KT, Kosmidis MH, Sayers MD: Symptomatology and the prediction of social skills acquisition in schizophrenia. Schizophr Res October(8):59–68, 1992

Newnan OS, Heaton RK, Lehman RAW: Neuropsychological and MMPI correlates of patients' future employment characteristics. Percept Mot Skills 46:635–642, 1978

Overall JE, Gorham DR: The Brief Psychiatric Rating Scale. Psychol Rep 10:799–812, 1962

Paulsen JS, Heaton RK, Sadek JR, et al: The nature of learning and memory impairments in schizophrenia. J Int Neuropsychol Soc 1:88–99, 1995

Penn DL, Van der Does AW, Spaulding WD, et al: Information processing and social cognitive problem solving in schizophrenia: assessment of interrelationships and changes over time (abstract). J Nerv Ment Dis 181:13–20, 1993

Penn DL, Mueser KT, Spaulding W, et al: Information processing and social competence in chronic schizophrenia. Schizophr Bull 21:269–281, 1995

Penny NH, Mueser KT, North CT: The Allen Cognitive Level Test and social competence in adult psychiatric patients. Am J Occup Ther 49:420–427, 1995

Rogers DGC: Schizophrenia: a neuropsychological perspective, in The Cognitive Disorder of Psychiatric Illness: A Historical Perspective. Edited by Panelis C, Nelson HE, Barnes TR. New York, Wiley, 1996, pp 19–30

Schooler NR, Hogarty GE, Weissman MM: Social Adjustment Scale II (SASII), in Resource Materials for Community Health Evaluators (Publ No ADM 79-328). Edited by Hargreaves WA, Attkisson CC, Sorenson JE. Washington, DC, U.S. Department of Health, Education and Welfare, 1979, pp 290–330

Seidman LJ, Pepple JR, Faraone SV, et al: Wisconsin Card Sorting Test performance over time in schizophrenia. Preliminary evidence from clinical follow-up and neuroleptic reduction studies. Schizophr Res 5:233–242, 1991

Silverstein ML, Fogg L, Harrow M: Prognostic significance of cerebral status: dimensions of clinical outcome. J Nerv Ment Dis 179:534–539, 1991

Slater E, Beard AW, Glithero E: The schizophrenia-like psychoses of epilepsy. Br J Psychiatry 109:95–150, 1963

Sohlberg MM, Mateer CA: Prospective Memory Process Training (PROMPT). Puyallup, WA, Association for Neuropsychological Research and Development, 1986

Sohlberg MM, Mateer CA: Introduction to Cognitive Rehabilitation: Theory and Practice. New York, Guilford, 1989

Spaulding WD, Sullivan M, Weiler M, et al: Changing cognitive functioning in rehabilitation of schizophrenia (abstract). Acta Psychiatr Scand Suppl 90: 116–124, 1994

Spring B, Ravdin L: Cognitive remediation in schizophrenia: should we attempt it? Schizophr Bull 18:15–20, 1992

Strauss JS, Carpenter WT: The prediction of outcome in schizophrenia, I: characteristics of outcome. Arch Gen Psychiatry 27:739–746, 1972

Strauss JS, Carpenter WT: The prognosis of schizophrenia: rationale for a multidimensional concept. Schizophr Bull 4:56–67, 1978

Strauss JS, Carpenter WT, Bartko JJ: The diagnosis and understanding of schizophrenia, III: speculations on the processes that underlie schizophrenic symptoms and signs. Schizophr Bull 1:61–69, 1974

Torrey W, Becker D, Drake R: Rehabilitation day treatment vs supported employment, II: consumer, family and staff reactions to a program change. Psychosocial Rehabilitation Journal 3:67–75, 1995

Townes BD, Martin DC, Nelson D, et al: Neurobehavioral approach to classification of psychiatric patients using a competency model. J Consult Clin Psychol 53:33–42, 1985

Trotter S, Minkoff K, Harrison K, et al: Supported work: an innovative approach to the vocational rehabilitation of persons who are psychiatrically disabled. Rehabilitation Psychology 33:27–37, 1988

van Os J, Fahy TA, Jones P, et al: Increased intracerebral cerebrospinal fluid spaces predict unemployment and negative symptoms in psychotic illness: a prospective study. Br J Psychiatry 166:750–758, 1995

Weaver LA, Brooks GW: The use of psychomotor tests in predicting the potential of chronic schizophrenics. Journal of Neuropsychiatry 5:170–180, 1963

Wechsler D: Wechsler Adult Intelligence Scale—Revised. San Antonio, TX, Psychological Corporation, 1981

Zec RF, Parks RW, Gambach J, et al: The executive board system: an innovative approach to cognitive-behavior rehabilitation in patients with traumatic brain injury, in Handbook of Head Trauma: Acute Care to Recovery. Edited by Long JC. New York, Plenum, 1992, pp 219–230

Index

*Page numbers printed in **boldface** type refer to tables or figures.*